D1474821

THE FUNCTION AND MECHANICS OF NORMAL, DISEASED AND RECONSTRUCTED MIDDLE EARS

THE FUNCTION AND MECHANICS OF NORMAL, DISEASED AND RECONSTRUCTED MIDDLE EARS

Proceedings of the Second International Symposium on
Middle-Ear Mechanics in Research and Otosurgery,
held in Boston, MA, USA, October 21st-24th, 1999

edited by

John J. Rosowski, PhD
Saumil N. Merchant, MD

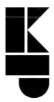

Kugler Publications/The Hague/The Netherlands

ISBN 90 6299 181 5

Distributors:
For the U.S.A. and Canada:
Library Research Associates, Inc.
474 Dunderberg Road
Monroe, NY 10950
Telefax (914) 782 3953

For all other countries:
Kugler Publications
P.O. Box 97747
2509 GC The Hague, The Netherlands
Telefax (+31.70) 3300254

© Copyright 2000 Kugler Publications
All rights reserved. No part of this book may be translated or reproduced in any form by print,
photoprint, microfilm, or any other means without prior written permission of the publisher.
Kugler Publications is an imprint of SPB Academic Publishing bv, P.O. Box 97747
2509 GC The Hague, The Netherlands

TABLE OF CONTENTS

Midde-ear reconstruction

SECOND INTERNATIONAL SYMPOSIUM ON MIDDLE EAR MECHANICS IN RESEARCH AND OTOSURGERY

Special topic: chronic otitis media

October 21st-24th, 1999, Massachusetts Eye and Ear Infirmary, Boston, MA, USA

Sponsors
Harvard Medical School, Department of Continuing Education
Massachusetts Eye and Ear Infirmary, Department of Otolaryngology

Symposium Directors
Saumil N. Merchant, MD
John J. Rosowski, PhD

Organizing Committee
Richard L. Goode, MD, Stanford University Medical Center, Stanford, CA
Prof. Dr med. Karl-Bernd Hüttenbrink, Carl Gustav Carus University, Dresden, Germany
David J. Lim, MD, House Ear Institute, Los Angeles, CA
Robert H. Margolis, PhD, University of Minnesota, Minneapolis, MN
Joseph B. Nadol, Jr, MD, Harvard Medical School, Boston, MA

Harvard Faculty
Barbara Herrmann, PhD, Massachusetts Eye and Ear Infirmary
Margaret Kenna, MD, Children's Hospital Medical Center
Trevor McGill, MD, Children's Hospital Medical Center
Michael J. McKenna, MD, Massachusetts Eye and Ear Infirmary
William T. Peake, ScD, Massachusetts Eye and Ear Infirmary
Dennis S. Poe, MD, Massachusetts Eye and Ear Infirmary
Steven D. Rauch, MD, Massachusetts Eye and Ear Infirmary
Michael E. Ravicz, MS, Massachusetts Eye and Ear Infirmary
Christopher Shera, PhD, Massachusetts Eye and Ear Infirmary
Aaron Thornton, PhD, Massachusetts Eye and Ear Infirmary
Susan E. Voss, PhD, Massachusetts Eye and Ear Infirmary
Howard Zubick, PhD, Longwood Otolaryngology

Guest Faculty

Paul Avan, MD, PhD, University of Clermont-Ferrand, France

Richard A. Chole, MD, PhD, Washington University, St Louis, MO

Willem F. Decraemer, DSc, University of Antwerp, Belgium

William J. Doyle, PhD, University of Pittsburgh School of Medicine, Pittsburgh, PA

Prof. Dr med. Ugo Fisch, University of Zurich, Switzerland

A. Julianna Gulya, MD, National Institute on Deafness and Other Communication Disorders, Bethesda, MD

Kiyofumi Gyo, MD, Ehime University School of Medicine, Ehime, Japan

John W. Hamilton, FRCS, Gloucestershire Royal Hospital, Gloucester, UK

Dr-Ing. Herbert Hudde, Ruhr University, Bochum, Germany

Shyam M. Khanna, PhD, Columbia University, New York, NY

Michael M. Paparella, MD, University of Minnesota, Minneapolis, MN

Sunil Puria, PhD, Stanford University, Stanford, CA

James M. Robinson, FRCS, Gloucestershire Royal Hospital, Gloucester, UK

Mirko Tos, MD, University of Copenhagen, Denmark

Hiroshi Wada, PhD, Tohoku University, Japan

Financial support

National Institute on Deafness and Other Communication Disorders

Deafness Research Foundation

International Hearing Foundation

National Organization for Hearing Research

PREFACE

The Second International Symposium on Middle-Ear Mechanics in Research and Otosurgery was co-sponsored by the Department of Otolaryngology of Massachusetts Eye and Ear Infirmary and the Department of Continuing Medical Education of Harvard Medical School, and was held in Boston, Massachusetts, on October 21st-24th, 1999. The symposium was attended by 190 participants from 20 countries, and featured oral and poster presentations, as well as panel discussions concerning the function and mechanics of the normal, diseased, and reconstructed middle ear.

The impetus for the symposium came from the successful First International Symposium on Middle-Ear Mechanics in Research and Otosurgery organized by Prof. Dr med. Karl-Bernd Hüttenbrink in Dresden, Germany in September, 1996. There was near unanimous opinion amongst the participants that the first meeting had a positive impact in both the basic science and clinical arenas and that it would be worthwhile organizing a second meeting. The objective of the second symposium was to bring together clinicians and basic scientists interested in middle ear mechanics with special emphasis on chronic otitis media. The symposium was targeted toward otolaryngologists, audiologists and basic scientists, as well as toward students of these disciplines. Fruitful collaboration between these disciplines can do much to improve the diagnosis and therapy of middle ear disease. Basic scientists are not generally familiar with the pathogenesis and hearing outcomes of middle ear disease, and clinicians often do not fully understand the mechanical and acoustical constraints on the ear that result from middle ear disease and its treatment. Even within the narrow confines of basic research, there are groups that investigate the biology of middle ear disease, and there are other groups that investigate only the physics and acoustics of the middle ear.

The symposium brought together a well-represented faculty of experts in middle ear acoustics, middle ear biology and clinicians, to give overviews and to present state-of-the-art information within their respective areas. Emphasis was on free exchange of ideas between clinicians and basic scientists, as well as education of the two groups. Chronic otitis media was chosen to ensure a worthwhile exchange of views on a critical clinical topic. Another goal of the symposium was to encourage students and young investigators to become familiar with cutting edge research and with unsolved research challenges.

This book is a compilation of symposium papers that were submitted for possible publication, and that successfully underwent scientific peer review. The book is organized into six sections covering various aspects of the mechanics and function of normal, diseased and reconstructed middle ears.

The six papers on *the normal ear* include discussions of the homeostatic control of middle ear gases via eustachian tube function, measurements and models of sound transduction in the normal middle ear, and middle ear measurement techniques for both the clinic and the laboratory.

The four papers on *the diseased middle ear* discuss the pathology of chronic otitis media and clinical tests of middle ear function in pathological ears.

The five papers on *middle-ear mechanics in the diseased ear* discuss the effect of pathology on middle ear sound transmission via models and measurements.

The ten papers on *middle-ear reconstruction* describe surgical techniques, and the postsurgical hearing results of several common middle ear reconstructive procedures.

The five papers on *middle-ear mechanics in reconstructed ears* use measurements and models to describe how different reconstructive procedures affect middle ear function.

Finally, four papers in *new areas of research* describe the latest efforts in implantable hearing aids and the use of laser vibrometry in the clinic.

We gratefully acknowledge the support provided in the organization of the symposium and the publication of its proceedings by the National Institute on Deafness and Other Communication Disorders, the Deafness Research Foundation, the International Hearing Foundation, and the National Organization for Hearing Research.

John J. Rosowski, PhD
Saumil N. Merchant, MD
Boston, Massachusetts, USA, July, 2000

THE NORMAL MIDDLE EAR

MIDDLE EAR PRESSURE REGULATION

William J. Doyle

Department of Otolaryngology, Children's Hospital of Pittsburgh and the University of Pittsburgh School of Medicine, Pittsburgh, PA, USA

Anatomical abbreviations

ME	middle ear = protympanum + tympanic cavity + mastoid air cells
ET	eustachian tube
TM	tympanic membrane
mTVP	tensor veli palatini muscle
mLVP	levator veli palatini muscle

Operators

$E(M)$	expected value of M
$\Sigma(M)$	sum of M over physiological gases
$\delta(M)$	change in M
$|M|$	absolute value of M
Eff	efficiency

Physical variables

R	gas constant
T_c	temperature of compartment c (time invariant)
V_c	volume of compartment c (time invariant)
$P_c(t)$	total pressure of compartment c at time t
$N_{cg}(t)$	number of moles of gas g for compartment c at time t
$P_{cg}(t)$	pressure of gas g for compartment c at time t
F_c	blood flow for compartment c
A_c	surface area of compartment c

ΔP_{am}	pressure difference between environment and middle ear
$\Delta P_{crit}1$	critical pressure difference between middle ear and environment for hearing loss

Supported in Part by a grant from the National Institutes of Health (DC 01260)

Address for correspondence: William J. Doyle, PhD, Department of Pediatric Otolaryngology, Children's Hospital of Pittsburgh, 3705 Fifth Avenue, Pittsburgh, PA 15213, USA. email: Docdoyle@ix.netcom.com

The Function and Mechanics of Normal, Diseased and Reconstructed Middle Ears, pp. 3–21
edited by J.J. Rosowski and S.N. Merchant
© *2000 Kugler Publications, The Hague, The Netherlands*

ΔPcrit2   critical pressure difference between middle ear and tissue for pathology
ΔPcrit2'   critical pressure difference between middle ear and environment for
             pathology

Introduction

The middle ear (ME) is a bridged airspace within the petrous temporal bone
that can be functionally subdivided into three communicating compartments:
the anterior protympanum or osseous portion of the eustachian tube (ET); the
intermediate tympanic cavity which contains the ME ossicles; and the posterior
mastoid air cells. For hearing, the ME functions as an acoustic coupler that
amplifies and transfers environmental sound energy (pressure waves in a gas)
captured as vibrations of the tympanic membrane (TM) to the inner ear (pressure waves in a fluid) where the energy is presented as vibrations of the oval
window. Because the effectiveness of this energy transfer depends, in part, on
the mechanical impedance of the system, damping the vibrational amplitudes
of the TM, oval window and/or round window compromises efficiency. Thus,
pressure imbalances between ME and ambient environment that restrict TM
response to ambient sound energy and/or the presence of fluid within the usually
gas filled ME that restricts movements of both the TM and round window
cause a decreased energy transfer which is perceived as a hearing loss.
    Because the ME is usually isolated from direct communication with the en-
vironment, the functionally requisite pressure equilibrium is intrinsically un-
stable and is disturbed continuously by normal fluctuations in ambient barometric pressure. Also, for air breathing animals, passive mechanisms alone cannot
maintain ambient ME pressures because diffusive gas exchange has the net
effect of driving total pressure to equilibrium with that of the surrounding tissues, an approximate 50 mmHg deficit with respect to environment[1,2]. Therefore, to maintain an air-filled ME at near ambient pressure, a conceptually simple,
yet functionally elegant mechanism for ME pressure regulation has evolved.
There, the ME is opened intermittently to the environment allowing for gradient driven gas transfers that reset ME pressure to near ambient[3].
    In this presentation, the various factors that contribute to ME pressure regula-
tion are reviewed and evaluated critically. To that end, ME pressure regulation is
defined broadly as consisting of those mechanisms that promote a negligible expected value for the ME to ambient pressure differential (i.e., E(ΔPam)→0 mmHg).

Processes that affect middle ear pressure

For the majority of its surface area, the ME airspace is bounded by mucosally
covered bone, and consequently that airspace can be described as a non-collapsible
(ignoring the minor volume changes caused by TM retraction and mucosal swell-

ing), biological gas pocket. By the general gas law (*i.e.*, Pme=RTmeNme/Vme), the pressure (Pme) of the non-collapsible ME at constant temperature (Tme) is a direct function of the contained gas volume (Nme/Vme) and transfers of gas volume to or from the ME change its pressure (*i.e.*, δPme=(RTme/Vme)δNme).

As shown in Figure 1, the 'healthy' ME can potentially exchange gas with each of four adjacent compartments; *i.e.*, the local blood via gas transfers across the mucosa, the inner ear via transfers across the round window, the environment via transfers across the TM and the nasopharynx via transfers across the ET[4]. Gas exchange across each of the first three routes is a passive, bi-directional, diffusive process, and the expected value of total ME pressure for each route is the sum of the ME-compartment equilibrium partial-pressures of the component gases (*i.e.*, E(Pme)=Σ(E(Pmeg)) over all physiological gases). Of the three passive exchange routes, only transTM exchange promotes an expected ME-ambient pressure differential of 0 mmHg (*vis à vis* E(ΔPam) ≈ −50 mmHg for trans-mucosal and trans-round window exchanges). In contrast, gas exchange across the ET is a bi-directional, total pressure gradient dependent transfer of mixed gas that in the more usual situation requires active, muscle assisted tubal openings[3]. As for the transTM route, gas exchange across the ET has an expected ME-ambient pressure differential of approximately 0 mmHg and, by definition, both exchange routes are potentially pressure regulating.

ME pressure regulation by transTM exchange

The TM is a three-layered membrane that bounds the tympanic cavity on its lateral aspect and isolates that space from the environment of the external ear canal. Its

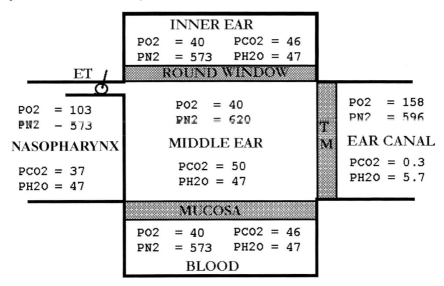

Fig. 1. Cartoon showing the four compartments that can exchange gas with the ME, and the partial pressures of the physiological gases for each compartment. Values taken from Felding *et al.*[4] and Hergels and Magnuson[84].

two bounding surfaces are covered with the cell type characteristic of the lining of the respective cavities (mucosa medially, keratinized squamous epithelium laterally) and these layers sandwich an inner layer composed mainly of collagen fibers[5].

The rate of transTM volume gas exchange is a function of the partial-pressure differentials of the gases in the ME and external canal, the diffusivity and solubility of those gases in the TM and the surface area and thickness of the structure. While many of these parameters have not been measured directly in either humans or animals, experiments have shown that the TM is permeable to different gases[6-8]. However, the volume rate of gas exchange across the TM is very slow, and these transfers cannot under normal circumstances balance the net volume gas loss to blood by the trans-mucosal exchange route[8]. This observation shows that transTM gas exchange is not an effective regulator of ME pressure, a conclusion supported by the large measured gas partial-pressure differentials between ME and environment for both normal ears and for ears with a dysfunctional ET[4,9,10], and by the clinical need to perforate the TM to relieve significant ME-environment pressure differentials during periods of ET dysfunction (*i.e.*, myringotomy, tympanostomy tube insertion).

ME pressure regulation by transET exchange

The ET extends from the posterio-lateral nasopharyngeal wall to the protympanum of the ME. Morphologically, the ET resembles a guttered conduit with a fixed, rigid superio-medial cartilaginous wall and a compliant inferio-lateral membranous wall[11] (*see* Fig. 2). The lumen of the tube is lined with a modified respiratory mucosa continuous with that of the nasopharynx anteriorly and that of the protympanum posteriorly[12]. The submucosa is relatively thick containing lymph channels and numerous blood vessels, the latter of which were shown to be responsive to a variety of vasoactive stimuli[13-15]. The superior aspect of the ET cartilage lies within a bony cradle (sulcus tubarius) along the cranial base, to which it is attached by connective tissue[11]. Extant periluminal, tissue overpressure (measured in normal subjects to be on the order of 4-12 mmHg) collapses the ET lumen causing the isolation of the ME airspace (*i.e.*, a closed gas pocket)[16,17]. For this reason, the ET usually represents only a potential communication between ME and nasopharynx, and an active opening mechanism is required to realize that potential.

Most likely because of anatomical differences between animal species and the inaccessibility of the ET to direct study, the mechanism of tubal opening in humans is still debated. However, consensus holds that the tensor veli palatini muscle (mTVP) is primarily responsible for tubal opening, while the levator veli palatini muscle (mLVP) may have an accessory role[18]. The triangularly shaped mTVP was shown to be directly continuous with the tensor tympanii muscle of the tympanic cavity, and to be structurally and functionally subdivided into lateral (mTVP proper) and medial (dilator tubae) bundles[11]. The basal aspect of the lateral bundle originates from the cranial base and lateral aspect of the tubal cartilage along its entire length.

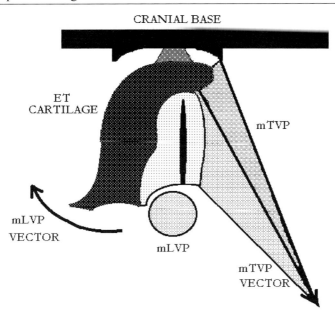

Fig. 2. Drawing showing the relationships of the ET, cranial base and paratubal muscles in cross-section. mLVP and mTVP vector arrows indicate their within plane movement during contraction. Note that mTVP contraction will displace the lateral wall of the tube inferio-laterally thereby opening the lumen. mLVP contraction can rotate the ET cartilage medio-superiorly creating a more favorable alignment for the inferior component of the mTVP vector. (*See* text for details, superior is to the top and medial is to the left in the figure.)

The tendonous apex of the muscle inserts into the fixed hamular process and/or the palatal aponeurosis. The medial bundle originates from the posterior one-third of the length of the membranous wall of the ET, and its fibers converge to a tendon that blends and fuses with that of the lateral bundle at its insertion. The mLVP lies along the domed floor of the ET and is bounded medially by the lower most extension of the tubal cartilage. That muscle originates from the inferior aspect of the petrous temporal bone and inserts into the soft palate[11].

Most simply, the ET lumen is opened by contraction of the mTVP during swallowing, yawning and other activities, wherein the medial bundle displaces the membranous wall of the ET inferio-laterally[18]. More complex mechanisms have been suggested that, while recognizing the primacy of mTVP contractions in tubal opening, also require medial displacement and/or medial rotation of the tubal cartilage, translations that are effected by the synchronous contraction of the mLVP (*see* Fig. 2)[19]. Irrespective of the specific mechanics, the transient, muscle assisted openings of the ET expose the ME gas pocket to the environment of the nasopharynx (*i.e.,* near ambient pressure). This allows for the passive, total pressure gradient driven, bolus transfer of mixed gas between the ET and environment. Because these transfers decrease the ME-ambient pressure gradient, active ET opening is by definition pressure regulating.

Other proposed mechanisms of middle ear pressure regulation

An emerging concept in the area of ME physiology is the hypothesized ability of the ME mucosa to regulate and stabilize ME pressure in the absence of a well functioning ET (sometimes referred to as 'the other ventilatory function')[20-25]. That presumed function implies that gas transfer across or gas production by the ME mucosa can, under physiological conditions, stabilize ME pressure in the absence of bolus gas re-supply during ET openings. The proponents of that hypothetical function cite experimental results that show increasing ME pressure during sleep or after maneuvers that cause the rapid development of ME underpressure as evidence of mucosal pressure generation[20-25]. However, it was demonstrated previously that the experimental conditions under which increasing ME pressure is realized always cause a positive blood to ME partial-pressure gradient for those physiological gases that have a relatively high trans-mucosal exchange rate. Thus, the ME pressure increase is more simply explained as a diffusively driven equilibration of the imposed gradient(s)[26]. Indeed, simple mathematical models of diffusive gas exchange that simulate the experimental conditions reproduce the apparently counter-intuitive experimental results without recourse to exotic pressure generating mechanisms[26,27].

To understand the mechanism responsible for the epiphenomenon, two facts need to be appreciated. First, the experimentally measured, relative rate of trans-mucosal inert gas exchange is orders of magnitude less than that predicted by the solubility and permeability of the reactive gases (*i.e.*, at identical partial-pressure gradients, the exchanges of CO_2 and O_2 between ME and blood are very much faster than the trans-mucosal exchange of N_2)[28-30]. Second, for the normal ME and the ME with a poorly functioning ET, the gas partial-pressures of O_2, CO_2 and H_2O are in approximate equilibrium with blood, while the N_2 partial-pressure exceeds that of blood by approximately 50 mmHg[4,9,10]. Consequently, the expected rate of ME pressure decrease in the absence of ET openings is dependent on the N_2 trans-mucosal exchange rate, and is therefore very slow. For this reason, the short term kinetics of ME pressure change is dominated by established ME-blood, partial-pressure gradients for O_2, CO_2 and/or H_2O.

In that regard, increasing ME pressure during sleep epochs[20,21] is readily explained by the blood to ME transfer of CO_2 consequent to the increased blood CO_2 partial-pressures caused by the suppression of respiratory drive during sleep. Less obvious is the explanation for the increasing ME pressure observed after inducing a ME underpressure by sniffing, or by swallowing at relatively negative ambient pressure[23,25]. For those situations, the rapid (<1 second) development of a ME underpressure is a unique signature for trans-ET transfer of a volume of ME gas to the nasopharynx. Because this loss of gas volume is distributed over the component gases in proportion to percent composition, the pre-existing ME-blood equilibrium conditions for O_2, CO_2 and H_2O are disturbed by the maneuvers. The subsequent ME pressure increased is caused by the transfer of these gases from the blood to ME which re-establishes their equilibrium values[26,27]. Consistent with this explanation is the agreement between the observed and predicted magnitudes of the post-maneuver ME pressure increase. There, for passive blood to ME gas transfers, the maximum pressure increase is limited by the magnitudes of the ME partial-pressure change in the fast exchange gases, and in specific, by the product of absolute value of the total initial pressure loss ($\mid$ Pme(t=0)–Pme(–δt) $\mid$, where δt$\rightarrow$0) and the pre-maneuver fractional representation (Pmeg(–δt)/Pme(–δt)) of the fast exchange gases (*i.e.*, Pme(max)–Pme(t=0) = $\mid$ Pme(0)–Pme(–δt) $\mid$ (Pmeco2 (–δt)+Pmeo2(–δt)+Pmeh2o(–δt))/Pme(–δt)))[27]. In no experiment has this theoretical limit to the post maneuver pressure increase been exceeded. Thus, the experimental results represent short-term aberrations in the usual course of decreasing ME pressure caused by the slow trans-mucosal exchange of N_2 and do not evidence ME pressure regulation.

There are no experimental data that evidence the ME mucosa as a regulator of ME pressure. A consideration of the applicable gas partial-pressure gradients (*see* Fig. 1) shows that passive, diffusive processes cannot maintain ambient ME pressure, and no active pressure generating mechanism for the ME mucosa that is well founded in physiology has been advanced. For these reasons, and because the behavior of ME pressure can be simulated accurately by mathematical models that include only gas exchange between the ME and nasopharynx during ET openings and the passive diffusive exchanges of gas between ME and blood, the hypothesis of pressure regulation by the ME mucosa must be rejected.

Consequences of middle ear pressure dysregulation

As described above, the majority of data supports only two exchange routes by which ME gas volume is changed under normal physiological conditions: *(1)* the bolus exchange of mixed gas between the nasopharynx and ME during ET openings; and *(2)* the diffusive exchange of gases between the ME and blood. Net gas exchange via these two routes is opposing, with the ET supplying mixed gas to the ME (nasopharyngeal composition) and trans-mucosal exchange depleting ME gas (primarily N_2).

Numerous past studies have determined the effect on ME pressure of preventing gas re-supply by the ET. The earliest studies showed that physical obstruction of the ET in animals provoked the sequential development of ME underpressures, mucosal inflammation and serous effusion[31-34]. Later experimental protocols using primates did not violate the patency of the ET lumen, but rather impaired the function of the mTVP muscle[35-38]. The resultant failure of ET opening (described as functional ET obstruction) caused an identical sequence of events leading from the progressive development of ME underpressure to ME effusion. Importantly, the effusion and abnormal pressures resolved with recovery of mTVP muscle function[38].

In more recent studies, magnetic resonance imaging was used to visualize the changes in the ME mucosa and airspace after inducing functional ET obstruction by botulinum paralysis of the mTVP in monkeys[38,39]. The results showed a rela-tively slow, progressive development of ME underpressures over a period of days. Increased mucosal permeability to fluids was observed at ME underpressures of approximately –14 mmHg and effusion occurred at a critical underpressure of ap-proximately –20 mmHg (ref. ambient). In both monkeys and chinchillas, experi-mentally created, acute ME underpressures were shown to cause vascular responses and effusion accumulation at those underpressures[40,41].

These results support the classic mechanism relating ET dysfunction to the de-velopment of ME effusion as described by Politzer[42] and more completely devel-oped by others[43,44]. That mechanism, the *hydrops ex vacuo* theory, consists of four causally related events: *(1)* the unabated absorption of ME gas; *(2)* a resultant ME underpressure; *(3)* an increased permeability of the mucosal vasculature to fluids; and *(4)* a transudation of mucosal fluid into the ME space. More specifically, a failure in ET openings prevents the re-supply of gas to the ME. Because of the large ME-blood partial-pressure gradient for N_2, diffusive exchange of that gas reduces the total ME gas volume, thereby driving total ME pressure to lower val-ues. In turn, the decreasing ME pressure causes a developing gradient between the hydrostatic pressure of the surrounding mucosa (maintained at approximate ambi-ent pressure) and the total gas pressure of the ME airspace. At certain gradient magnitudes (critical pressure differentials), fluids escape from the vasculature into the mucosa, and at larger gradients the mucosal epithelium becomes permeable to those fluids allowing for spillage into the ME airspace (development of effusion)[45,46].

Efficiency of middle ear pressure regulation

As described above, both a large ME-ambient pressure difference and the presence of a ME effusion (precipitated at a critical ME-tissue pressure gradient) will com-promise the acoustic coupling function of the ME and cause a conductive hearing loss[42,47]. Effective ME pressure regulation will maintain the absolute value of the ME-ambient pressure gradient at less than the critical value for a conductive hear-ing loss (ΔPcrit1) and the ME-tissue pressure gradient in excess of the critical value that precipitates effusion (ΔPcrit2). Because hydrostatic tissue pressure tracts ambient pressure (Ptis=Pamb + K, where K is a constant), both critical gradients can be expressed in terms of ME and ambient pressures. There, efficient ME pres-sure regulation can be described for each of the two critical values by the following equations:

E(Pme–Ptis)=E(Pme–Pamb–K)> ΔPcrit2 or E(Pme–Pamb)> ΔPcrit2'; where ΔPcrit2' = ΔPcrit2+K; and | (Pme–Pamb) | <ΔPcrit1

Note that the ME-ambient pressure difference that causes a conductive hearing loss by TM deformation is much less than that required to precipitate effusion and therefore, | ΔPcrit2'| >| ΔPcrit1| . Below, a physical model of ME pressure regula-tion is presented, and this concept of efficiency is refined.

Consider the physical model of ME gas exchange presented in Figure 3. There, the three primary exchange compartments are modeled as boxes with relative effective volumes of ambient environment >>blood>ME. Initially, each box contains a certain volume of fluid which represents the gas volume for the compartment. The ambient compartment is fitted with a syringe that allows for volume change to simulate the expected changes in barometric pressure, and is separated from the ME compartment by a pressure valve representing the ET. The pressure within the ET valve (Pet) represents the periluminal tissue pressure and is controlled by a syringe that usually maintains a relative overpressure (ref. ambient; (*i.e.,* Pet=Pamb+Pc)). The ME and blood compartments communicate via a valved drain which represents the trans-mucosal exchange pathway. The height of the fluid level in each box corresponds to the compartment pressure, the height of the mast on the float corresponds to the difference between tissue and ambient pressures, and the depth of the keel corresponds to the magnitude of underpressure (ref. ambient) that causes ME pathology. In the model, volume fluid exchange between compartments corresponds to volume gas exchange.

As configured, the fluid level of the ME compartment will decrease to that of the drain (fluid level of the blood compartment) passing through the level of the float's keel where pressure regulation fails and system function is severely compromised.

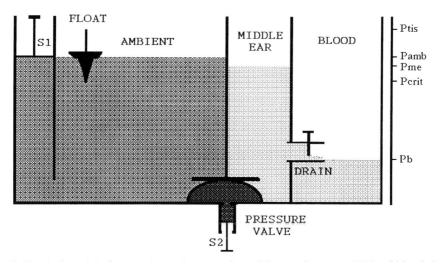

Fig. 3. Physical model of gas exchange between the ambient environment, ME and blood. The three compartments are modelled as boxes shown in cross-section, the ET is modelled as a pressure valve, and the ME to blood exchange route is modelled as a drain interposed between the respective compartments. Volumes of the ambient and blood boxes are much greater than that for the ME box. Initially, the boxes are filled to a specified level with a volume of fluid representing contained gas volume. The height of the fluid level in each box corresponds to the compartment pressure, the height of the mast on the float corresponds to the difference between tissue and ambient pressures, and the depth of the keel corresponds to the magnitude of underpressure (ref. ambient) that causes ME pathology. Fluid flow between compartment simulates gas flow and the behavior of the fluid levels (Pamb, Pme and Pb) in the model simulates the predicted change in gas pressure for the respective compartments over time (*see* text for details).

Alternatively, the ET valve can be periodically opened by withdrawing from its syringe (active ET opening) and decreasing valve pressure to less than ambient. This allows for fluid flow between the large volume ambient compartment and the limited volume ME compartment, thereby effecting a reduction in the difference in fluid levels for those compartments (*i.e.*, pressure equalization).

For this system, effective pressure regulation minimizes the difference over time in the pressures of the ambient and ME compartments (E(Pme–Pamb)= E(ΔPam)→0). Most simply, this can be accomplished by adjusting the pressure in the ET valve to less than ambient. There, the ET valve would be continuously open, gas would readily exchange between ME and ambient compartments and the inter-compartmental pressure difference would be maintained at 0. However, the simple elegance of that solution to ME pressure regulation is betrayed by the relative complexity of the ET opening mechanism in humans and animals. Indeed, the clinical presentation of such a condition is the patient with a patulous ET[48]. Such individuals report disturbing autophonia as well as annoying, ambiguous sensations of ME pressure, and are 'at risk' for acute bacterial infections of the ME.

Many patients with patulous ETs induce ME underpressure by 'sniffing'[49-51] which, in the model, corresponds to a rapid but transient decrease in the pressure of the ambient compartment. Because of the open ET, this is accompanied by a decrease in the pressure of the ME compartment. During the transition from ambient to less than ambient pressures, a relative overpressure in the ET develops which causes it to close. At that point, the two compartments no longer communicate, and the ET is exposed to a relative overpressure at its ambient communication and to a relative underpressure at its ME communication. The latter maintains ET closure and quasistable ME underpressures that can be of sufficient magnitude to precipitate pathology. Clinically, patients that regularly induce ME underpressures by 'sniffing' are 'at risk' for otitis media and for complications of ME pressure dysregulation such as cholesteatoma[50,51]. Thus, the maximum efficiency of the ET in ME pressure regulation is compromised by its concurrent function of protecting the ME from nasopharyngeal pressures and pathogens. As with pressure dysregulation, failure of the protective function can lead to the development of a ME effusion.

For these reasons, the ET is usually closed to optimize its protective function, but opens intermittently to fulfil its pressure regulating function. The volume of gas transfer with each opening of the tube depends on the extant (ME-nasopharyngeal) pressure gradient, the resistance of the ET to airflow at maximum dilation, and the duration of the opening[18,52,53]. The effectiveness of a single tubal opening with respect to pressure equalization depends on the extant pressure gradient, the volume gas transferred and the total ME volume. The importance of these variables to the efficiency of ME pressure regulation can be appreciated by considering the behavior of the model system while varying select parameters.

Figure 4a shows the ambient (Pamb) and ME (Pme) compartmental pressures over time for one model configuration. The critical underpressure (ΔPcrit2') at which effusion develops is also depicted. There, volume gas flow between ME and blood (fixed drain diameter) and the frequency of ET openings are held constant, and the duration of each ET opening allows for total equilibration of the pressure difference between the ambient and ME compartments. Under those conditions, ambient pressure shows oscillations caused by changes in barometric pressure (varying syringe 1 position), and ME pressure shows a progressive decrease attributable to N_2 exchange with blood that is periodically interrupted by ET openings (ETo). For this system, the efficiency of pressure regulation can be expressed in terms of the area of the ME-ambient pressure deviation (Ama, shaded area in Fig. 4), and that of the ambient-critical underpressure deviation (Aac, shaded area + white area in Fig. 4), and explicitly as: Eff=(1–Ama/Aac)×100%. Holding other variables constant, an increasing frequency of ET openings increases system efficiency to the limit of 100% for a continuously open ET (*see* caveat discussed above).

Figures 4b-d show the effects on system efficiency of decreasing the frequency of ET openings (b), decreasing the volume of gas transferred with each ET opening (c), and increasing the volume rate of gas transfer to blood (d) while holding the other variables constant. Of note, all three changes clearly decrease system efficiency (*vis à vis* that characterizing the system presented in Fig. 4a).

The behaviors depicted in the figures emphasize the incompleteness of the presented definition of efficiency. Specifically, no weighting is given to the percent of time at which the ME-ambient pressure difference is less than the critical value for pathology, though this is expected to be a predictive determinant of pressure dysregulation. Moreover, the definition is idealized and cannot be applied to clinical data sets. There, sampling of ME pressures is usually of low frequency measured as samplings per hour, day, week or month[54,55]. While methodologies for the continuous measurement of ME pressure were described recently[56], they are not likely to be used for other than experimental purposes because of the invasiveness of the monitoring system. Nonetheless, as a theoretical construct, this definition is useful for comparing the pressure regulating efficiencies of the ME system under different assumptions regarding the constraining parameters.

Factors that influence the efficiency of middle ear pressure regulation

A major criticism of current testing methodologies designed to measure ET function is their lack of prognostic value with regard to the expected consequences of diagnosed dysfunction. This diagnostic failure can be attributed, in the main, to two factors; the lack of appreciation for system dynamics that moderate the efficiency of pressure regulation, and the failure to concurrently assess the demand placed upon the ET for re-supply of gas. Indeed, individuals are often assigned to a ET function class based upon a single measurement[57-60], and no methods are in clinical use for concurrently assessing the rate of inert gas exchange across the ME mucosa. Below, the expected effects of rate buffering, feedback modulation and pathology on the efficiency of ME pressure regulation are reviewed. This illustrates the dynamic changes that occur over time in both the supply and demand

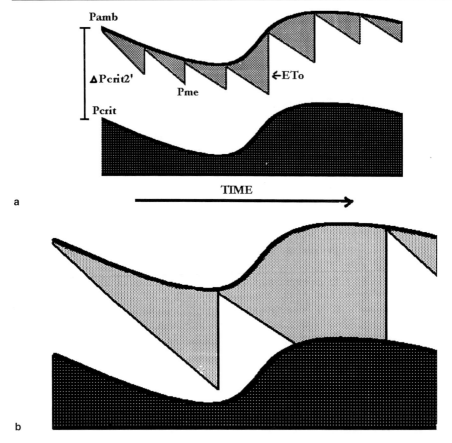

Fig. 4. Behavior over time of the ambient (labelled Pamb) and ME (labelled Pme) pressures, and the critical underpressure causing ME effusion (labelled ΔPcrit2') predicted by the physical model shown in Figure 3 under conditions of slow oscillations in the ambient pressure, a fixed drain diameter (transmucosal exchange rate), a fixed ET opening (labelled ETo) frequency, and ET opening times sufficient to equilibrate the pressures in the ME and ambient compartments *(a).* Also shown are the predicted system behaviors after decreasing the frequency of ET openings *(b),* decreasing the volume flow across the ET *(c)* and increasing the gas exchange rate (drain diameter) *(d).* Shaded area depicts the difference in pressures for the ambient and ME compartments. System efficiency can be defined as a function of the ratio of the shaded area to the sum of the shaded and white areas below the line labelled Pamb *(see* text for details).

aspects of ME pressure regulation, and documents the need for repeated measurement to achieve diagnostic reliability.

Rate buffering

Transient ME over and underpressures can be created by TM displacements, and if sufficiently large, these will decrease the efficiency of acoustic transfer by increasing the impedances of the TM and round window. To maximize acoustic transfer efficiency, these pressure fluxes must be minimized, a condition favored by a large

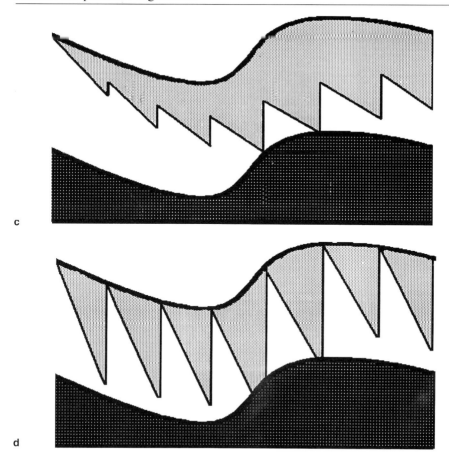

Fig. 4c, d.

ratio of ME volume to TM displacement volume. In that regard, a large mastoid volume (*vis à vis* the tympanic cavity) can serve the ME as a pressure buffer by damping the relatively large, TM induced pressure fluxes expected for the tympanic cavity in isolation.

A large volume mastoid was suggested also to buffer the rate of ME pressure decrease caused by trans-mucosal gas exchange[60-68]. There, the mastoid would behave as a volume gas reserve, thereby decreasing the rate of pressure change consequent to the continuous removal of a standard volume of gas (trans-mucosal N_2 exchange). If that hypothesis is correct, the volume of the mastoid would be directly related to the efficiency of ME pressure regulation. However, more recent computational analyses question the validity of that hypothesis and suggest that efficiency is inversely related to mastoid volume[27,69].

Logically, the mastoid will serve as a gas reserve if and only if the ratio of the volume of N_2 transferred across the mastoid mucosa to mastoid volume is less than that for the tympanic cavity. Geometrical considerations show this requirement to be extremely restrictive with respect to mucosal perfusion rates of the different regions of the ME, and to be rather unlikely[27]. Specifically, while the tympanic cavity is not partitioned, the mastoid volume is subdivided into numerous communicating air cells, each bounded by mucosa covered bone. For that geometry, the surface area to volume ratio of the mastoid is much greater than that of the tympanic cavity. Because inert gas exchange across the ME mucosa was shown to be primarily perfusion limited[28-30], the gas exchange rate of N_2 is directly related to the volume blood flow within the mucosa which is an expected function of surface area. Consequently, the mastoid will serve as a gas reserve only if the volume blood flow per unit surface area is much less than that of the tympanic cavity, with the condition explicitly defined by the inequality: $(Fm/Am)/(Ft/At)<(At/Vt)/(Am/Vm)$; where F is blood flow; A, surface area; and V, volume for the mastoid (m) and tympanic cavity (t). This restriction requires that the blood flow per unit surface area of the mastoid be orders of magnitude less than that of the tympanic cavity, a condition not supported by experiment[69]. Thus, the hypothesized gas reserve function of the mastoid is not consistent with existing data, and a small volume mastoid may create conditions favoring a low rate of ME-blood N_2 exchange, *i.e.*, greater efficiency of ME pressure regulation.

Possible feedback mechanisms

With the exceptions of developmental changes and the acute effects of concurrent disease, most past studies considered ET function to be static. However, experimental evidences suggest that the efficiency of the pressure regulating function of the ET is characterized by patterned rhythms and fluctuations. For example, one study reported that the duration of tubal openings with swallowing showed changes that were synchronized to the nasal cycle[70]. Experiments in monkeys documented changes in the closing pressure of the ET in response to changes in ME gas composition[71,72].

Also, for most individuals, the ability to reduce ME pressure by 'sniffing' is episodic[49-51]. These results are interpretable as reflecting controlled fluctuations in the periluminal pressures that usually serve to maintain a closed tubal lumen (*see* Fig. 3). Alternatively, anatomical studies that documented continuity between the tensor tympanii muscle and mTVP[11], and those describing sensory fibers within the ME mucosa that synapse with nerves that innervate the mTVP[73], suggest mechanisms for physiological modulation of the tonus of the primary muscle that effects ET opening.

While not proved, the above listed observations show that the efficiency of ME pressure regulation may be modulated by feedback mechanisms with sensory elements that include baroreceptors, chemoreceptors and stretch receptors, and effector elements that include the submucosal vasculature of the ET and mTVP tonus. Such feedback systems could fine tune ET function for efficient re-supply of gas during times of increased demand. Complementary systems may exist that down regulate the demand for gas re-supply by decreasing the rate of mucosal perfusion and thus the rate of trans-mucosal N_2 exchange. These possibilities need to be more fully studied in future experiments.

Pathology

While constitutively poor ET function imposes a strict limitation on the efficiency of ME pressure regulation, certain pathologies and diseases can temporarily or permanently decrease efficiency by reducing gas re-supply to the ME, increasing gas efflux from the ME (increasing demand), or both. For example, enlarged adenoids or nasopharyngeal carcinomas extending into the Fossa of Rosemuller can increase peritubal pressures and thereby prevent tubal openings despite active mTVP function[74,75]. Children born with certain craniofacial abnormalities, including cleft palate, often have altered mTVP and mLVP muscle vectors and insertions that impair their function in tubal opening[76,77]. Also, upper respiratory inflammation caused by nasal allergic reactions or by virus infections causes a concurrent impairment in the tubal opening mechanism, most probably mediated by reflex increases in the periluminal tissue pressure and/or extension of the inflammation into the tubal lumen[78-82].

While the normal ME mucosa consists of a single cell layer and a very thin submucosa, the ME mucosa inflamed by bacterial or viral infection or by persistent ET obstruction is characterized by marked edema and hyperemia[83]. These pathologies increase the thickness of the mucosal barrier and the volume of local blood flow by orders of magnitude. The edema may have a limiting effect on diffusive gas exchange by increasing barrier thickness, while the hyperemia will increase the rate of trans-mucosal N_2 exchange and thus, the rate of ME pressure decrease.

Summary

Experimental results and theory support the broad aspects of ME pressure regulation outlined above, but this remains a much debated and poorly understood aspect of physiology. Frustrating advancements in this area is the hypothesized role of ME pressure dysregulation in the pathogenesis of otitis media and related diseases. In that regard, philosophies based upon clinical impressions often preceded empirical demonstrations of principal, and validation experiments were often poorly designed, lacked falsifiable hypotheses and generated ambiguous results. In this review, an attempt was made to: *(1)* disassociate observation from clinical implication; *(2)* discuss the available data within the context of accepted physiological principals; *(3)* outline those hypothesized aspects of ME pressure regulation that currently lack sufficient data for support or refutation; *(4)* emphasize the need to concurrently assess the supply and demand aspects of pressure regulation; and *(5)* present a working framework for describing the efficiency of ME pressure regulation. The latter may prove useful in developing and testing hypotheses related to the physiological and pathological modulation of ME pressure regulation, and also, hypotheses regarding the direct consequences of dysregulation (decreased efficiency). In turn, the adoption by all investigators of strict hypothesis testing approaches can bring clarity to this interesting aspect of ME physiology.

Acknowledgments

I thank my colleagues at the Children's Hospital of Pittsburgh who collaborated on many of the studies reviewed in this report. I would also like to thank my colleagues who served on the Middle Ear Physiology and Pathophysiology Panel convened last June for their input into many of the presented ideas, though all errors and omissions are my own.

References

1. Piiper J: Various models for analysis of the absorption of inert gases from gas cavities in the body. Respir Physiol 9:74-85, 1970
2. Ranade A, Lambertsen CJ, Noordergraaf A: Inert gas exchange in the middle ear. Acta Otolaryngol (Stockh) 371:1-23, 1980
3. Bluestone CD, Doyle WJ: Eustachian tube function: physiology and role in otitis media. Ann Otol Rhinol Laryngol 94(Suppl 20):1-60, 1985
4. Felding JU, Rasmussen JB, Lildholdt T: Gas composition of the normal and ventilated middle ear cavity. Scand J Clin Lab Invest 47(Suppl 186):31-41, 1987
5. Lim DJ: Human tympanic membrane. Acta Otolaryngol (Stockh) 70:176-186, 1979
6. Elner A: Gas diffusion through the tympanic membrane: a model study in the diffusion chamber. Acta Otolaryngol (Stockh) 69:185-191, 1970
7. Riu R, Flottes L, Bouche J, Le Den R: La Physiologie de la Trompe d'Eustache. Paris: Librairie Arnette 1966
8. Doyle WJ, Alper CM, Seroky JT, Karnavas WJ: Exchange rates of gases across the tympanic membrane in rhesus monkeys. Acta Otolaryngol (Stockh)118:567-573, 1998
9. Hergels L, Magnuson B: Human middle ear gas composition studied by mass spectrometry. Acta Otolaryngol (Stockh) 110:92-99, 1990
10. Hergils L, Magnuson B: Middle ear gas composition in pathologic conditions: mass spectrometry in otitis media with effusion and atelectasis. Ann Otol Rhinol Laryngol 106:743-745, 1997
11. Rood SR, Doyle WJ: The morphology of the tensor veli palatini, tensor tympani and dilator tubae muscles. Ann Otol Rhinol Laryngol 87(2):202-211, 1978
12. Sadé J: Middle ear mucosa. Arch Otolaryngol 84:137-143, 1966
13. Shotts RF, Jackson RT: Changes in the patency of the dog's eustachian tube induced by histamine and antihistamines. Arch Otolaryngol 96:57-61, 1972
14. Jones JS, Sheffield W, White LJ, Bloom MA: A double-blind comparison between oral pseudoephedrine and topical oxymetazoline in the prevention of barotrauma during air travel. Am J Emerg Med 16(3):262-264, 1998
15. Malm L, Tjernstrom: Drug-induced changes in Eustachian tube function. Ear Nose Throat J 77:778-782, 1998
16. Bluestone CD, Beery QC, Andrus WS: Mechanics of the Eustachian tube as it influences susceptibility to and persistence of middle ear effusions in children. Ann Otol Rhinol Laryngol 83(Suppl 11):27-36, 1974
17. Bylander A, Tjernstrom O, Ivarsson A: Pressure opening and closing functions of the Eustachian tube by inflation and deflation in children and adults with normal ears. Acta Otolaryngol (Stockh) 96(3/4):255-268, 1983
18. Cantekin EI, Doyle WJ, Reichert TJ, Phillips DC, Bluestone CD: Dilation of the Eustachian tube by electrical stimulation of the trigeminal nerve. Ann Otol Rhinol Laryngol 88:40-51, 1979

19. Rood RS, Doyle WJ: The nasopharyngeal orifice of the auditory tube: implications for tubal dynamics. Cleft Palate J 19:119-128, 1982

20. Hergils L, Magnuson B: Morning pressure in the middle ear. Arch Otolaryngol Head Neck Surg 111:86-89, 1985

21. Bylander A, Ivarsson A, Tjernstrom O et al: Middle ear pressure variations during 24 hours in children. Ann Otol Rhinol Laryngol 94(Suppl 20):33-35, 1985

22. Hergils L, Magnuson B: Middle-ear pressure under basal conditions. Arch Otolaryngol Head Neck Surg 113:829-832, 1987

23. Hergils L, Magnuson B: Regulation of negative middle ear pressure without tubal opening. Arch Otolaryngol Head Neck Surg 114:1442-1444, 1988

24. Buckingham RA: Patent Eustachian tube in the underaerated middle ear: a paradox. Ann Otol Rhinol Laryngol 97:219-221, 1988

25. Miura M, Takahashi T, Honjo I et al: Influence of the gas exchange function through the middle ear mucosa on the development of sniff-induced middle ear disease. Laryngoscope 108:683-686, 1998

26. Doyle WJ: Increases in middle ear pressure resulting from counter-diffusion of oxygen and carbon dioxide into the middle ear of monkeys. Acta Otolaryngol (Stockh) 117:708-713, 1997

27. Doyle WJ: Mucosal surface area determines the middle ear pressure response following establishment of sniff induced underpressures. Acta Otolaryngol (Stockh) 119:695-702, 1999

28. Doyle WJ, Seroky JT: Middle ear gas exchange in rhesus Monkeys. Ann Otol Rhinol Laryngol 103:636-645, 1994

29. Doyle WJ, Seroky JT, Alper CM: Gas exchange across the middle ear mucosa in monkeys: estimation of exchange rates. Arch Otolaryngol Head Neck Surg 111:887-892, 1995

30. Doyle WJ, Alper CM, Seroky JT: Trans-mucosal inert gas exchange constants for the monkey middle ear. Auxus Nasus Larynx 26:5-12, 1999

31. Proud GD, Odoi H: Effects of Eustachian tube ligation. Ann Otol Rhinol Laryngol 79:30-32, 1970

32. Reiner CE, Pulec JL: Experimental production of serous otitis media. Ann Otol Rhinol Laryngol 78:880-887, 1969

33. Senturia BH, Carr CD, Ahlvin RC: Middle ear effusions: pathologic changes of the muco-periosteum in the experimental animal. Ann Otol Rhinol Laryngol 71:632-647, 1962

34. Tos M: Experimental tubal occlusion. Acta Otolaryngol (Stockh) 92:51-61, 1981

35. Paparella MM, Hiraide F, Juhn SK, Kaneko Y: Cellular events involved in middle ear fluid production. Ann Otol Rhinol Laryngol 79:766-779, 1970

36. Cantekin EI, Bluestone CD, Saez C, Doyle WJ, Phillips DC: Normal and abnormal middle ear ventilation. Ann Otol Rhinol Laryngol 86(Suppl 41):1-15, 1977

37. Doyle WJ: Functional Eustachian tube obstruction and otitis media in a primate model. Acta Otolaryngol (Stockh) Suppl 414:52-57, 1984

38. Casselbrant ML, Cantekin EI, Dirkmaat D, Doyle WJ, Bluestone CD: Experimental paralysis of the tensor veli palatini muscle. Acta Otolaryngol (Stockh) 106:178-185, 1988

39. Alper CM, Tabari R, Seroky JT, Doyle WJ: Magnetic resonance imaging of the development of OM with effusion caused by functional obstruction of the ET. Ann Otol Rhinol Laryngol 106:422-431, 1997

40. Swarts JD, Alper CM, Seroky JT, Chan KH, Doyle WJ: In vivo observation with MRI of middle ear effusion in response to experimental underpressures. Ann Otol Rhinol Laryngol 104:522-528, 1995

41. Alper CM, Ardic FN, Doyle WJ: The effects of changing middle ear pressure and gas partial pressure on mucosal blood flow and vascular permeability in the chinchilla. Auxus Nasus Larynx 27:105-111, 2000

42. Politzer A: Lehrbuch der Ohrenheilkunde fur Prachtische Arzte und Studierende. Stuttgart: Ferdinand Enke Verlag 1878

43. Van Dishoeck HAE: Negative middle ear pressure and losses of hearing in tubal catarrh. Acta Otolaryngol (Stockh) 29:303-312, 1940

44. Flisberg K, Ingelstedt A, Ortegren U: On middle ear pressure. Acta Otolaryngol (Stockh) 182:43-56, 1963

45. Hiraide F, Eriksson H: The effects of the vacuum on vascular permeability of the middle ear. Acta Otolaryngol (Stockh) 85:10-16, 1978

46. Lamkin R, Axelsson A, McPherson D, Miller J: Experimental aural barotrauma: electro-physiological and morphological findings. Acta Otolaryngol (Stockh) Suppl 335: 1975

47. Fria TJ, Cantekin EI, Eichler JA: Hearing acuity of children with otitis media with effusion. Arch Otolaryngol 111:10-16, 1985

48. Munker G: The patulous Eustachian tube. In: Munker G, Arnold W (eds) Physiology and Pathophysiology of Eustachian Tube and Middle Ear, pp 113-118. New York, NY: Thieme-Stratton Inc 1980

49. Magnuson B: On the origin of the high negative pressure in the middle ear space. Am J Otolaryngol 2:1-12, 1981

50. Magnuson B: Tubal opening and closing ability in unilateral middle ear disease. Am J Otolaryngol 2:199, 1981

51. Falk B, Magnuson B: Evacuation of the middle ear by sniffing: a cause of high negative pressure and development of middle ear disease. Otolaryngol Head Neck Surg 92:312-318, 1984

52. Cantekin EI, Doyle WJ, Bluestone CD: A comparison of normal Eustachian tube function in the rhesus monkey and man. Ann Otol Rhinol Laryngol 91:179-184, 1982

53. Cantekin EI, Saez CA, Bluestone CD et al: Airflow through the eustachian tube. Ann Otol Rhinol Laryngol 88:603-612, 1979

54. Bylander A: Middle ear pressure variations during 24 hour in children. Ann Otol Rhinol Laryngol 94:(Suppl 120):335-342, 1985

55. Moody SA, Alper CM, Doyle WJ: Daily tympanometry in children during the cold season: association of otitis media with upper respiratory tract infections. Int J Ped Otolaryngol 45:143-150, 1998

56. Tideholm B, Carlborg B, Jonsson S, Bylander-Groth A: Continuous long-term measurements of the middle ear pressure in subjects without a history of ear disease. Acta Otolaryngol (Stockh) 118:369-374, 1998

57. Bylander A: Comparison of Eustachian tube function in children and adults with normal ears. Ann Otol Rhinol Laryngol 89:20, 1980

58. Bylander A, Tjernstrom O, Ivarsson A, Andreasson L: Eustachian tube function and its relation to middle ear pressure in children. Auris Nasus Larynx 12(Suppl 1):43-45, 1985

59. Stenstrom C, Bylander-Groth A, Ingvarsson L: Eustachian tube function in otitis-prone and healthy children. Int J Pediatr Otorhinolaryngol 21:127, 1991

60. Diamant M, Rubensohn G, Walander A: Otosalphingitis and mastoid pneumatization. Acta Otolaryngol (Stockh) 49:381-388, 1958

61. Goto T, Kaieda T: The relation of the middle ear pneumatization and the catarrhal otitis media. J Otorhinolaryngol Soc Jpn 61:897-899, 1958

62. Hadas E, Sadé J: Prognosis in secretory otitis media relative to pneumatization. Arch Otolaryngol 225:39-44, 1979

63. Sederberg-Olsen JF, Sedeberg-Olsen AE, Jensen AM: The prognostic significance of the air volume in the middle ear for the tendency to recurrence of secretory middle ear condition. Int J Pediatr Otorhinolaryngol 5:179-187, 1983

64. Nakano Y, Sato Y: Prognosis of otitis media with effusion in children and the size of the mastoid air cell system. Acta Otolaryngol (Stockh) Suppl 471:56-61, 1990

65. Sadé J: The correlation of middle ear aeration with mastoid pneumatization: the mastoid as a pressure buffer. Eur Arch Otorhinolaryngol 249:301-304, 1992

66. Bayramoglu I, Ardic FN, Kara CO, Ozuer MZ, Katircioglu O, Topuz B: Importance of

mastoid pneumatization on secretory otitis media. Int J Pediatr Otorhinolaryngol 40:61-66, 1997

67. Sadé J, Fuchs C: Secretory otitis media in adults: I. The role of mastoid pneumatization as a risk factor. Ann Otol Rhinol Laryngol 105:643-647, 1996

68. Sadé J, Fuchs C: Secretory otitis media in adults: II. The role of mastoid pneumatization as a prognostic factor. Ann Otol Rhinol Laryngol 106:37-40, 1997

69. Doyle WJ: Experimental results do not support a gas reserve function for the mastoid. Int J Ped Otolaryngol 2000 (in press)

70. Leclerc JE, Doyle WJ, Karnavas W: Physiological modulation of Eustachian tube function. Acta Otolaryngol (Stockh) 104:500-510, 1987

71. Shupak A, Tabari R, Swarts JD, Doyle WJ, Bluestone CD: Effects of middle ear oxygen and carbon dioxide tensions on Eustachian tube ventilatory function. Laryngoscope 106:(2)221-224, 1996

72. Shupak A, Tabari R, Swarts JD, Bluestone CD, WJ Doyle: Effect of systemic hyperoxia on eustachian tube ventilatory function. Laryngoscope 107:1409-1413, 1997

73. Eden AR, Gannon PJ: Neural control of middle ear aeration. Arch Otolaryngol Head Neck Surg 113:133-137, 1987

74. King AD, Kew J, Tong M, Leung SF, Lam WW, Metreweli C, Van Hasselt CA: Magnetic resonance imaging of the Eustachian tube in nasopharyngeal carcinoma: correlation of patterns of spread with middle ear effusion. Am J Otol 20:69-73, 1999

75. Takahashi H, Honjo I, Fujita A: Endoscopic findings at the pharyngeal orifice of the Eustachian tube in otitis media with effusion. Eur Arch Otorhinolaryngol 253:42-44, 1996

76. Doyle WJ, Cantekin EI, Bluestone CD: Eustachian tube function in cleft palate children. Ann Otol Rhinol Laryngol 89(Suppl 68):34-40, 1980

77. Doyle WJ, Reilly JS, Jardini L, Rovnak S: The effect of palatoplasty on the function of the Eustachian tube in cleft palate children. Cleft Palate J 23:68-80, 1986

78. Doyle WJ, Friedman R, Fireman P, Bluestone CD: Eustachian tube obstruction after provocative nasal antigen challenge. Arch Otolaryngol 110:508-511, 1984

79. Skoner DP, Doyle WJ, Boehm S, Fireman P: Late phase Eustachian tube and nasal allergic responses associated with inflammatory mediator elaboration. Am J Rhinol 2:155-162, 1988

80. Doyle WJ, Alper CM, Buchman C, Moody SA, Skoner DP, Cohen S: Illness and otological change provoked by experimental upper respiratory virus infection. Laryngoscope 109:324-327, 1999

81. Doyle WJ, Skoner DP, Fireman P, Seroky JT, Green I, Ruben F, Kardatzke DR, Gwaltney JM: Rhinovirus 39 Infection in allergic and non allergic subjects. J Allergy Clin Immunol 89:968-978, 1992

82. Doyle WJ, Skoner DP, Hayden F, Buchman C, Seroky JT, Fireman P: Nasal and otologic effects of experimental Influenza A virus infection. Ann Otol Rhinol Laryngol 103:59-69, 1994

83. Chan KH, Swarts JD, Doyle WJ, Wolf GL: Assessment of middle ear status during experimental otitis media using magnetic resonance imaging. Arch Otolaryngol 117:91-95, 1991

84. Hergels l, Magnuson B: Nasal gas composition in humans and its implications on middle ear pressure. Acta Otolaryngol (Stockh) 118:697-700, 1998

NEW INSIGHTS INTO VIBRATION OF THE MIDDLE EAR

Willem F. Decraemer[1] and Shyam M. Khanna[2]

[1]Biomedical Physics Department, University of Antwerp, RUCA, Antwerp, Belgium; [2]Department of Otolaryngology, Columbia University, New York, NY, USA

Abstract

To investigate the relationship between the motion of the malleus, incus and stapes in the middle ear of the cat, the three-dimensional (3D) vibrations of the three ossicles were measured in the same ear utilizing a confocal heterodyne interferometer. Each ossicle was treated as a separate rigid body and its motion was calculated individually. The motion parameters derived from this calculation were combined to animate a 3D model of the complete middle ear.

While the malleus vibration changed from simple, nearly hinged motion at low frequencies to very complex motion at higher frequencies, the stapes moved in a predominantly piston-like way. The incus transforms the complex malleus motion into the simple motion of the stapes. The incudo-stapedial joint plays a major role in this complex transmission mechanism.

It is accepted that the ossicles rotate around a fixed axis and function as mechanical levers. The authors' precise vibration measurements on malleus do not confirm this theory.

Keywords: middle ear, mechanics, ossicles, vibration, interferometer

Introduction

The function of the middle ear is that of an impedance transformer between the low input impedance of the middle ear at the air-tympanic membrane interface

This research was supported by the Emil Capita Fund, NOHR, National Science Research Foundation of Belgium, and Research Funds of the University of Antwerp (RUCA).

This study was performed in accordance with PHS Policy on Humane Care and Use of Laboratory Animals, the NIH Guide for the Care and Use of Laboratory Animals, and the Animal Welfare Act (7 U.S.C. et seq.); the animal use protocol was approved by the Institutional Animal Care and Use Committee (IACUC) of Columbia University, New York, NY.

Address for correspondence: Willem Decraemer, University of Antwerp, RUCA, Groenenborgerlaan 171, B-2020 Antwerpen, Belgium. *email:* wimdec@ruca.ua.ac.be

The Function and Mechanics of Normal, Diseased and Reconstructed Middle Ears, pp. 23–38
edited by J.J. Rosowski and S.N. Merchant
© *2000 Kugler Publications, The Hague, The Netherlands*

(large displacement velocity combined with small pressure) and a high output impedance at the stapes footplate-perilymph interface (small displacement velocity combined with large pressure). Part of this transformer action is classically attributed to a lever formed by the ossicles. It is commonly believed that the ossicles rotate about a fixed axis, which runs through the anterior process of the malleus and the end of the short process of the incus. Some of the authors who contributed to the adoption of this hypothesis include: Helmholtz[1], Bárány[2], Dahman[3,4], Stuhlman[5], Fumagalli[6], von Békésy[7], Wever and Lawrence[8]. At different times it was noted that, at higher frequencies, the 'lever ratio of the middle ear' did not remain fixed[9-14], which was argued to be slippage in the joints between the ossicles, or a shift of the fixed rotation axis.

In a series of papers, we have clearly shown that the malleus of cat does not vibrate around a fixed axis[15-19], but that the motion changes with frequency, and that all three-dimensional (3D) components of translation and rotation are present. A fixed rotation axis at any frequency is seen only occasionally. Even the instantaneous rotation axis does not remain fixed within a cycle. More recently, we also investigated the motion of the stapes[20-22]. As in our studies of malleus vibration, we did not assume any preferential direction of stapes motion, but measured the full 3D components of the stapes vibration at three points. It was found that the stapes moves predominantly as a piston in the oval window, but that smaller rocking modes of the footplate are also present.

In this paper, to investigate how the middle ear converts and couples complex malleus motion to a simple stapes motion, we measured the 3D motion of the three ossicles in the same ear, using a heterodyne interferometer. Each ossicle was treated as a separate rigid body, and its motion was calculated individually. The motion parameters derived from this calculation were combined to animate a 3D model of the complete middle ear.

Material and preparation

It is not practical to measure the 3D vibrations of the three ossicles in the middle ear in living animals due to the lack of visual access. The ossicles lie deep in the middle ear, partly hidden by the walls of the complexly-shaped middle ear or by ligaments, and they further obstruct each other from view. Therefore, a fresh temporal bone model was developed. Even in the temporal bone, a good approach that allows visualization of all three ossicles, is hard to find. We have developed a novel preparation that allows good optical access to the malleus and reasonably good access to incus and stapes, while it leaves the septum intact.

The experiments were performed on fresh temporal bones from cats with clear tympanic membranes, weighing between 1.9 and 2.5 kg. After the cats had been deeply anesthetized and sacrificed, both temporal bones were extracted and examined. Only those middle ears with no bleeding in the middle

ear cavity were used. Both left and right ears were utilized for the measurements.

The external ear was removed, leaving about 1 cm of the end of the external
ear canal. A tight fitting conical ear insert was placed in the remaining ear
canal for attaching the sound system. The middle ear cavity was opened from
the ventral side, near the attachment of the base of the conical tensor tympani
muscle to the middle ear wall. The muscle ligament extending to the anterior
process of the malleus handle was cut and removed. The hole was enlarged to
a maximum, taking care not to damage any structures such as the annulus, or to
dislocate the incudo-malleolar joint, and preventing bone debris from falling
into the middle ear. Looking through this opening (Fig. 1) we can see the larger
part of the side of the manubrium, from the thin part at the umbo to the thick
part near the malleus neck. Only a small part of the incus close to the lenticular
process can be seen. The stapes head and upper part of both crura can also be
observed. The lower part of the crura and the footplate of the stapes remain
hidden behind a bony rim, and vibrations could not be measured there.

When the middle ear is opened and the medial mucous side of the tympanic
membrane is exposed to the air, it dries out quickly. This is a well-know problem in middle ear research. We provided extra humidity in the middle ear by
placing tiny pieces of wet paper towel on the floor of the middle ear cavity and
resealing the middle ear cavity with a microscope cover slip. This cover slip
was held with a ring of soft modelling clay pressed around the cavity opening.
To equalize pressure differences between the middle ear cavity and the ambient
room, a small capillary tube (PE 10, length 6 cm) was conducted through the
modelling clay. This novel middle ear preparation has the advantage that the
middle ear acoustics are minimally changed, since the cavity is practically unaltered in volume and closed during the measurements, and that the bony sep-

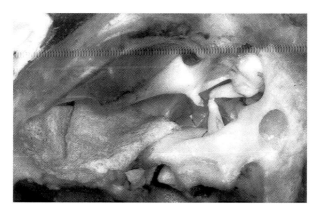

Fig. 1. Photograph of the middle ear of a cat taken through the opening made in the wall of the
middle ear. From top to bottom, we can first see the white structure of the malleus (M) with the
anterior process (AP) pointing towards the camera (the ligament was severed), then part of the
incus (I) and stapes (S) with its front and rear leg. The footplate is hidden in a bony niche.

tum is also kept in place. The total preparation time was approximately three hours.

Equipment and measuring procedure

Vibration measurements

After orientating the temporal bone for the best view of the ossicles, it is glued with dental cement onto a metal tube (4 cm long, 2 cm diameter). This tube has a C-mount, which is screwed into a piezoelectric device originally designed for precise microscope object lens focusing (PI, P 721.10). A rod attached to the piezo device is clamped in the object holder of the interferometer. The object mounting system of the interferometer is suspended within two nested goniometers. These allow a change in the observation angle of any selected point in two orthogonal planes by rotation of the object around the focal point[16]. The point of rotation of the two goniometers is adjusted to coincide precisely with the focal point of the microscope-interferometer objective lens. Therefore, rotation of the goniometers does not shift the point of observation. Three translation stages equipped with micrometer reading scales allowed precise changes in the x, y and z planes of the laser beam's position. Stepper motors, which can be controlled from a computer, activate the two rotations and the three translations.

An acoustic transducer with a probe microphone is tightly coupled to the insert placed in the ear canal in order to apply sound and measure its pressure[23]. The acoustic system and the temporal bone are mounted on the same post and move together as the position or the observation direction is changed. The measuring equipment and procedure have been described previously[15].

At the start of the experiment, the interferometer is focused on a point on the head of the stapes, about a tenth of a mm below the incudo-stapedial joint. Using pure-tone stimuli with reasonably moderate sound pressures (between 80 and 90 dB), frequency responses are repeatedly measured with the heterodyne interferometer at this same position until we obtain a stable response.

Then vibration is measured at a large number of frequencies at a set of points spread over the visible parts of the three ossicles (six to seven points per ossicle). Coordinates of the observation points are stored, so that we can later return to these points using the stepper motors under computer control.

After the first set of measurements over the three ossicles has been completed, with the goniometers set at their mid positions, the measurements are repeated at four different viewing angles, chosen by changing either the vertical or horizontal goniometer position as far as possible up and down. Maximal change in angle was about ±15°, beyond this limit the interferometer beam was blocked by the bulla wall. Sound pressures were measured simultaneously with a probe microphone whose tip was at the end of the metal ear insert, a few mm in front of the tympanic membrane.

In order to define the position of the middle ear ossicles in the experimental reference system, a set of anatomical coordinates was determined by focusing the laser spot on a large number of points spread over the ossicles while recording the x, y and z coordinates of the different points. This anatomical tracing was performed with the goniometer set to the mid position.

Three-dimensional ossicular chain model

Using a high resolution computer tomograph (Skyscan 1072 X-Ray Microtomograph), the temporal bone of one of the experiments was scanned. The malleus, incus and stapes were individually segmented using the software package Surfdriver. 3D reconstructions of the three ossicles were finally produced in the form of triangulated objects.

In order to align the computer tomography (CT)-generated model with the position of the ossicles during the experiment, we first rotated the model within the Surfdriver environment to obtain a rough visual alignment. Then, we applied an Iterative Closest Point (ICP) algorithm[24] registration procedure for final alignment. Figure 2 shows the triangulated model after this alignment on a color coded, 3D plot. The color is proportional to surface height, which can be useful for distinguishing the motion of some locations in the subsequent

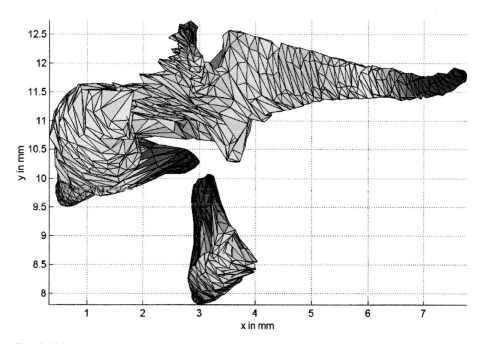

Fig. 2. Triangulated 3D model of the ossicular chain after registration of the position of the ossicles during the experiment. The motion parameters determined from the experimental data can be applied directly to animate the model. The ossicles are shown with a color code proportional to surface height. This can be useful for distinguishing the motion of some locations in the subsequent figures of moving ossicles (Figs. 3 to 6).

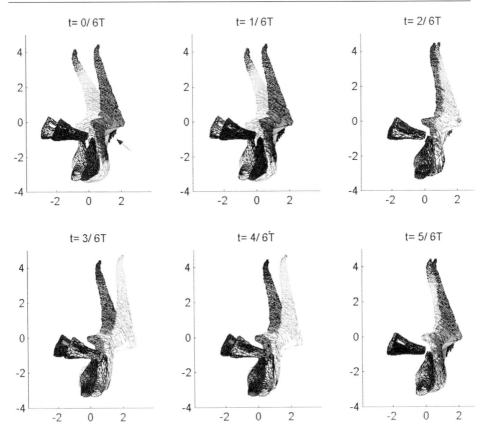

Fig. 3a. Six panels illustrating the motion of the cat ossicular chain at 290 Hz. The 3D plots are shown from a viewpoint that gives a more or less posterior-to-anterior view of the ossicles. In each of the panels, we have plotted the resting position of the chain (dark, color-shaded), as well as its displaced position (lighter, meshed) at t = 0, T/6, 2T/6 ... 5/6T, as indicated at the top. The scaling factor for the displacements is 1500.

figures that show the moving ossicles (Figs. 3 to 6). The gap between the incus and stapes head is normally filled by a fibrous ligament, which is invisible on the CT microscan.

Methods

Rigid body motion calculation

To describe the motion of a rigid body mathematically, we use a stationary, inertial reference frame O_{xyz} attached to the set up (right-handed system with x-axis horizontal to the right, y-axis vertical up, z-axis along observation direction). The general motion of a rigid body may be decomposed in a rotation about the origin O, followed by a global translation of the body. Consequently

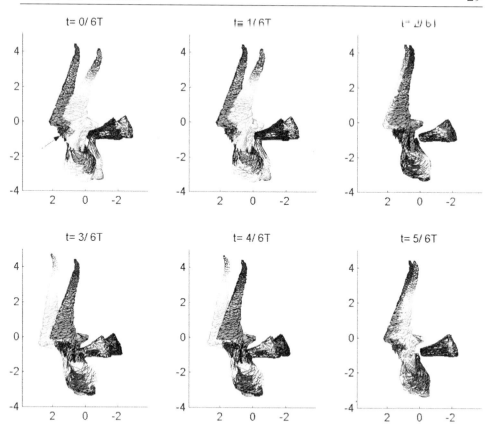

Fig. 3b. The same motion with a viewing direction opposite to that of Figure 3a. The malleus and incus vibrate as one block while the incus moves with a piston-like motion. *See* text for further interpretation of the motion.

the velocity of a point P_i of the rigid body (here the malleus, incus or stapes) can be written as

$$\mathbf{v_i(t)} = \mathbf{v_t(t)} + \mathbf{\Omega(t)} \times \mathbf{r_i} \tag{1}$$

$\mathbf{v_i(t)}$:   velocity of P_i with components v_x, v_y, v_z

$\mathbf{v_t(t)}$:   velocity of the global translational motion component, with components $v_{O'x}, v_{O'y}, v_{O'z}$

$\mathbf{\Omega(t)}$:   angular velocity of the rigid body rotating about O with components $\Omega_x, \Omega_y, \Omega_z$

$\mathbf{r_i}$:   rest-position vector of point P_i with components x,y,z

$\mathbf{\Omega(t)} \times \mathbf{r_i}$: velocity of the rotational motion component of P_i relative to O_{xyz}

In our experiments, we use a harmonic sound stimulus and, as a consequence, all functions of time t become harmonic.

We can write **v** as **ds/dt** and **dΩ** as **dΘ/dt**, so that multiplying both sides of

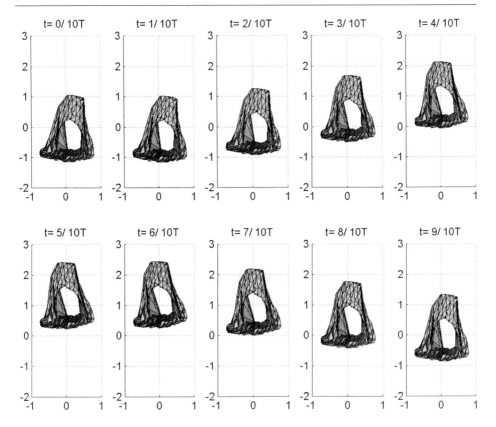

Fig. 4. The motion of the incus is shown in an 'intrinsic' reference system, with the y-axis from the center of the footplate (system origin) to the top of the stapes head, and the x- and y-axes along the long and short axes of the footplate, respectively. Ten consecutive phases of the motion at 0.3 kHz (compare Fig. 3) are shown. Tilting of the footplate is present around both its long and short axes, but this must be regarded as a second order effect superimposed on the dominant motion perpendicular to the oval window. *Fig. 4a.* Frontal view.

equation (1) by dt, we end up with an equation between infinitesimal linear and angular displacements

$$ds_i(t) = ds_t(t) + d\Theta(t) \times r_i \qquad (2)$$

The middle ear vibration amplitudes are small (of the order of 10^{-8} m), so that equation (2) can be used to describe the experimental displacements. In what follows, the differential notation will be further used to denote very small but finite displacements.

With the interferometer, we can only observe the component of vibration along the interferometer viewing direction. When the object is rotated using the goniometers, we can observe vibration from a different viewing direction. Using the vibration measured from the five different observation directions, we can cal-

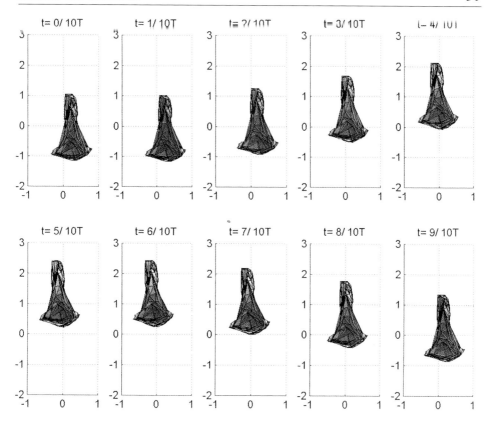

Fig. 4b. Motion of the stages at 0.3 kHz. Sideways view.

culate the x,y,z components of the motion parameters $ds_t(t)$ and $d\Theta(t)$. As these parameters are all harmonic functions of time, we obtain three amplitudes and three phase angles for the translation and three amplitudes and three phase angles for the rotation. This procedure is repeated for each experimental frequency.

Animation of the three-dimensional model

It is hard to describe how a body moves in three dimensions unless the motion itself can be shown, and then it becomes self-explanatory. We use animations to show the motion of the 3D model. To construct such animation, we use the motion parameters extracted from the experimental vibration data, and calculate the positions of the triangulated model at a number of equally spaced intervals during a cycle (Figs. 3, 5 and 6). It is obvious that the microscopic displacements must be magnified by a large factor in order to make them visible in the mm scale used to plot the ossicles. A computer can then be used to show the 3D model going through its sequential positions. These animations can be viewed from different viewpoints so that all aspects of the motion can be studied. On a printed page we can only show a 'still' animation, a series of different stages of the object during the cycle. The Internet

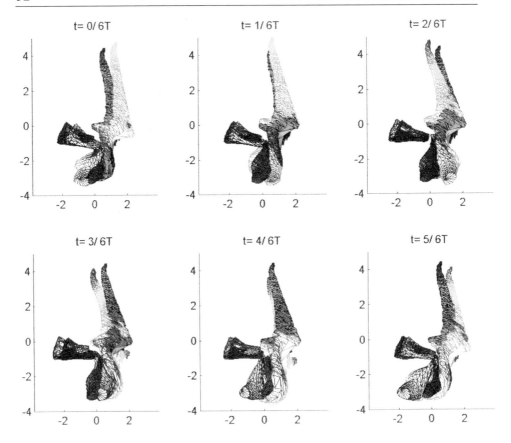

Fig. 5a. Ossicular chain motion at a frequency of 5 kHz. This Figure is organized similarly to Figure 3. The scaling factor for the displacements is now 4500. Slippage in the malleus-incus joint can now be seen. The incus motion is quasi unchanged from that seen at low frequencies.

can play a perfect complementary role to classical printing when the animations are put on a web page. The realization of such a page under the name of one of the authors (WFD) is in preparation.

Results

Frequency responses of the different motion parameters are not too instructive as the motion is too complex, and will therefore not be shown. A simple look at the very different trends in these plots tells us that the motion will change significantly with frequency. We cannot show the motion at all frequencies that were measured, but will give some typical examples to illustrate the variation of the vibration mode with frequency.

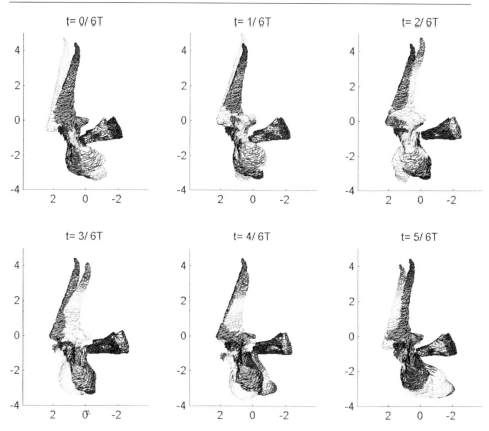

Fig. 5b. Ossicular chain motion at 5 kHz in an anterior-to-posterior view.

Motion at 0.3 kHz

Figure 3a illustrates the sequence of motion of the cat ossicular chain at 300 Hz in six panels (at t = 0, T/6, 2T/6 ... 5/6T). In each of the panels, we have plotted the resting position of the chain (dark, color shaded) and its displaced position (lighter, meshed). The displacements have been magnified by a factor of 1500. The 3D plots are shown from a viewpoint that gives an approximate posterior-to-anterior view of the ossicles in Figure 3a. In Figure 3b the ossicles have been rotated by 180 degrees. The motion of the ossicles in the plane of the paper can be seen directly as the change in the position of the ossicles (lighter color) with reference to the stationary image (dark color). The representation of the motion perpendicular to the plane of the paper is harder to interpret. We see how, during the cycle, the manubrium moves at times in front of its stationary image (Fig. 3a, t = 5T/6) and is then hidden behind it (Fig. 3b, t = 2/6T). The posterior process of the incus (the very tip of it was missed during the CT scan) points towards us at the bottom of the figure, the stapes points to the left in the middle (Fig. 3a), and the manubrium points vertically up. The anterior mallar process is partially visible in panels 1 and 2 as the red blob under the lateral process of the manubrium (indicated by an arrow in the top left panel). It remains almost stationary during the cycle. The sequences of the panels in Figures 3a and 3b show that the malleus and incus move as one block. The stapes does not move solidly along with the two other ossicles, but performs a nearly linear motion along a direction from the center of its footplate through its head. The posterior tip of the incus moves in the same direction as the stapes, which means that a fixed rotation axis not is observed. The angle between the incus and the plane of the crura of the stapes is constantly changing during the cycle.

The motion of the stapes was studied in more detail by plotting its position as a time sequence (Fig. 4) for t = 0, 1/10T, 2/10T, ... 9/10T , in a frontal (Fig. 4a) and a sideways view (Fig. 4b). The displacements are also shown for a frequency of 300 Hz, and have been magnified by a factor of 1500. The footplate motion is predominantly piston-like with some tilt along the major and minor axes.

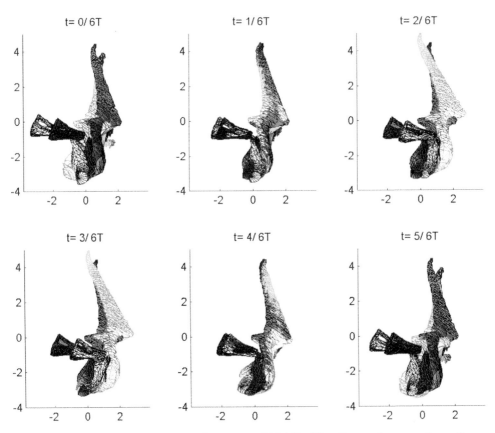

Fig. 6a. Ossicular chain motion at a frequency of 10 kHz. The slippage between the malleus and incus is more pronounced than at 5 kHz (Fig. 5). The malleus motion has become very complex, with the umbo and footplate vibrating almost in opposing phase. As for the stapes, this is still moving in a dominantly piston mode.

Motion at 5 kHz

The motion of the ossicles at 5 kHz is shown in Figure 5. The displacement has now been scaled up by a factor of 4500. Compared to the motion at 300 Hz, the motion of the malleus and incus at 5 kHz is more complex, since some relative motion between the malleus and incus can be observed. The anterior process of the malleus is no longer stationary and the excursion of the posterior incudal process has become larger than at the low frequency. The stapes motion remains qualitatively unchanged. Once again, the angle between the incus and the plane of the crura of the stapes is changing continuously.

Motion at 10 kHz

Figure 6 illustrates the motion at 10 kHz, again with a scaling factor of 4500. The strong coupling in motion between the malleus and incus is now completely lost. It is remarkable that the phase between umbo displacement and footplate displacement is quite different from that at 0.3 and 5 kHz. At this frequency, while the

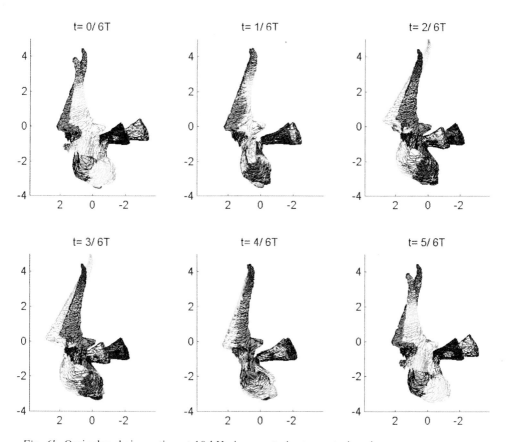

Fig. 6b. Ossicular chain motion at 10 kHz in an anterior-to-posterior view.

umbo moves medially, the stapes moves out of the oval window. As seen in the 3D animation, the motion of the malleus has now become very complex. The motion of the ossicular chain is far from being a hinged motion. However, the stapes continues to move in a simple, mainly piston-like way. Again, the angle with the incus keeps changing during the cycle.

Discussion

At low frequencies, the motion of the middle ear chain is characterized by the malleus and incus moving as one fixed block, and a stapes that moves quasi piston-like in a direction perpendicular to the oval window. During the cycle, the angle between the crura of the stapes and the incus is continually changing. The anterior mallar process remains almost fixed, while the posterior incudal process vibrates back and forth. These two points are believed to define the stationary rotation axis.

At high frequencies, the stapes motion remains qualitatively unchanged and 'piston-like'. The coupling between the malleus and incus is gradually lost. The phase of vibration between, for example, umbo and footplate is strongly frequency-dependent. At low frequencies, inward motion of the umbo produces an inward motion of the footplate, while at 10 kHz, the same motion of the umbo produces an outward motion of the footplate.

The joints between the malleus and incus allow for their differences in motion. The thin connection between the incus and stapes (Fig. 7) forms a coupling with multiple degrees of freedom, which makes it possible to have a complex motion of the incus resulting in a simple motion of the stapes.

Conclusions

The middle ear is a mechanical system that must efficiently couple sound energy from the ear canal to the inner ear. At the input of this system, the malleus is found to change vibration mode with frequency, and the vibrations occur in all three dimensions. At the output of the middle ear, a stapes motion perpendicular to the footplate is most efficient for moving the fluid in the cochlea. The stapes vibrates in this mode from low to very high frequencies. To make it possible to couple the complex malleus motion at the input to the simple stapes motion, the middle ear uses a construction with three ossicles and intermediate joints. The joint between the malleus and the incus mainly allows a rotation perpendicular to the joint surfaces. The joint between the incus and the stapes is more like a point-to-point contact, and allows many degrees of freedom. The result of both connections is that the middle ear transfers a large variety of malleus motion, which may even become very complex, into simple and quasi, invariably piston-like vibration at its output. The 3D vibrations of the malleus are due to the geometry of the coupling with the tympanic membrane and the modes of the membrane vibrations. If only a single

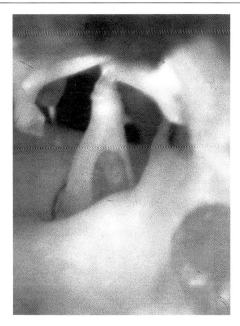

Fig. 7. The connection between the malleus and incus in greater detail. The fibrous band can be seen to be very thin in the direction of the plane of the two crura, and somewhat broader in the opposite direction. This makes up for an almost point-to-point contact between incus and stapes which allows many degrees of freedom. It must play an important role in the mechanism of the middle ear, which converts a complex malleus motion at its input into a simple stapes motion at its output.

mode of vibration was utilized, the frequency response would have maxima and minima associated with this mode. Combining different modes smoothes the overall frequency response of the middle ear system.

References

1. Helmholtz H: The mechanism of the ossicles of the ear and membrana tympani (translation). Originally published in German in Plfügers Arch Physiol Vol 1, Bonn 1869
2. Bárány E: A contribution to the physiology of bone conduction. Acta Otolaryngol (Stockh) Suppl 26, 1938
3. Dahman H: On the physiology of hearing: experimental studies on the mechanics of the ossicular chain, as well as on the behaviours of tones and air pressure I. Zeitschr Hals Nas Ohrenhlk 24:462-498 [in German], 1929
4. Dahman H: On the physiology of hearing: experimental studies on the mechanics of the ossicular chain, as well as on the behaviours of tones and air pressure II-IV. Zeitschr Hals Nas Ohrenhlk 27:329-368, discussion 398-402 [in German], 1930
5. Stuhlman O Jr.: The nonlinear transmission characteristics of the auditory ossicles. J Acoust Soc Am 9:119-128, 1937
6. Fumagalli Z: Ricerche morfologiche sull'apparato di trasmissione del suono (sound conducting apparatus: a study of morphology). Arch Ital Otol Rinol Laringol 60 Suppl 1, 1949

7. Békésy G: Experiments in Hearing. New York, NY: McGraw Hill Book Co 1960
8. Wever EG, Lawrence M: Physiological Acoustics. Princeton, NJ: Princeton University Press, Princeton, 1954
9. Guinan JJ, Peake WF: Middle-ear characteristics of anesthetized cats. J Acoust Soc Am 41:1237-1261, 1967
10. Gundersen T, Høgmoen K: Prosthesis in the ossicular chain. Arch Otolaryng 96:416, 1972
11. Gundersen T, Høgmoen K: Holographic vibration analysis of the ossicular chain. Acta Otolaryngol (Stockh) 82:16-25, 1976
12. Feenstra L, Vlaming MSMG: Laser interferometry with human temporal bones. Adv Oto-Rhino-Laryngol 37:36-38, 1987
13. Guyo K, Aritomo H, Goode R: Measuring of the ossicular vibration ratio in human temporal bones by use of a video measuring system. Acta Otolaryngol (Stockh) 103:87-95, 1987
14. Brenkman CJ: Sound transfer characteristics of the middle ear. Thesis, University Leiden 1986
15. Decraemer WF, Khanna WM, Funnell WRJ: Malleus vibration mode changes with frequency. Hearing Res 54:305-318, 1991
16. Decraemer WF, Khanna SM, Funnell WRJ: Modelling the malleus vibration as a rigid body motion with one rotational and one translational degree of freedom. Hearing Res 72(1/2):1-18, 1994
17. Decraemer WF, Khanna SM: Malleus motion modelled as rigid body motion. Acta Oto-Rhino-Laryngol Belg 49:139-145, 1995
18. Decraemer WF, Khanna SM: Malleus vibrations in the cat ear are three dimensional. In: Proceedings of the Diversity in Auditory Mechanics, Berkeley, CA, pp 115-121. 1996
19. Decraemer WF, Khanna SM: Vibrations on the malleus measured through the ear canal. In: Hüttenbrink KB (ed) Proceedings of Middle Ear Mechanics in Research and Otosurgery, Dresden, September 19-22, 1996, pp 32-39. 1997
20. Decraemer WF, Khanna SM: Three-dimensional vibration of the stapes measured with a heterodyne interferometer. In: Tomasini EP (ed) Vibration Measurements by Laser Techniques: Advances and Applications, Vol 3411, pp 550-563. SPIE 1998
21. Decraemer WF, Khanna SM: Measurement and modelling of the three-dimensional vibrations of the stapes in cat. In: Abstracts of the Symposium on Recent Developments in Auditory Mechanics, Sendai, Japan, pp 20-21, 1999
22. Decraemer WF, Khanna SM: Vibration in the cat middle ear. In: Proceedings of the 15th Brazilian Congress of Mechanical Engineering, COBEM 99, CD-rom (Sonopress, Brazil), pp 1-12. 1999
23. Stinson MR, Khanna SM: Spatial distribution of sound pressure and energy flow conditions in the ear canals of cats. J Acoust Soc Am 96(1):170-180, 1994
24. Besl PJ, McKay ND: A method for registration of 3D shapes, IEEE Trans Pattern Anal Machine Intell 14(2):239-256, 1992

CIRCUIT MODELS OF MIDDLE EAR FUNCTION

Herbert Hudde and Christian Weistenhöfer

Institute of Communication Acoustics, Department of Electrical Engineering and Information Sciences, Bochum, Germany

Abstract

Comprehensive simulation of the vibrations occurring in the middle ear can only be obtained by using general numerical methods such as finite element (FE) algorithms. However, such procedures are very time consuming. If transfer functions are to be calculated, computing times typically of several hours are necessary. Therefore, harmonic analysis by means of FE algorithms is not well-suited if the effects of parameter changes are to be investigated. In this paper, the benefits of circuit models are discussed. Whereas one-dimensional (1D) circuit models can only reproduce the basic properties of the middle ear, three-dimensional (3D) circuit models allow a functional analysis that includes spatial vibrations. Since circuit models are unable to describe mechanical continua, such as the tympanic membrane, results of finite element computations have to be recalculated to provide corresponding 3D circuit elements. After this has been done, calculations using the 3D circuit are carried out within half a minute. The ossicular vibrations for air conduction and the middle ear component of bone conduction are calculated to provide examples of possible applications.

Keywords: middle ear, circuit models, air conduction, bone conduction, spatial vibrations

Introduction

Like almost every other biological system, the middle ear includes constituents that are rather complicated in shape and structure. Therefore, it is quite obvious that only general numerical procedures, such as finite element (FE) methods, are capable of modelling the vibrations at arbitrary locations in detail[1-4]. The main disadvantage of FE methods is the vast amount of computing time and storage capabilities needed. In particular, if the focus is placed on the functional analysis of the middle ear function, the computing time of FE programmes seriously hampers the investigations. For such an analysis, it is necessary to observe the effect of parameter changes within acceptable computing time in-

Address for correspondence: Herbert Hudde, PhD, Institute of Communication Acoustics IC1/132, Ruhr-Universität Bochum, D-44780 Bochum, Germany. *email:* hudde@ika.ruhr-uni-bochum.de

The Function and Mechanics of Normal, Diseased and Reconstructed Middle Ears, pp. 39–58 edited by J.J. Rosowski and S.N. Merchant
© *2000 Kugler Publications, The Hague, The Netherlands*

tervals. Running times of several hours that occur when using FE methods make the analysis much more difficult, or almost impossible.

On the other hand, it is not necessary to recalculate all the vibrations of the eardrum and the ossicles at hundreds or thousands of points after each change of a parameter. The spatial vibrations of the ossicles, including their suspension by ligaments and muscles, can be fairly accurately described by three-dimensional (3D) circuit models which only use several selected points on the ossicles. The eardrum is the only part that cannot be accurately described by circuit elements, because it is an inhomogeneous continuum system vibrating in many superimposed modes. An effective solution can be obtained by combining the advantages of FE methods and circuit models (see *Three-dimensional circuit modelling*).

Common circuit models, based on the electroacoustical and electromechanical analogies, are one-dimensional (1D). Such models cannot reproduce vibrations that change their form with frequency. Therefore, the applicability of such 1D models is limited to comparatively simple investigations. We were able to expand the usual 1D circuits to 3D ones[5]. No deeper insight into the mathematical details can be provided here, but instead a short overview of the potentials of 1D and particularly 3D circuit models will be given.

One-dimensional circuit modelling

The use of 1D models for describing the middle ear is justified by the fact that the input (pressure and volume velocity in the ear canal at some distance from the eardrum) and output (pressure and volume velocity in the vestibule at some distance from the stapes footplate) of the middle ear are one-dimensional in good approximation. At the start of middle ear research, the vibrations of the human ossicles were also assumed to be essentially one-dimensional. The ligamentum mallei anterior and ligamentum incudis posterior (Fig. 1) were believed to form a suspension that resulted in a simple rotational movement of the malleus/incus unit about the 'main axis'. The stapes was assumed to move like a piston, *i.e.*, translationally in direction '1' of the reference base depicted in Figure 1. Today, we know that, in fact, complicated spatial vibrations arise[6].

In Figure 2, the most important features of the electroacoustical and electromechanical analogies are summarized using two simple example circuits. The effects of acoustical and mechanical compliant elements, masses, and dampers are described by circuit elements analogous to inductors, capacitors, and resistors. The first well-established circuit model of the middle ear, including the coupling to the ear canal, was published by Zwislocki[7] in 1962. Up until now, a wide variety of such 1D circuits have been developed. A thorough review of these models, including not only the ear canal, but also the scattering and diffraction of sound at the head, has been published by Rosowski[8].

The main problem of all these models is that many of the circuit elements do not

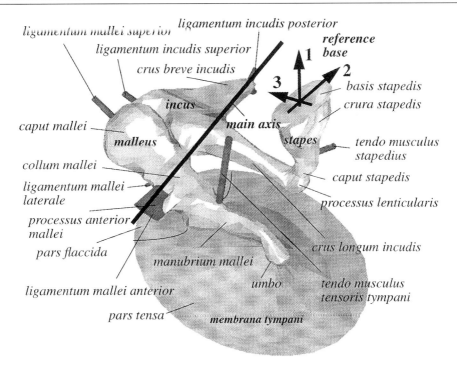

Fig. 1. Eardrum, auditory ossicles and ligaments. At low frequencies, movement of the malleus and incus is essentially rotation around the main axis established by the ligamentum mallei anterior and the ligamentum incudis posterior. Also shown is the reference base used for all 3D calculations: the main direction '1' is perpendicular to the stapes footplate. Only this component essentially contributes to the finally perceived sound. The lateral directions '2' and '3' refer to the long and short axes of the footplate.

truly correspond to physical elements. Actually, the ossicles change their vibrational behavior with frequency, and the eardrum behaves as a continuum which cannot be described by lumped elements. While the ear canal can be represented quite well by a corresponding electrical analogue, namely a 'transmission line', the eardrum vibrates in a multi-modal manner. As a consequence, most of the 1D circuit elements are more or less fictive, *i.e.*, either their values change with frequency, or they must be approximated by several elements which cannot be physically interpreted, or they must be supplemented by nonphysical factors[9]. Moreover, such models cannot correctly describe the effect of changes in the middle ear. For instance, an otosclerotic blocking of the stapes alters not only the load impedance at the processus lenticularis, but also many other elements, because the vibrational modes of the eardrum and the ossicles have changed. However, 1D circuit elements can be adapted to fit measured transfer functions. Therefore, 1D circuits can be used to effectively describe basic transfer characteristics of the middle ear. It is possible to reproduce several frequency responses, such as input impedance, stapes displacement and vestibular pressure for a given eardrum pressure with a single set

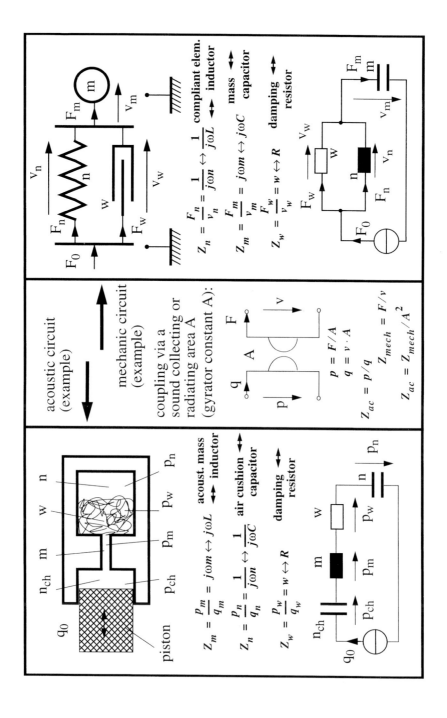

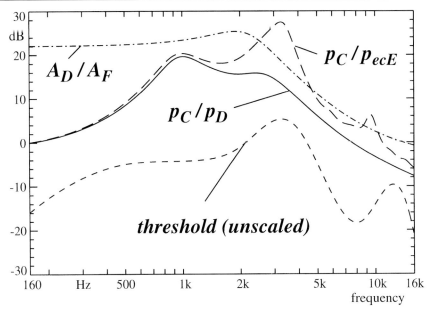

Fig. 3. Pressure transfer function p_C/p_D of the middle ear from the drum (D) to the vestibulum in the cochlea (C). Comparison to the effective (frequency dependent) area ratio A_D/A_F between the drum and stapes footplate shows that the decrease in the pressure gain at high frequencies is mainly determined by this 'transformer'. If the pressure transfer function refers to the pressure of an external sound source p_{ecE}, the additional gain due to ear canal resonance can be observed. Comparing this to the free-field threshold of hearing, reveals an obvious correlation between the hearing threshold and the pressure transfer function p_C/p_{ecE}.

←

Fig. 2. Electroacoustical and electromechanical (translational) analogies represented by simple examples. In acoustical circuits, the pressure p corresponds to a voltage u, the volume velocity q to a current i. In mechanical circuits, we consider the velocity v to be an analogue of a voltage, and the force F to be an analogue of a current. On the left, an acoustical structure driven by a piston is considered: the idealized piston produces a volume velocity q_0 independent of the load. This is represented by an ideal current source without internal impedance (circle with horizontal line). The other elements are taken into account using acoustic impedances Z (complex ratio of pressure to volume velocity, unit Nsm^{-5}). No wave effects are considered here: only lumped elements are used in the example. Acoustic chambers are characterized by a compliance n (unit m^5/N, analogue of a capacitor), acoustic masses m (unit kg/m^4, analogue of an inductor), and acoustic frictional damping w (unit Nsm^{-5}, analogue of a resistor). In the example, all the elements are connected in series. Therefore, there is only a common volume velocity $q = q_0 = q_{ch} = q_m = q_w = q_n$ in analogy to an electric current. On the right, a translationally vibrating mechanical structure driven by an ideal force source F_0 (again an analogue of a current source) is depicted. The other elements are represented by mechanical impedances (complex ratio of force to velocity, unit Ns/m). The elements, connected in parallel and in series, are a spring with a compliance n (unit m/N, analogue of an inductor), a mass (unit kg, analogue of a capacitor), and a damping element w (unit Ns/m, analogue of a resistor). In the example, force F_0 is split into the two forces F_w and F_n acting on the damping element and the spring. These are then combined again to drive the mass m ($F_m = F_0$). Obviously, the structure of the original mechanical arrangement is preserved in the circuit model. Unfortunately, this leads to an analogy of mechanical impedances to electrical admittances and *vice versa*. This is the reason why a gyrator, and not a transformer, is necessary for coupling acoustical and mechanical circuits via an area A which can then act as a sound collecting or sound radiating area. The alternative choice of an electromechanical analogy, F ↔ u, v ↔ i, leads to dual structures with loops converted into nodes and *vice versa*.

of model parameters. The pressure gain of the middle ear and the combined outer and middle ear, according to our 1D model[9], are shown in Figure 3.

Three-dimensional circuit modelling

Because of the fictive character of many circuit elements, 1D circuit models cannot be applied if the effects of changes in geometrical and mechanical parameters are to be investigated. 3D models are also needed for a deeper functional understanding. It seems that the change in spatial movements should not be interpreted as irrelevant deviations from the simple low frequency mode that are caused by the imperfect suspension of the ossicles. It is quite probable that the rolling movements of the ossicles can be considered a design principle that makes biomechanic systems insensitive to parameter changes and, therefore, robust with respect to all kinds of environmental factors. Such questions can be easily examined using a 3D circuit model.

In such a model spatial forces (F), torques (M), translational (v) and rotational (Ω) velocities at different points are taken into account. The components (i = 1, 2, 3) of all these quantities are indicated according to the reference frame depicted in Figure 1. Torques and forces are combined to set up the vector of a generalized force T which has six components. This and the corresponding definition of a generalized velocity S are shown in the upper panel of Figure 4.

Defining the generalized forces T and velocities S is the first step towards developing a pseudo-1D representation of 3D circuits. Figure 4 shows how an impedance matrix and a generalized chain-matrix can be defined and represented by corresponding circuit elements. The generalized velocity is analogous to an electric voltage, the generalized force to a current. The simple electrical scalar operations of 1D circuits have to be replaced by corresponding matrix operations describing the 3D circuit. A theoretical basis (a publication is in preparation) could be developed that uniquely specifies these matrix operations. Using this theory, arbitrarily composed 3D circuits can be depicted like 1D circuits, but treated mathematically as 3D circuits.

The most simplified form of a 3D circuit model of the middle ear is represented in Figure 5. The model explicitly contains the manubrium reference point M_{ref} in the middle of the coupling area between the manubrium and the eardrum, the center of gravity $C_{m,i}$ of the malleus/incus unit, a point I_{pl} at the processus lenticularis (incus), and a point at the caput stapedii (S_{cs}). As the ossicles are assumed to be rigid in this simplified model, the complete movements of the ossicular chain are determined by the movements at these points.

The vibrations of the eardrum are condensed in the eardrum source (T_0, Z_0) which is calculated by an FE programme. In contrast to the volume velocity source q_0 and the force source F_0, in Figure 2 the eardrum source contains an internal impedance matrix Z_0. Therefore, the generalized force T_M^{ref} acting on the manubrium reference point is dependent on the ossicular load. This step, connecting the

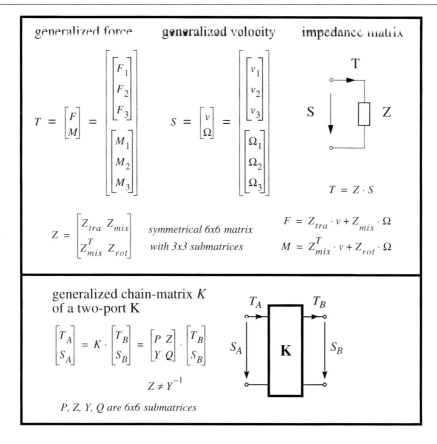

Fig. 4. Upper panel: For defining the 3D relations between different points in a vibrating linear system, the force vector F and the torque vector M are combined to set up the vector of the generalized force T. Also, the translational (v) and the rotational (Ω) velocities are combined. These set up the vector of the generalized velocity S. Using these generalized quantities, a 6×6 impedance matrix Z can be defined at a given point. The matrix is partitioned into 3×3 submatrices which describe a purely translational part (Z_{tra}), a purely rotational part (Z_{rot}), and a mixed part (Z_{mix}). The superscript T means taking the transpose of a matrix. In a reciprocal system, the impedance matrix is symmetrical. *Lower panel:* Two points A and B of a system are related by a generalized 12×12 chain-matrix K which can be partitioned into four 6×6 submatrices. Submatrices Z and Y function like an impedance or admittance matrix. Several relationships between the submatrices can be proved in the case of a reciprocal system.

FE generated source to the input port of the 3D circuit model of the ossicles, sets up the already mentioned combination of FE calculations and circuit models.

The essential assumption to be made is that the vibrational pattern of the eardrum is not greatly changed by the parameter changes in the ossicular chain. If that were the case, the eardrum source would change too. The source has to be computed only once under conditions specified by the normal ossicular chain. In 1D circuits, the two elements of an equivalent source (T_0, Z_0) are usually calculated by regarding the port without load (no force) and the one for the short-circuit case (no

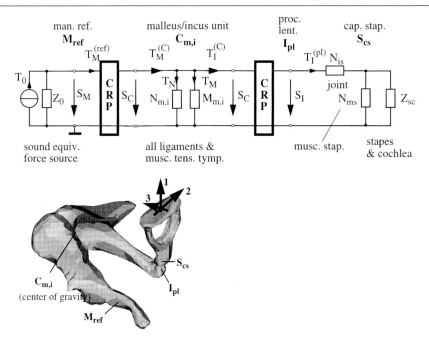

Fig. 5. Basic 3D middle ear model, represented as a pseudo-1D circuit. In this circuit, the generalized forces and velocities at only four points completely describe the vibrations of the total ossicular chain. All the ossicles are assumed to be rigid bodies. The grounding symbol means that the velocities are referred to a resting reference point. The point M_{ref} is in the center of the coupling area between the eardrum and manubrium. $C_{m,i}$ denotes the common center of gravity of the malleus/incus unit without taking into account an incudomalleal joint. The acoustical source is converted into a generalized force source, including an internal impedance matrix Z_0. The two boxes 'CRP' describe a 'change of reference point' on a rigid body which is treated using a corresponding generalized chain-matrix. The impedance matrix $N_{m,i}$ represents the total elastic lossy suspension of the malleus/incus unit referred to the center of gravity, $M_{m,i}$ represents the inertial matrix, as given in Weistenhöfer and Hudde[10]. Between the points at the processus lenticularis (I_{pl}) and the caput stapedius (S_{cs}), a joint N_{is} is taken into account. Z_{sc} denotes the impedance matrix of the stapes and cochlea referred to the stapes head, N_{ms} represents the musculus stapedius.

velocity). However, this procedure cannot be applied if the source is not fully constant, but is to some extent dependent on the load. The short and open circuits are extreme cases where many real sources are not completely constant if they are described as a simple Thevenin or Norton equivalent source. The problem can be solved by using two loads which do not differ very much from the 'normal' load.

In the case of the eardrum, two loads are not sufficient to obtain the complete source since the simple impedance of 1D circuits is replaced by a 6×6 impedance matrix and the internal source T_0 is a vector with six elements. Seven different loads are needed to be able to calculate the complete source, including the impedance matrix. Again, the loads used for the calculations should not represent extreme cases, such as completely clamping the manubrium, but should be fairly close to the normal ossicular load.

Once the source has been calculated, the effect of changing various parameters of the ossicles and their suspension can be investigated quickly. Therefore, 3D circuits provide an effective method for calculating the sensitivity of system properties (transfer functions, modes of vibrations) with respect to different parameters. As only very small changes are used for these calculations, the assumption of a constant source is uncritical. However, larger parameter changes can also be expected to have only a moderate influence on the eardrum source, or at least on its effect on the transfer characteristics of the middle ear – an assumption soon to be checked out.

As an example of application, the spatial vibrations of the ossicles for the frequencies 100, 1000, and 2000 Hz are presented in Figure 6. The model confirms the essentially rotational movement of the malleus/incus unit at low frequencies. Here, by means of the two ligaments that form the main axis (Fig. 1), the suspension mainly governs the movement of the ossicular chain. As the center of gravity of the malleus/incus unit is rather close to the main axis, the center of gravity only moves a little compared to points like the processus lenticularis or the stapes footplate.

At higher frequencies, the inertial forces of the ossicular masses become increasingly important compared to the elastic forces of the suspension. Therefore, it can be expected that the simple rotation about the main axis is no longer maintained. On the other hand, a rotation about the center of gravity of the malleus/incus unit would be particularly favorable at higher frequencies, because the effective mass of the ossicles would be kept small. Actually, such a rotation is to a certain extent supported by the form of the malleus and incus. Most of the common mass is concentrated near the center of gravity, and the exciting forces of the air-conducting path act at a certain distance from the center of gravity (in the center of the manubrium).

The second and third panels of Figure 6 show that, above the main middle ear resonance at about 800 Hz, the simple rotation gives way to movements that exhibit a rolling or tilting character. Also, the center of gravity and the whole main axis (Fig. 1) vibrate significantly. At 2000 Hz, the absolute displacement of the center of gravity almost equals the displacement at 100 Hz, but when compared to the displacement of the stapes footplate, it has increased from 12% to 38%. Thus, there is some evidence to suggest that the mass distribution of the malleus and incus, and the eccentric point of application of the force exerted by the tympanic membrane, can help to stabilize the rotational movement at higher frequencies to some extent, but cannot prevent the ossicular chain from moving with increasing frequency in an increasingly irregular fashion.

Middle ear component of bone conduction

The effect of the vibrating bony walls of the middle ear cavities on the stapes vibration is referred to as the middle ear component of bone conduction. This com-

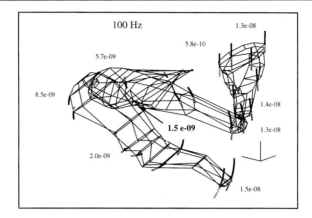

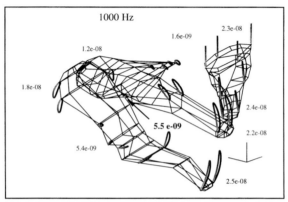

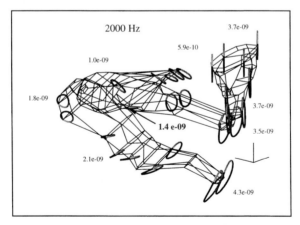

Fig. 6. Spatial vibrations of the ossicles at different frequencies. The movements of different points on the ossicles and of the center of gravity of the malleus/incus unit are represented by their vibrational paths. These paths are seen in the same perspective as the ossicles. The graphical representation is normalized to a constant vibration of the stapes footplate. In order also to provide quantitative insight, the magnitude of the vibrations should be indicated by a single number. In fact, the vibrational magnitude of a certain point does not vary sinusoidally. Therefore, instead of a peak value, only an effective value can be given. The effective displacement of different regions is given as a number indicating the displacement in nm for an excitation of 1 Pa pressure at the eardrum. The bold number between the malleus and incus refers to the center of gravity (arrow).

prises excitation of the ossicular chain via its elastic suspensions (eardrum, ligaments, muscles) and the effect of the additional sound pressure in the middle ear
cavities caused by the vibrating walls. In this paper, only the first fraction, the
inertial bone conduction, is considered.

The transmission of forces onto the ossicles via elastic elements (the 'inertial
component') is schematically depicted in Figure 7. In general, the points where the
elastic elements are attached to the wall of the tympanic cavity ($P_{tc,k}$) vibrate with
different magnitudes and phases. These mixed translational-rotational velocities
set up the stimulating input signals in the following investigations. Therefore, they
can be represented by ideal velocity sources $S_{0,k}$.

In general, the tympanic cavity walls vibrate in a complex manner which can
only be calculated by means of numerical algorithms such as FE programmes. If
this task is to be carried out, the complete skull must be described by an FE model
and coupled to the 3D circuit of the middle ear at all points common to both models. We are presently developing such programmes. In this study, the tympanic
cavity is assumed to be completely stiff. Therefore, the vibrations at different points
can be calculated from the prescribed vibration at one point. In fact, only a very
special case is considered here, namely that the whole tympanic cavity has simply
been translationally shaken.

The necessary changes made to the 3D circuit model are elucidated in Figure 8

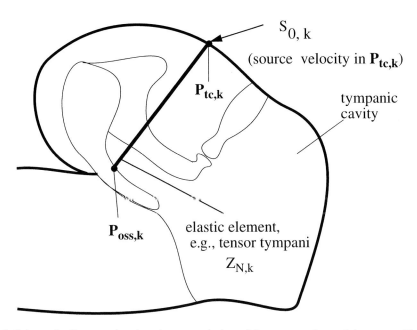

Fig. 7. Schematic diagram showing the transmission of forces onto the ossicles, caused by the
vibrating walls of the tympanic cavity. The ligaments or muscles (the figure shows the tensor
tympani schematically) are attached at points $P_{tc,k}$ at the tympanic cavity wall, and at points
$P_{oss,k}$ on the ossicles. They are described by impedance matrices $Z_{N,k}$ which contain 3D elastic
and frictional properties, and the position in space. The vibration of the tympanic cavity wall is
represented by ideal velocity sources $S_{0,k}$ at the different points $P_{tc,k}$.

in a schematic way. Somewhere in the air-conduction path, the generalized force T_0 acts at a point P_1 on a mass (impedance matrix Z_M with respect to the point P_1) suspended by a spring (impedance matrix Z_N between the points P_1 and P_2). The point P_0 represents a resting reference. In the upper left arrangement of Figure 8, the point P_2, which may represent a point on the tympanic cavity wall, is also resting. The force T_0 has to drive both the mass and the spring. Therefore, in the circuit it 'flows through' the parallel connection of both impedances Z_N and Z_M. If the point P_2 is now considered to be moving (upper right panel), the points P_0 and P_2 no longer coincide in the corresponding circuit. The source S_0 excites the series impedance of Z_N and Z_M instead of the parallel impedance.

The impedance Z_N can be considered the internal impedance of a general velocity source (S_0, Z_N). This source can be converted into an equivalent force source consisting of the internal force source $T_{S0}=Z_N \cdot S_0$ and the internal impedance Z_N. This relation is formally the same as that known from 1D circuits, but, of course, here a matrix multiplication has to be applied. Both sources can be combined to form a force source $T_0'=T_0+Z_N \cdot S_0$. The resulting equivalent circuit is identical to

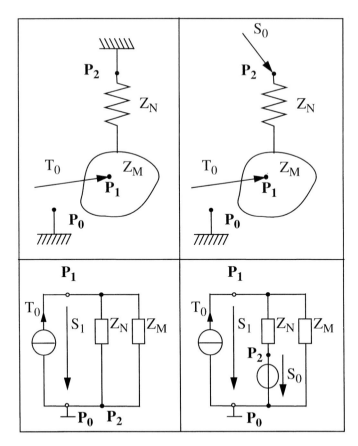

Fig. 8. Schematic diagram used to obtain representation of vibrating tympanic cavity walls in 3D circuits (*see* text).

the circuit depicted in the lower left panel if the force source T_0 is replaced by T_0'. Thus, all the contributions of the different suspending elements can be represented by additional force sources at new ports, corresponding to the points where the ligaments and muscles are attached to the ossicles. In a final step, the sources at the new ports can be converted into equivalent sources acting at the ports that are used in the model, by applying the CRP ('change of reference point') operation used in Figure 5. In conclusion, the effect of vibrating tympanic cavity walls can be described by additional force sources at the ports chosen for the analysis. A rather general 3D circuit model, including excitation of the ossicles in this way via the elastic suspensions, is shown in Figure 9. Here, the bending of the ossicles is also approximated by lumped 'joints' between two stiff masses. The resulting 3D circuit allows the ossicular vibrations to be calculated by fast, standard operations, requiring computing times of less than half a minute.

The properties of the middle ear regarding the inertial bone conduction component can be expressed in terms of certain transfer functions which relate exciting vibrations of the tympanic cavity to the generated output at a point of interest. In order to compare measured data and model predictions, or to obtain valuable data with respect to middle ear mechanics, the exciting vibrations of the tympanic cavity should be as simple as possible. The only type of excitation that can be realized in a broad frequency range is a shaking movement of the whole tympanic cavity. Such translational vibrations can be generated by means of commercial vibration exciters. In experiments, we use temporal bone preparations which are reduced to a rather small bony part constituting little more than the tympanic cavity. This preparation can be positioned on a small shaker head.

One experiment investigates the vibration of the stapes footplate. The components of the stapes velocity $v_{st} = (v_{st1}, v_{st2}, v_{st3})^T$ are measured by means of a laser vibrometer in the frame given in Figure 1. The most meaningful results are obtained when the preparations are excited one after the other in the directions of this frame. The three excitations can be combined to set up an input velocity vector $v_{tc} = (v_{tc1}, v_{tc2}, v_{tc3})^T$ of the tympanic cavity. The measurement for each input component yields three output components. All the results can be expressed by a 3×3 'bone conduction transfer function matrix' H_{bc} defined by $v_{st} = H_{bc} \cdot v_{tc}$. The diagonal elements of this matrix describe the stapes vibrations in the same directions as the excitation, the off-diagonal elements show the effect in the two orthogonal directions. A non vanishing off-diagonal element indicates that a fraction of the driving force must be deflected due to inertial effects and/or the lack of symmetry in the elastic suspensions.

The experiments described above can also be simulated using the 3D circuit model in Figure 9. In this way, the thick continuous lines in Figure 10 were calculated. The other three lines show the results of these measurements. These are part of a series of measurements that have been, and are at present being, performed in order to determine the element parameters of the complete 3D circuit model. Obviously some of the off-diagonal elements are not well reproduced by the model in its present form.

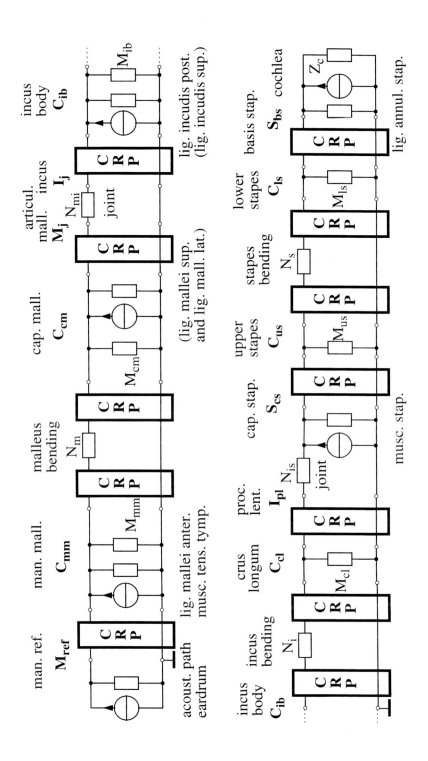

The approximate unity gain of the diagonal elements at low frequencies means that the ossicles almost follow the stimulating vibrations. With increasing frequency, the inertial effects of the ossicles produce an increasing velocity difference, resulting in a decrease in the transfer function. The off-diagonal elements start at small values. This is explained by very small forces occurring at low frequencies. Only if noticeable inertial forces arise, can they be deflected in lateral directions. At high audio frequencies, the transfer functions decrease or remain almost constant.

If the bone-conducted sound that is actually perceived is to be investigated, only the stapes movement in the main direction 1 has to be considered. The other movements approximately act as dipole sources with little influence on the vestibular pressure. Therefore, only the first row of the bone conduction matrix is of interest in this context:

$$V_{st,1} = H_{bc,11}V_{tc,1} + H_{bc,12}V_{tc,2}\ H_{bc,13}V_{tc,3}$$

However, it is not the stapes vibration itself, but the difference between the stapes and the wall vibration in direction 1 that governs the vestibular pressure. This leads to:

$$\Delta v_{st,1} = v_{st,1} - v_{tc,1} = (H_{bc,11}-1)v_{tc,1} + H_{bc,12}v_{tc,2} + H_{bc,13}v_{tc,3}$$

Therefore the elements $H_{bc,11}-1$, $H_{bc,12}$, and $H_{bc,13}$ are shown in Figure 11 in order to show the bone conduction elements that actually determine the perceived sound if the tympanic cavity is shaken in directions 1, 2, and 3. As expected, excitation in the main direction (i=1) produces the highest bone conduction. If we examine the

←

Fig. 9. 3D circuit of the middle ear, including the inertial component of bone conduction and approximately taking into account the bending of the ossicles. The ports correspond to points on the ossicles. The input port M_{ref} belongs to the manubrium reference point in the center of the coupling area between the eardrum and manubrium, the output port S_{bs} denotes a central point under the footplate (basis stapedii). In general, the notation of the ports indicates the name of the ossicle (M: malleus; I: incus; S: stapes) or a center of gravity (C). The additional indices more specifically indicate the location (*see* captions in figure). All the ossicles are divided into two parts with partial masses (M) and centers of gravity. They are coupled via lumped elastic elements (N_m, N_i, N_s) approximating the bending of the ossicles. Moreover, the two joints, between the malleus and incus, and between the incus and stapes, are modelled by elastic elements (N_{mi}, N_{is}). If appropriate data are available, losses can be added. The force source at M_{ref} represents the acoustic drive converted into the mechanical quantities and the inertial bone conduction component caused by the eardrum. All the other sources represent pure bone conduction components which are transformed to the point (or port) under investigation. The origin of these sources is given in the captions below the source symbols. The CRP two-ports provide the transformation from one port to another. For instance, the first CRP allows the input source at M_{ref} to be transformed into the center of gravity of the manubrium (C_{mm}). After such a transformation, both sources can be combined by simply adding the internal force sources, and also the internal impedances. In this way, the circuit can be reduced step by step. Thus, the quantities at each port (and therefore each transfer function that is of interest) can easily be calculated – if necessary analytically.

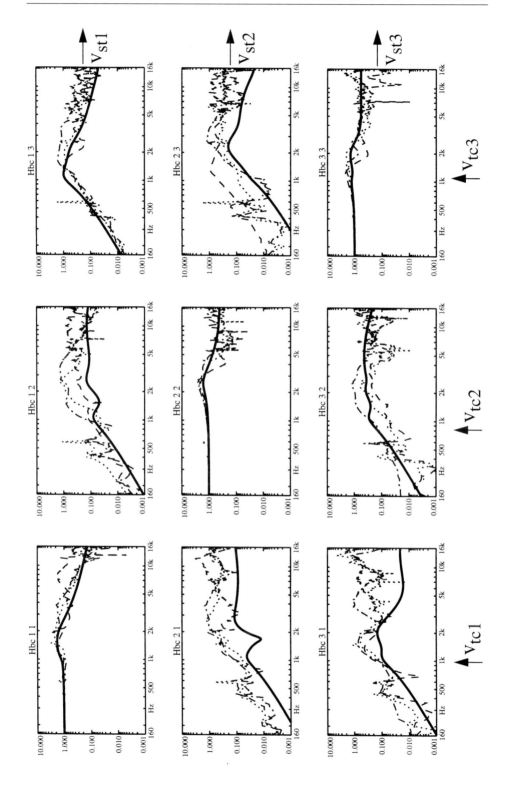

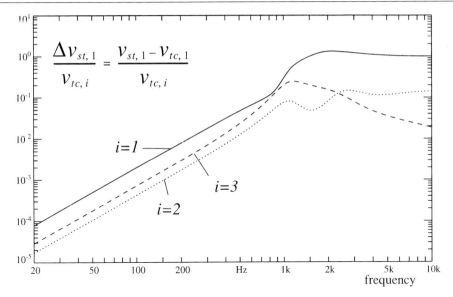

Fig. 11. Hearing-related bone conduction transfer functions for excitation in the three base directions 1, 2, 3 (*see* Fig. 1). The three elements describe the effect on the difference in the vibration of the stapes and the tympanic cavity in the main direction 1. The loading cochlea is taken into account.

velocity difference in direction 1 instead of the stapes velocity, this leads to the same 40 dB/dec increase at low frequencies that occurs in the other directions. At high frequencies, it approaches unity. Here, the full sensitivity is effective in the main direction 1: the tympanic cavity wall velocity dominates the relative stapes movement, because the movement of the stapes diminishes as a result of inertial forces.

In order to rate the significance of the middle ear bone conduction, the relative stapes vibration must be compared to stapes vibrations generated via air conduction (Fig. 12). The curves for i=1, 2, and 3 represent the absolute accelerations of the tympanic cavity walls in the three directions that produce the same (relative) stapes vibration as would be generated via the air conduction path at the threshold of hearing. To this end, the minimum audible field (MAF) according to ISO 226 was taken into account. This provides the free-field pressure $p_{ff,th}$ at the threshold as a function of frequency. This pressure has to be transformed into a corresponding stapes acceleration $a_{st,1}$, which can be converted into corresponding accelerations

←

Fig. 10. Bone conduction transfer function matrix H_{bc} of the middle ear without cochlea. This matrix gives the stapes velocity $v_{st} = (v_{st1}, v_{st2}, v_{st3})^T$ as a result of shaking the tympanic cavity as a whole in three orthogonal directions. The stapes velocity and exciting vibrations also refer to the base 1,2,3 given in Figure 1. If the three exciting vibrations v_{tc1}, v_{tc2}, v_{tc3} are combined to form an input vector v_{tc}, the bone conduction transfer matrix can be defined by $v_{st} = H_{bc} \cdot v_{tc}$. The thick lines represent the model predictions, while the others show the results of measurements. Only the magnitudes of the frequency responses are shown.

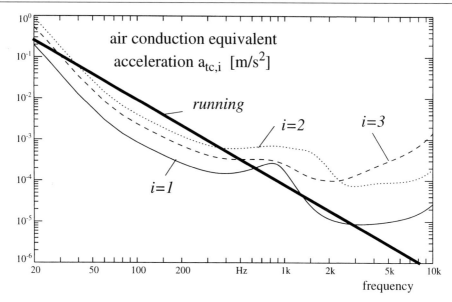

Fig. 12. Bone conduction velocity thresholds corresponding to the transfer functions in Figure 11. The curves represent the translational tympanic cavity accelerations in the three base directions that produce the same stapes vibration as would occur in the case of air conduction at the threshold of hearing. For comparison, a rough estimate of the acceleration when running on hard ground is also represented (thick line).

of the tympanic cavity $a_{tc,i}$ in the three base directions i using the velocity ratios (which equal the acceleration ratios) of Figure 11.

The most inaccurate step of this comparison is estimating the transfer function $a_{st,1}/p_{ff,th}$. In principle, our 1D model[9] is able to give an estimate of this transfer function if the head-related transfer function (HRTF) for the front direction is also taken into account. But the HRTF and, more particularly, the ear canal transfer function are problematic with respect to resonance. Also, the MAF curves include both transfer functions, although they are averaged over many subjects. Therefore, the resonance, particularly in the ear canal, appears broader in these curves than in any individual case (see Fig. 3). This means that the use of a mean ear canal, as provided in our 1D model, cannot cancel the ear canal resonance of the MAF curves.

As the actual details of the mean transfer function $a_{st,1}/p_{ff,th}$ are not very important for the comparison made in Figure 12, no effort was made to calculate this more exactly. Instead, we eliminated the ear canal resonance from the MAF curves (we simply took smoothed curves) and used the free-field pressure as the input of the middle ear model at the eardrum. For comparison, a rough estimate of the skull velocities produced when running on hard ground is depicted, which is based on measurements of our own. Figure 12 suggests that the inertial middle ear component of bone conduction caused by running is only weakly perceived. The main contribution is produced by the translational excitation in direction 1, which is common to the stapes footplate.

Concluding remarks

The main advantage of 3D circuit models over FE methods is that they require very little computing time (and storage capabilities). 3D circuit models are able to simulate spatial movements of the ossicular chain for air and bone conduction if the acoustic or mechanical excitation is known in terms of the source elements of the circuit model. In this case, frequency responses can usually be obtained within about half a minute. However, the excitation involves multi-modal continuum systems in both cases (the eardrum or the complete skull), which have to be dealt with using FE methods. Therefore, the 3D circuit has to be complemented with FE methods. The results of the time-consuming FE calculations are expressed as equivalent 3D sources which only need to be computed once. This makes the combined usage of 3D circuits and FE calculations very effective.

The results reported in this paper are based on very simple 3D sources: for air conduction, the stiffness matrix of the tympanic membrane provided in Beer *et al.*[11] and the rough source approximation given in Hudde and Weistenhöfer[5], were used. The internal impedance matrix was supplemented by losses that comply with the parameters of our 1D model[9]. For calculating the bone conduction transfer functions, velocity sources without internal impedances were taken into account. In future, the sources will be calculated using FE models of the eardrum and the skull which we are presently developing.

For more realistic calculations, the ossicles should not be assumed to be completely rigid. To achieve this, 3D circuits can be refined by using more lumped elements. In fact, the bending of ossicles has already been included in the circuit by means of an elastic 3D element in each ossicle. The accuracy finally achieved is a product of the correctness of the parameters and the model structure.

FE models are more general than 3D circuit models. So what use do 3D circuits have when they can only approximately describe the actual vibrations in the middle ear?

Firstly, pure FE models are also based on many assumptions involving the structure and properties of middle ear components. Perhaps the approximate character of FE models is not as obvious as that in 3D circuits. But, in fact, present FE models of the middle ear cannot provide correct results: a direct comparison of measured and FE-calculated vibrations is often unconvincing, although sophisticated parameter identification procedures have been used.

On the other hand, a middle ear model is not usually utilized to predict the behavior of an individual ear. This task could be considered valuable when preparing for middle ear surgery. But the mechanical and geometrical parameters of an individual ear to be reconstructed are never exactly known in practice, and, moreover, they are considerably changed by surgery. In order to understand the middle ear function or to optimize surgical techniques, the typical (and not the individual) effects of parameter changes or manipulations on transfer characteristics have to be simulated. Such functional analyses are ideal fields for applying 3D circuit models.

Acknowledgment

This work was supported by grants from the Deutsche Forschungsgemeinschaft.

References

1. Wada H, Metoki T, Kobayashi T: Analysis of dynamic behavior of human middle ear using a finite-element method. J Acoust Soc Am 92:3157-3168, 1992
2. Beer HJ, Bornitz M, Hardtke HJ, Schmidt R, Hofmann G, Vogel U, Zahnert Th, Hüttenbrink KB: Modelling of components of the human middle ear and simulation of their dynamic behaviour. Audiol Neuro-Otol 4:156-162, 1999
3. Eiber A: Mechanical modeling and dynamical behavior of the human middle ear. Audiol Neuro-Otol 4:170-177, 1999
4. Prendergast PJ, Ferris P, Rice HJ, Blaney AW: Vibro-acoustic modelling of the outer and middle ear using the finite-element method. Audiol Neuro-Otol 4:185-191, 1999
5. Hudde H, Weistenhöfer C: A three-dimensional circuit model of the middle ear. ACUSTICA/acta acustica 83:535-549, 1997
6. Decraemer WF, Khanna SM, Funnell WRJ: Malleus vibration mode changes with frequency. Hearing Res 54:305-318, 1991
7. Zwislocki J: Analysis of the middle-ear function. Part 1: Input impedance. J Acoust Soc Am 34:1514-1523, 1962
8. Rosowski JJ: Models of external- and middle-ear function. In: Fay RR, Popper AN (eds) Auditory Computation, Springer Handbook of Auditory Research, Springer, New York, Berlin, Heidelberg 1996
9. Hudde H, Engel A: Measuring and modeling basic properties of the human middle ear and ear canal. Part 3: Eardrum impedances, transfer functions, and complete model. ACUSTICA/acta acustica 84:1091-1108, 1998
10. Weistenhöfer C, Hudde H: Determination of the shape and inertia properties of the human auditory ossicles. Audiol Neuro-Otol 4:192-196, 1999
11. Beer H-J, Bornitz M, Drescher J, Schmidt R, Hardtke H-J, Hofmann G, Vogel U, Zahnert T, Hüttenbrink K-B: Finite element modelling of the human eardrum and applications. In: Hüttenbrink K-B (ed) Middle Ear Mechanics in Research and Otosurgery, Proceedings of an International Workshop, Dresden, pp 40-47, 1997

THE NORMAL PRESSURE-VOLUME RELATIONSHIP OF THE MIDDLE EAR SYSTEM AND ITS BIOLOGICAL VARIATION

Michael Gaihede and Jesper Kabel

Department of Otolaryngology, Holstebro Central Hospital, Holstebro, Denmark

Abstract

The dynamic non-linear mechanical behavior of the middle ear system (MES) can be described by ear canal pressure changes in response to controlled volume displacement of the tympanic membrane. This study demonstrates the derivation of such a pressure-volume relationship (PVR) in terms of a standard PVR ± 1 SD, which expresses mean properties and biological variation based on individual recordings in 76 normal ears. These PVRs are accurately expressed in a condensed form by fifth order polynomia. Such mathematical expressions only apply to the stimuli parameters and conditions of the current method, but they can form the basis for future extensions to derive constitutive equations describing the general physical properties of the MES. This can be useful in predictions of middle ear mechanical behavior and modelling. Further possibilities are discussed, including the derivation of an expression describing the static PVR, together with the possibilities of describing stiffness and compliance functions of the MES.

Keywords: hysteresis, compliance, stiffness, ear canal pressure, tympanic membrane volume displacement, constitutive equations

Introduction

The mechanical properties of the tympanic membrane (TM) and the structures of the middle ear are fundamental in the research of hearing. Most of this research has been dedicated to investigations on the acoustic transmission function, whereas there are only few studies on larger pressure changes[1]. The human ear may be subject to such larger pressure changes in the range of kPas due to environmental factors (aviation, high buildings, diving), but physiological factors also make a contribution.

Address for correspondence: Michael Gaihede, MD, Department of Otolaryngology, Head and Neck Surgery, Aalborg Hospital, DK-9000 Aalborg, Denmark. *email:* mgaihede@dadlnet.dk

The Function and Mechanics of Normal, Diseased and Reconstructed Middle Ears, pp. 59–70
edited by J.J. Rosowski and S.N. Merchant
© *2000 Kugler Publications, The Hague, The Netherlands*

Positive middle ear pressures (P_m) of up to 3.33 kPa may result from nose blowing, while sniffing can induce negative P_ms of up to –0.67 kPa[2]. Changing the body position from sitting to supine also affects the P_m, resulting in a mean increase of 0.22 kPa[3]. Physiological factors also include the effects of middle ear gas exchange, which in normal subjects can result in positive morning P_ms of up to 1.65 and 2 kPa[4,5], while negative P_ms in the range of –1 to –4 kPa are found in patients with tubal dysfunction. Such negative P_ms are considered to be a pathogenetic factor in otitis media with effusion, and they are also held responsible for the development of TM retraction, atelectasis, and cholesteatoma[6].

The behavior of the middle ear system (MES) in response to such pressure loads exhibits two common biomechanical characteristics: non-linearity and hysteresis. These properties have previously been demonstrated in a study in which the pressure-volume relationship (PVR) of the normal human MES was measured[7], *i.e.*,

$$P_{ec} = f(V_{tm})$$

P_{ec} refers to the ear canal pressure measured as a function of continuous dynamic volume displacements of the TM (V_{tm}). The MES is defined as the assembly of the TM, the ossicles (including ligaments, joints, and tendons), the P_m, the middle ear mucosa, and the air volume of the middle ear including the mastoid.

The purpose of the present study was to demonstrate the derivation of a more general description of the normal MES by constructing a standard PVR based on previous individual measurements in the normal group[7]. This was accomplished by calculating the mean PVR from individual recordings together with the mean PVR ±1 SD, which reflects its biological variation. These PVRs could be described by fifth order polynomia, which are used to summarize the typical mechanical properties of the normal MES. The standard PVR constructed in this way only represents deformation characteristics, which are limited by the stimuli parameters and conditions of the current method, but the results and principles demonstrated can form the basis for future studies. Such studies, taking into account more variables (volume amplitude, strain rate, P_m), can lead to the establishment of constitutive equations, which will form a more complete description of the MES deformation characteristics. The benefits of such equations are discussed, together with further possibilities, which include the derivation of an equation describing the static PVR and equations describing stiffness and compliance functions.

Material and methods

Instrument and individual recordings

TM volume displacements were created by a pump and transmitted to the ear canal by a stiff tube system. The tube system, including the ear canal, was filled with water, which was used to avoid any delay between volume and pressure changes, since this medium is incompressible for practical purposes. Volume displacements were sinusoidal with a frequency of 0.14 Hz (period time, 7.14 sec) and an amplitude of ±20 mm^3. The resulting changes in P_{ec} were measured by a transducer, and signals of volume and pressure data were fed into an AD converter connected to a 386 PC. Data were sampled ten times during 10 msec. These samples were averaged by the computer to decrease measurement errors and the averaged data were stored. Another similar sampling procedure was repeated after 30 msec, and the result for a full deformation cycle should be a total set of (7.14 sec/((10+30) $\times$ 10^{-3} sec) 178 pressure and volume coordinates. However, a smaller variation in the total number of coordinates registered was found between the individual recordings, so that only 165 coordinates were constantly available.

The details of the instrument and the measuring procedure have been described elsewhere[7]. However, it should be noted that, in each individual ear, the method includes the recordings of up to 32 continuous deformation cycles, which are separated automatically from each other by the computer. Each of these separate cycles represents PVR recordings with slightly different appearances, reflecting slightly different relative starting positions of the TM deformation. Among these recordings, one specific PVR is identified based on the most symmetrical behavior and defined by a symmetry indicator (SI) $\simeq 0$[7]. This implies that the pressure distances from the center of the PVR at $V_{tm} = 0$ mm^3 to each of its extremes (P_{max} and P_{min}) are identical.

The symmetric PVR has been argued to represent the neutral position of the TM, since it is characteristic that it exhibits a minimum hysteresis (*i.e.*, energy loss) in response to deformations compared with PVRs in adjacent positions[7]. Further, the symmetric PVR has a P_{ec0} (P_{ec} at $V_{tm} = 0$ mm^3 for the decreasing curve of the PVR), which corresponds to the P_m measured by tympanometry in decreasing direction implying that $P_{ec0} = P_m$[7]. This symmetric recording was previously used to determine the mechanical variables characterizing each individual ear[7], and similarly it was used in the present study for further calculations. In all cases, the symmetric PVR was determined only after five or more deformation cycles (on average, 17), so that the MES had been preconditioned to ensure repeatability of the experiments[7].

The normal group and derivation of the mean PVR

Thirty-nine healthy younger adults (mean age, 29 years; SD, 4.2) without previous middle ear disorders, were enrolled. Otomicroscopy and tympanometry were normal in all cases. In two ears, complete sealing of the ear probe failed. Thus, 76 individual symmetric PVRs, described each by 165 coordinates of pressure and volume, were available. For each of the corresponding numbers of coordinates (1 to 165), the means of the 76 pressure and volume values were calculated, resulting in 165 averaged coordinates. The data around each mean were normally distributed, and the SD could be used to describe the variation. It should be noted that initially we calculated the mean PVRs from the 38 right and 38 left ears separately, but since they coincided exactly, the data from right and left ears were pooled simply to describe the mean PVR from 76 ears.

From these 165 averaged coordinates the standard PVR was constructed. Since the relationship exhibits hysteresis, *i.e.*, it depends on the direction of volume and pressure change, functions were fitted separately for the decreasing and increasing curves of the PVR. Similarly, curves were constructed and fitted separately describing the pressure variation by ±1 SD.

The sampling of the independent variable (V_{tm}) was also subject to variation, which was very small due to its dense sampling at high rates. Thus, the mean SD of the volume data was only 0.47 mm^3 (range, 0.16-0.86 mm^3) and will not be commented on further.

Results

Figure 1 shows the standard PVR illustrated by the averaged sampling points. For an easier comparison with earlier studies (see later), the dependent variable (P_{ec}) is illustrated on the abscissa, while the independent variable (V_{tm}) is shown on the ordinate. The decreasing and increasing parts of the PVR could accurately be described by two fifth order polynomia, which are also illustrated in Figure 1. Their mathematical expressions appear in Table 1 (equations 1 and 4).

The mechanical variables previously used for the individual description of the PVR were also determined for the standard PVR in Figure 1[7]. Hysteresis, which is the energy equivalent of the circumscribed area, was measured by planimetry and corresponded to 20.78 µJ. Compliance, which is determined by the slope of the tangential line of the decreasing curve in the area of $V_{tm} = 0±5$ mm^3, was 25.27 mm^3/kPa. The pressure range, *i.e.*, the difference between P_{max} and P_{min}, was 3.70 kPa, and P_{ec0} was –0.19 kPa.

Figure 2 shows the standard PVR and the variation of the P_{ec} illustrated by lines of –1 SD for the decreasing curve of the PVR and +1 SD for its increasing curve. The fifth order polynomia fits of ±1 SD are depicted in Table 1 for both the decreasing and increasing functions (equations 2, 3, 5, and 6).

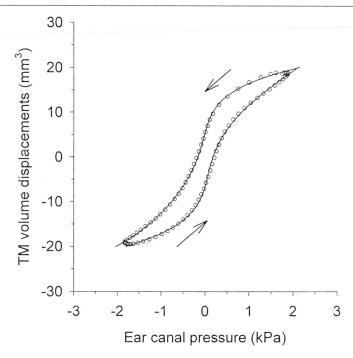

Fig. 1. The standard PVR is shown by the averaged sampling points (circles). For the sake of clarity, only every second sampling point is illustrated. Positive and negative volumes correspond to medial and lateral displacement of the TM, respectively. Arrows indicate the direction of volume and pressure change. Solid lines illustrate the polynomial fits of decreasing and increasing curve (Table 1, equations 1 and 4).

Table 1. The PVR curves and their fifth order polynomial fits

Curve	Equation
1. Decreasing mean curve	$-1.6579 \times 10^{-1} +3.6859 \times 10^{-2} \times V_{tm} -1.9465 \times 10^{-3} \times V_{tm}^{2}$ $+7.6764 \times 10^{-5} \times V_{tm}^{3} +6.2155 \times 10^{-6} \times V_{tm}^{4} +2.2814 \times 10^{-7} \times V_{tm}^{5}$
2. Decreasing mean curve -1 SD	$-4.2073 \times 10^{-1} +3.6651 \times 10^{-2} \times V_{tm} -2.5039 \times 10^{-3} \times V_{tm}^{2}$ $+1.3525 \times 10^{-4} \times V_{tm}^{3} +4.4569 \times 10^{-6} \times V_{tm}^{4} +8.0552 \times 10^{-8} \times V_{tm}^{5}$
3. Decreasing mean curve $+1$ SD	$8.9149 \times 10^{-2} +3.7068 \times 10^{-2} \times V_{tm} -1.3892 \times 10^{-3} \times V_{tm}^{2}$ $+1.8282 \times 10^{-5} \times V_{tm}^{3} +7.9740 \times 10^{-6} \times V_{tm}^{4} +3.7572 \times 10^{-7} \times V_{tm}^{5}$
4. Increasing mean curve	$1.7705 \times 10^{-1} +3.4355 \times 10^{-2} \times V_{tm} +2.2388 \times 10^{-3} \times V_{tm}^{2}$ $+1.3214 \times 10^{-4} \times V_{tm}^{3} -5.7622 \times 10^{-6} \times V_{tm}^{4} +6.6360 \times 10^{-8} \times V_{tm}^{5}$
5. Increasing mean curve -1 SD	$-1.0468 \times 10^{-1} +3.0699 \times 10^{-2} \times V_{tm} +1.3105 \times 10^{-3} \times V_{tm}^{2}$ $+4.4035 \times 10^{-5} \times V_{tm}^{3} -5.8953 \times 10^{-6} \times V_{tm}^{4} +3.1593 \times 10^{-7} \times V_{tm}^{5}$
6. Increasing mean curve $+1$ SD	$4.5878 \times 10^{-1} +3.8011 \times 10^{-2} \times V_{tm} +3.1670 \times 10^{-3} \times V_{tm}^{2}$ $+2.2024 \times 10^{-4} \times V_{tm}^{3} -5.6290 \times 10^{-6} \times V_{tm}^{4} -1.8321 \times 10^{-7} \times V_{tm}^{5}$

The general equation of the polynomia: $P_{ec} = \alpha_0 + \alpha_1 V_{tm} + \alpha_2 V_{tm}^{2} + \alpha_3 V_{tm}^{3} + \alpha_4 V_{tm}^{4} + \alpha_5 V_{tm}^{5}$. Units are kPa for P_{ec} and mm^3 for V_{tm}

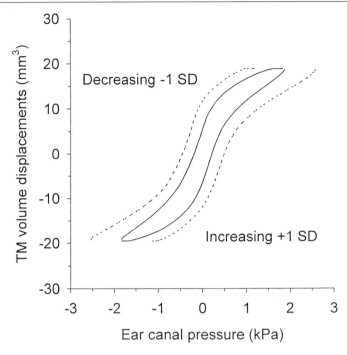

Fig. 2. The standard PVR is illustrated by solid lines. The biological variation is depicted by dashed lines: *left line* representing the decreasing curve –1 SD, and *right line* the increasing curve +1 SD (Table 1: equations 2 and 6). For the sake of clarity, +1 SD for the decreasing and –1 SD for the increasing curve have been omitted.

Discussion

The mean PVR function can also be described in terms of the same variables as those used for individual recordings. If the mean PVR function is to work as a standard, these variables should be similar to the means of the variables found in individual curves, which have been reported previously (mean hysteresis, 21.25 µJ; compliance, 26.25 mm³/kPa; P_{range}, 3.74; P_{ec0}, –0.21 kPa)[7]. These figures agree well with the characteristics of the standard PVR (Fig. 1), which indicates that the standard PVR is a reliable way of describing the typical mechanical properties of the MES.

Fitting of the polynomia to the sampling points included a compromise between the complexity of the equations and their agreement with the sampling points. We found that the fifth order polynomia used here was not too complicated and yet gave a sufficiently detailed agreement (Fig. 1). However, the curve fits are slightly closer to the center of the PVR at $V_{tm} = 0$ kPa and at the pressure extremes than the averaged sampling points (Fig. 1). At the middle pressures, the curve fits are slightly on the outside of the sampling points.

The standard PVR illustrated in Figure 1 describes the typical properties of the MES for normal ears, but it is limited by the stimuli parameters used by the

instrument and other methodological factors. Instrumental parameters of varia
tion include the volume amplitude, the rate of volume displacement, and the
rate pressure change. Other factors are the use of sinusoidal volume displacements, the use of only preconditioned and symmetric PVR curves, and, finally,
variations in the P_m may influence the position of the PVR on the pressure axis.

The volume amplitude was limited to ± 20 mm^3, which corresponded to a
mean pressure range of ± 1.85 kPa. This means that the description of the MES
behavior is restricted to this range and cannot be extrapolated due to non-linearity. The amplitude of ± 20 mm^3 was chosen in order to achieve an acceptable
large range of volume (and pressure) changes to give substantial information.
However, in a volume controlled system, the resulting pressure range would be
larger in ears with low compliance, and a risk for TM rupture may arise in such
ears, if the volume amplitude is too high. The present volume settings of the
instrument gave pressure ranges comparable to tympanometry, which were
considered safe.

Another factor may be related especially to the extremes of the PVR because of
variation in strain rate (rate of volume displacement). Since the volume displacement were sinusoidal ($V_{tm} = V_{max} \sin (\omega t)$), the strain rate could be described by
$dV_{tm}(t)/dt = V_{max} \omega \cos (\omega t)$, where V_{max} refers to the maximal amplitude (20 mm^3)
and $\omega = 2\pi f (= 0.88$ s^{-1}). Hence, the strain rate was not constant, but exhibited a
maximum around the origin of the PVR and approached 0 mm^3/sec towards the
volume turning point at the extremes of the PVR. When strain rate was close to 0
and eventually became 0, stress relaxation may occur for a moment. Stress relaxation is a common feature of biomechanical viscoelastic behavior, where stress decreases over time, when strain is held constant[8]. This was reflected by the small
almost horizontal zone of the PVR at the start of both its decreasing and increasing
curve (Fig. 1); in these regions, the volume displacement (strain) was almost constant, and the pressure (stress) decreased. If an amplitude of ± 30 mm^3 had been
used, the strain rate would have been larger in the regions of ± 20 mm^3 and stress
relaxation would not be likely to occur at this point. As a consequence, the mechanical behavior at the extremes of the curves may not be comparable to experiments, where other amplitudes are used. In general, however, stress-strain relationships are found to be insensitive to at least 10^3-fold changes in strain rate[8], which
means that the present curves should be representative of a large range of different
strain rates, and hence for most of the volume range.

Since the strain rate was not constant, the rate of pressure change was subject to
similar variation. From tympanometric studies, it is well known that increasing
rates of pressure change result in increasing compliance[9]. The mean rate of pressure change was 100 daPa/sec, which is comparable to tympanometric recordings,
but the rate depended on the compliance of the individual ear[7]. However, this effect
may also not be significant due to the earlier mentioned relative insensitivity of
stress-strain experiments to strain rate variations[8].

Since hysteresis is a time-dependent phenomenon, it would be influenced by
instrumental factors causing time delay. This was avoided by the instantaneous

change in direction of deformation due to the sinusoidal volume displacements, and an incompressible media (water) was used, where no time delay occurred between the deformation (volume) and the registration of pressure changes.

Preconditioning is another common biomechanical phenomenon found in stress-strain experiments, where compliance increases due to repeated cycles of loading and unloading until a *steady state* is reached usually after five to six cycles[8]. When *steady state* conditions are reached, the results are reproducible, and hence, data are usually presented in the biomechanical literature only after the specimens have been preconditioned[8]. Preconditioning has also been reported for the MES, where repeated tympanometries result in increasing compliance, until *steady state* and reproducibility is similarly reached after five measurements[10]. As a consequence, each individual experiment included in this study was also preconditioned by at least five repeated deformation cycles before determining the mechanical variables[7]. This means that the compliance of the MES reported here is higher than if only one initial recording had been used.

In Figure 2 the biological variation is illustrated by the range of ± 1 SD. From our previous study[7], we know that the appearance of the PVR and the mechanical variables are subject to individual variation, which is reflected by the interval shown in Figure 2. This interval allows a qualitative comparison between the standard PVR and any new recordings, which may coincide with the standard by falling within the range of ± 1 SD, or be outside the standard. It should again be noted, however, that the neutral position PVR of the individual recordings, which formed the basis of the present data, was based on a symmetrical behaviour of the PVR[7]. This means, as an example, that in a recording where P_{min} approaches -1 SD, a similar approach of P_{max} to $+1$ SD is assumed. This symmetric behavior must be complied with, when assessing the agreement of any future recordings with the normal range.

Variations in P_m should also be considered, since in cases of an abnormal P_m, the PVR will be displaced horizontally along the pressure axis corresponding to the magnitude of the P_m. Negative P_ms result in a correspondingly negative displacement of the PVR and *vice versa* (which will be reflected by a corresponding change in P_{ec0}). The normal group investigated in this study had similarly normal P_ms (mean, -10 daPa; SD, 26 daPa), but if cases with abnormal pressures are investigated, this abnormality should be corrected for.

Finally, the presented curves and their functions were limited by describing the properties of the MES only in a normal group. However, this can be used as a platform for future studies of patients with middle ear disorders. Preliminary clinical experiments have shown changes in the PVR related to such disorders, which are interesting for future studies in middle ear mechanics[11]. Sources of measurement errors and repeatability of the method have previously been described in detail[7].

A mean curve determined by the average polynomia between the two fits describing the increasing and decreasing curves in Figure 1 (Table 1: equations 1 and 4) can be interpreted as representing the static PVR. In a study by Elner *et al.*, the elastic properties of the MES were investigated by dynamic recordings of its

Table 2. Functions derived from the PVR

Curve	Equation
7. Static mean curve*	$5.6297 \times 10^{-3} + 3.5607 \times 10^{-2} \times V_{tm} + 1.4611 \times 10^{-4} \times V_{tm}^2$ $+1.0445 \times 10^{-4} \times V_{tm}^3 + 2.2665 \times 10^{-7} \times V_{tm}^4 + 1.4725 \times 10^{-7} \times V_{tm}^5$
8. Stiffness (decreasing)**	$3.6859 \times 10^{-2} - 3.8931 \times 10^{-3} \times V_{tm} + 2.3029 \times 10^{-4} \times V_{tm}^2$ $+2.4862 \times 10^{-5} \times V_{tm}^3 + 1.1407 \times 10^{-6} \times V_{tm}^4$
9. Stiffness (increasing)**	$3.4355 \times 10^{-2} + 4.4775 \times 10^{-3} \times V_{tm} + 3.9641 \times 10^{-4} \times V_{tm}^2$ $-2.3049 \times 10^{-5} \times V_{tm}^3 + 3.3180 \times 10^{-7} \times V_{tm}^4$

*The static mean curve was derived by calculating the average of the constants from equations 1 and 4

**The stiffness functions were derived by differentiation of equations 1 and 4; their general expression (with reference to the general expression in Table 1) is: $f'(V_{tm}) = dP_{ec}/dV_{tm} = \alpha_1 + 2\alpha_2 V_{tm} + 3\alpha_3 V_{tm}^2 + 4\alpha_4 V_{tm}^3 + 5\alpha_5 V_{tm}^4$
Units are kPa for P_{ec} and mm³ for V_{tm}

volume-pressure relationship (VPR), *i.e.*, V_{tm} was measured as a function of P_{ec}[12]. These measurements also exhibited hysteresis, although this was not quantitatively investigated. In the majority of ears, measurements could also be performed under static conditions, and it was found that the static VPR corresponded to the geometrical center of the decreasing and increasing parts of the dynamic VPR[12]. Hence, static results were constructed and reported from dynamic recordings. Similarly, the geometrical center of the standard PVR (Fig. 1) described by the mean polynomia of its decreasing and increasing parts represents a static PVR, which has been included in Table 2 (equation 7).

In Figure 3 this static standard mean PVR is illustrated, together with the static results of Elner *et al.* (Table III)[12]. Moreover, data are included from a study by Dirckx and Decraemer (Fig. 5; exact data have been provided by Dirckx), who measured static TM displacements in response to changes in P_m[1]. Another study by Flisberg *et al.*, investigating similar volume-pressure relations, has been omitted for reasons of clarity and because data are only accessible for lateral movements of the TM[13]. However, these results correspond well with the results of Elner *et al.*[12] and Dirckx and Decraemer[1].

Generally, there is close agreement between the three methods, although the PVR near $P_{ec} = 0$ kPa is steeper than the other two curves (Fig. 3). This property is reflected by a higher compliance for the static PVR (26.18 mm³/kPa). The compliance calculations from the results of Elner *et al.* is 18.57 mm³/kPa[12], while Dirckx and Decraemer reported a compliance of 19.5 mm³/kPa[1]. The higher compliance found in the present study may be the result of the preconditioning included in our methods.

Another difference between the methods is that the PVR exhibits symmetry around $V_{tm} = 0$ mm³, while in the two other studies the curves are slightly asymmetric (Fig. 3). The symmetry of the PVR is inherent to the present method, where symmetry is used to define the neutral position of the TM. The other studies

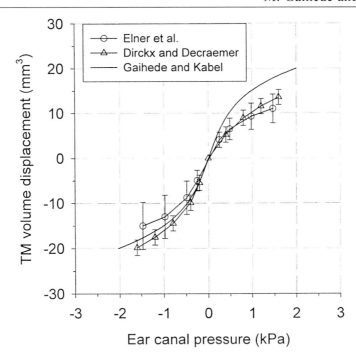

Fig. 3. The polynomial fit calculated for the static PVR. The results from previous static experiments have been illustrated for comparison. In the study by Elner *et al.*[12], points and error bars indicate the mean and SD of 101 normal subjects. The data of Dirckx and Decraemer[1] include the results from one normal temporal bone, where error bars illustrate the accuracy of the measurements. The P_ms reported by Dirckx and Decraemer have been converted to corresponding values of P_{ec}s.

defined this position in terms of a 0 pressure difference across the TM[1,12]. Such a definition was not possible in the current study, since the exact P_m was unknown. The preconditioning used in the present study is another factor that may increase symmetry.

From the polynomial descriptions of equations 1 and 4 (Table 1), we can estimate the stiffness of the MES as a function of V_{tm}, *i.e.*, $dP_{ec}/dV_{tm} = f(V_{tm})$ (Table 2: equations 8 and 9). These stiffness functions may also be described in relation to P_{ec}, *i.e.*, $dP_{ec}/dV_{tm} = f(P_{ec})$, when equations 1 and 8 (or 4 and 9) are combined. Since the reciprocal property of stiffness is compliance (dV_{tm}/dP_{ec}), this means that compliance can be described as functions of V_{tm} or P_{ec}. This has been demonstrated in Figure 4, where compliance of the MES is illustrated as a function of P_{ec} for both increasing and decreasing pressure. These functions resemble tympanometric recordings, where the compliance is low at the extremes of the P_{ec}, while showing a maximum around $P_{ec} = 0$ kPa. This is to be expected, since static compliance measured by tympanometry correlates significantly with the dynamic compliance measured by the PVR[7].

In conclusion, the validity of the standard PVR and its equations was justified

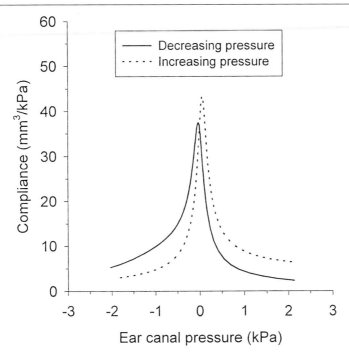

Fig. 4. Compliance (dV_{tm}/dP_{ec}) as a function of P_{ec}. The resemblance to a bidirectional tympanometric recording is obvious. For the decreasing curve, the peak appears at (–0.03 kPa; 37.40 kPa/mm³), while for the increasing curve, at (0.06 kPa; 43.31 kPa/mm³).

by the derivation from a substantial experimental material. Such expressions describe our results in a condensed form, and the principle of constructing the standard PVR can be extended by future studies to include more variables (volume amplitude, strain rate, effects of abnormal P_m), where the goal should be the establishment of constitutive equations. Such equations describe in a complete form the general physical properties of the MES, and make predictions of mechanical behavior possible in a continuum, which is more detailed than previous data at selected measuring points[1,12,13]. The standard PVR can also form a basis for future studies of pathological middle ear conditions[11], and finally, it can serve as a template for middle ear modelling. This was recently demonstrated in a study where a TM model was constructed with hysteresis and non-linear properties in accordance with the standard PVR and used to investigate the influence of variations in middle ear volume and pressure on tympanometric estimates of P_m[14].

Acknowledgments

This study was supported by The Foundation for Medical Scientific Research at the Hospitals in Ringkøbing, Ribe, and Sønderjylland Counties.

References

1. Dirckx JJJ, Decraemer WFS: Area change and volume displacement of the human tympanic membrane under static pressure. Hearing Res 62:99-104, 1992
2. Sakikawa Y, Kobayashi H, Nomura Y: Changes in middle ear pressure in daily life. Laryngoscope 105:1353-1357, 1995
3. Gaihede M, Kjær D: Positional changes and stabilization of middle ear pressure. Auris Nasus Larynx 25:255-259, 1998
4. Shinkawa H, Okitsu T, Yusa T, Yamamuro M, Kaneko Y: Positive intratympanic pressure in the morning and its etiology. Acta Otolaryngol (Stockh) Suppl 435:107-111, 1987
5. Hergils L, Magnuson B: Morning pressure in the middle ear. Arch Otolaryngol 111:86-89, 1985
6. Ars B, Decraemer W, Ars-Piret N: The lamina propria and cholesteatoma. Clin Otolaryngol 14:471-475, 1989
7. Gaihede M: Mechanics of the middle ear system: Computerized measurements of its pressure-volume relationship. Auris Nasus Larynx 26:383-399, 1999
8. Fung YC: Bioviscoelastic solids. In: Fung YC (ed) Biomechanics: Mechanical Properties of Living Tissues, 2nd edn, pp 242-273. New York, NY: Springer-Verlag 1993
9. Creten WL, Van Camp KJ: Transient and quasi-static tympanometry. Scand Audiol 3:39-42, 1974
10. Gaihede M: Tympanometric preconditioning of the tympanic membrane. Hearing Res 102:28-34, 1996
11. Gaihede M: Mechanical properties of the middle ear system investigated by its pressure-volume relationship. Introduction to methods and selected preliminary clinical cases. Audiol Neurootol 4:137-141, 1999
12. Elner Å, Ingelstedt S, Ivarsson A: The elastic properties of the tympanic membrane system. Acta Otolaryngol (Stockh) 72:397-403, 1971
13. Flisberg K, Ingelstedt S, Örtegren U: On middle ear pressure. Acta Otolaryngol (Stockh) Suppl 182:43-56, 1963
14. Gaihede M: Middle ear volume and pressure effects on tympanometric middle ear pressure determination: Model experiments with special reference to secretory otitis media. Auris Nasus Larynx 27:231-239, 2000

HUMAN MIDDLE EAR SOUND TRANSFER FUNCTION AND COCHLEAR INPUT IMPEDANCE

Ryuichi Aibara[1,2], Joseph T. Welsh[1], Sunil Puria[3] and Richard L. Goode[1,2]

[1]Department of Veterans Affairs Medical Center, Palo Alto; [2]Division of Otolaryngology – Head and Neck Surgery, Stanford University School of Medicine, Stanford University Medical Center, Stanford; [3]Stanford University Department of Mechanical Engineering, Stanford, CA, USA

Abstract

Middle ear sound transfer function (METF) and acoustic input impedance of the cochlea (Z_c) were measured in 12 fresh human temporal bones for the 0.05-10 kHz frequency range. METF was determined by two methods: middle ear sound pressure gain (GME) and the ear canal sound pressure to stapes footplate velocity transfer function (STF). The mean GME magnitude reached 23.5 dB at 1.2 kHz with a slope of approximately 6 dB/octave from 0.1-1.2 kHz and –6 dB/octave above 1.2 kHz. From 0.1-0.5 kHz, the mean GME phase angle was 51°, rolling off at –78°/octave above this frequency. The mean STF magnitude reached a maximum of 0.33 mm·s^{-1}/Pa at 1.0 kHz with nearly the same shape in magnitude and phase angle as the mean GME. Direct measurement of Z_c in human ears is reported here for the first time. The mean Z_c was virtually flat with a value of 21.1 acoustic GΩ MKS between 0.1 and 5.0 kHz. Above 5 kHz, the mean Z_c increased to a maximum value of 49.9 GΩ at 6.7 kHz. The mean Z_c angle was near 0° from 0.5-5.0 kHz, decreasing below 0.5 kHz and above 5 kHz with peaks and valleys.

Keywords: middle ear transfer function, middle ear sound pressure gain, cochlear input impedance, scala vestibuli sound pressure, stapes footplate velocity

Introduction

Several methods have been described for the measurement of the middle ear sound transfer function (METF) in human temporal bones with the cochlea intact[1-6]. The input parameter is universally the sound pressure level (SPL) at the ear canal surface of the tympanic membrane (TM), termed P_{ec}. The output parameter used varies, depending on the particular study; in intact human

Address for correspondence: Richard L. Goode, MD, Department of Veterans Affairs Medical Center, 3801 Miranda Avenue, MC 112-B1, Palo Alto, CA 94304, USA. *email:* goode@leland.stanford.edu

The Function and Mechanics of Normal, Diseased and Reconstructed Middle Ears, pp. 71–88
edited by J.J. Rosowski and S.N. Merchant
© *2000 Kugler Publications, The Hague, The Netherlands*

temporal bone measurements of METF, stapes footplate velocity (V_s) or scala vestibuli sound pressure near the stapes footplate (P_v) appear to be the best physiological choices. The ratio of V_s to P_{ec} is termed the ear canal sound pressure to stapes footplate velocity transfer function (STF), while the ratio of P_v to P_{ec} is termed the middle ear sound pressure gain (GME). Human GME has also been measured by comparing stapes displacement in response to a constant SPL before and after removal of the TM, malleus and incus[6]. Pressure gain estimates by Békésy[7], Onchi[8] and others[9,10], using different methods, have been reported as well. These methods have the disadvantage of requiring the middle ear to be removed or the cochlea drained to make the measurement.

Differences in human temporal bone METF results have been found by different investigators, particularly at the lower and higher test frequencies (reviewed by Goode et al.[11] and Puria et al.[12]). While these differences may be due to the wide range in normal middle ear function, particularly when small numbers of ears are tested, it is also possible that the measurement method is contributing to the differences.

The stapes footplate motion is, in general, a vector quantity with translational as well as rotational components. The piston-like translational component of the footplate V_s is generally assumed to be the primary determinant of stapes volume velocity and the input to the cochlea[13]. Thus, the STF measurement method assumes that stapes footplate volume velocity (V_s times the area of the footplate, A_{fp}) to be the appropriate input to the cochlea, so V_s is selected as the output parameter since A_{fp} is considered to be relatively constant. A laser Doppler vibrometer is usually used to make the measurement and the center of the footplate is chosen as the measurement site, based on the assumption that stapes movement is piston-like at physiological sound inputs and frequencies. Recent data from our laboratory suggest that stapes footplate movement is not entirely piston-like, but has an anterior-posterior rocking motion with rising frequency[14]; this may make measurement of stapes velocity at one site sub-optimal as the output measure of METF at higher frequencies (>2.0 kHz).

Sound pressure measured in the scala vestibuli has been reported to be a better output parameter[12], however, the measurement is more difficult to perform. Measurement of round window volume velocity, assumed to be the same as stapes volume velocity, has also been used but is not a direct measure[2].

Until now, no comparative measurements with these two methods have been made in the same human temporal bones. In addition, simultaneous measurement of stapes volume velocity and intracochlear sound pressure allows the direct measurement of human cochlear input impedance, an important measure that has only been previously measured indirectly. It is the purpose of this paper to describe experiments that compare the two METF methods in the same human ears, as well as to provide the direct measurement of human cochlear input impedance.

The complex acoustic input impedance of the cochlea, Z_c, is an important variable in our understanding of sound energy transfer through the middle ear into the cochlea. Zwislocki[15] defined the acoustic input impedance of the cochlea as 'the ratio of sound pressure produced in the scala vestibuli at the stapes footplate and the volume of perilymph the footplate displaces per unit time'. In other words, Z_c is the ratio of P_v to stapes footplate volume velocity, U_s, which is calculated by V_s times A_{fp}.

Direct measurements of the input impedance of the cochlea have been reported in the cat[16], guinea pig[17], and chinchilla[18]. However, only estimations of Z_c for humans have been reported by Merchant et al.[19] and Puria et al.[12], as well as theoretical predictions by Zwislocki[15,20] and Békésy[7]. Direct measurement of Z_c in human ears is reported here for the first time.

Material and methods

Measurement system

Measurements were performed using a SYSid 6.5 audio band measurement and analysis system (www.sysid-labs.com, Berkeley, CA, USA), a software program that interfaces with a DSP-16+ processing board (Ariel, Cranbury, NJ, USA) running on an IBM compatible PC. Simultaneous stimulus generation and response averaging are performed with the SYSid system, which extracts the amplitude and phase of the response at each frequency through Fast Fourier Transformation, or FFT.

A schematic of the measurement system is shown in Figure 1. Sound was presented at the lateral end of an artificial ear canal using an 83-13A/024 earphone (Tibbets Industries, Camden, ME, USA). Sound pressure in the ear canal (P_{ec}) was measured within 2 mm of the TM with an ER-7C probe-tube microphone (Etymotic Research, Elk Grove Village, IL, USA). Sound pressure in the scala vestibuli (P_v) was measured using an EPIL-127*-.13 D/R strain gauge (Entran, Fairfield, NJ, USA) modified for use as a hydrophone by placing a silicone seal on the tip of the sensor[12]. An OFV-302 and OFV 3000 Laser Doppler Vibrometer System (LDV) (Polytec, PI, Costa Mesa, CA, USA) was used to measure stapes footplate velocity (V_s). The LDV contained a 50-mm lens (Nikon, New York, NY, USA) to focus the helium-neon laser on a reflective target on the center of the stapes footplate. An articulating arm was connected to a joystick-operated beam-splitter, which was mounted over the lens of an operating microscope and reflected 95% of the laser beam onto the target. See Heiland et al.[14] for more details on the velocity measurement methods.

System calibration

The probe-tube microphone and the hydrophone were calibrated as follows. A sound level calibrator type 4230 (Brüel and Kjaer, Norcross, GA, USA) was

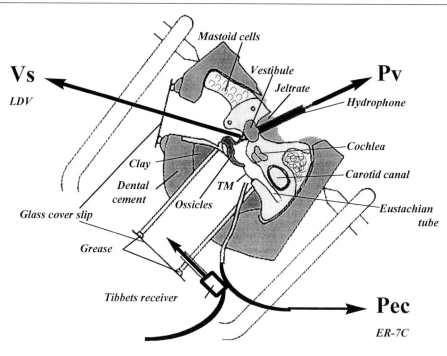

Fig. 1. Schematic of the measurement method.

used to calibrate a 1/8 inch reference microphone type 4138 (Brüel and Kjaer, Norcross, GA, USA) which had a flat response (±0.5 dB) and zero phase shift (±1°) in the 0.05-10 kHz frequency range. This reference microphone was then used to calibrate each microphone by comparing their response to that of the reference microphone at 0.05-10 kHz in a small 25-mm long cavity; the microphones were within 1 mm of the reference microphone. Due to its high impedance, the hydrophone's sensitivity is assumed to be the same in air and water. To check the calibration of the two microphones, the probe-tube microphone and hydrophone were placed together in a different 25-mm long cavity, 1 mm apart, and their responses were compared. The maximum deviation in magnitude was 1.0 dB at 1 kHz with a maximum deviation in phase of 15° at 10 kHz. The observed differences place a boundary on possible calibration errors in the measurement system.

The LDV system was calibrated by aiming the LDV at a target on top of an accelerometer type 4371 (Brüel and Kjaer, Norcross, GA, USA) that was attached to a mini shaker type 4810 (Brüel and Kjaer, Norcross, GA, USA). The response of the LDV was then compared to the accelerometer's, which had a known sensitivity and phase response between 0.05-10 kHz.

Postmortem materials

Twelve fresh human temporal bones, consisting of nine males and three females, ranging in age from 36-81 years with a mean of 67.9 years, were extracted from human cadavers within 48 hours of death using a Schuknecht bone saw at the time of autopsy. The cored specimens were wrapped in gauze, placed in a 100 ppm merthiolate in normal saline solution, and stored at 5°C. Measurements on individual bones were performed in one day within six days' postmortem. With the exception of one temporal bone, all were considered normal upon visual inspection using an operating microscope. One exception was made for a temporal bone where palpation of the umbo showed a stiffer malleus than normal. Since the footplate did not appear otosclerotic, only the cochlear input impedance measurement was used.

Temporal bone preparation and baseline measurements

Upon removal of attached connective tissue, the bony wall of the external ear canal was drilled down to 2 mm from the tympanic membrane annulus, keeping the posterior wall intact. A simple mastoidectomy and posterior hypotympanotomy were performed. The horizontal segment of the facial nerve and surrounding bone were removed to provide a good view of the stapes footplate, leaving the chorda tympani and stapedius muscle intact. After enlarging the internal auditory canal (IAC) to approximately 15×10 mm, the bone was drilled until a blue line over the vestibule was seen at a site lateral to the transverse crest and just superior to the singular foramen. The bone was then placed in a latex finger cot which kept the wet bone moist and thus prevented it from drying.

A plastic tube (8.5 mm internal diameter, 25 mm length) was attached around the bony ear canal opening using modelling clay so that the axis of the tube was perpendicular to the tympanic membrane. The Tibbets earphone was located at the lateral end of the tube for sound delivery. The probe-tube microphone was inserted into the tube for the sound pressure measurements. The tip of the probe-tube microphone was typically 1-2 mm from the tympanic membrane.

Except for the artificial ear canal and an opening in the mastoid for the laser beam, the remainder of the temporal bone was embedded in Hydrock dental cement (Kerr Co., Romulus, MI, USA), creating a solid specimen block. The cement edge of the mastoid opening was covered with Jeltrate (Dentsply Caulk Co., Milford, DE, USA); the opening provided a window that allowed the stapes footplate to be seen. The cemented bone was then secured in a temporal bone holder. Two 0.5-mm square pieces of reflective tape (3M, St Paul, MN, USA), weighing 0.04 mg, were placed; one on the lateral surface of the tympanic membrane over the umbo and the other on the center of the stapes footplate. Adhesive on the back of the targets kept them adhered to the umbo and footplate. Glass cover slips were placed over the mastoid opening and the lateral end of the ear canal sound assembly and held in place by silicone grease to prevent drying and create a good sound seal.

The earphone presented a stimulus consisting of 200 pure tones logarithmically spread from 0.024-25 kHz and ranging from 60-120 dB SPL at the TM, however, only the 0.05-10 kHz frequency range is reported here. The lower frequency limit is due to decreased signal-to-noise ratio and the upper frequency limit is due to microphone calibration limitations.

The stimulus was amplified using a D-75 power amplifier (Crown, Elkhart, IN, USA), fed through a 200-ohm resistor, then through the earphone to increase the high frequency response. The LDV output was amplified by 20 dB using the D-75 power amplifier. Sound-source attenuation and amplifier gains were chosen to minimize harmonic distortion. Although the noise floor varied with frequency, all data reported here had a signal-to-noise ratio greater than 10 dB. Responses from the ER-7C and LDV were then collected concurrently and the P_{ec} and related V_s data saved.

For the purpose of the experiment, the actual stapes footplate movement was considered to be predominantly piston-like and parallel to the motion of the umbo. Therefore, because the laser beam passed through the mastoid opening and was not perpendicular to the plane of the stapes footplate vibration, only a component of the actual movement of the stapes footplate was considered measured. The angle between the laser beam aimed through the ear canal perpendicular to the umbo target and the laser beam aimed at the stapes footplate target through the mastoid was measured using a protractor. The output of the LDV was divided by the cosine of that measured angle to determine the actual stapes footplate velocity, V_s. STF was then determined from the ratio V_s/P_{ec}, while the phase angle, $\angle$STF, was determined from the difference in phase between the outputs of the LDV and probe tube microphone.

Hydrophone insertion and measurement

After baseline measurements of STF, the temporal bone was orientated so the IAC was superior. After removing cement and latex to expose the IAC, the canal was filled with saline solution. The saline prevented the introduction of air bubbles while a 1.4-mm diameter opening was made with a fine pick just anterior and superior to the singular canal into the scala vestibuli. The saccule was moved aside using a fine pick so that the stapes footplate could be directly seen through this vestibular opening. The bone was placed in a temporal bone holder fixed to a vibration-reducing table. The hydrophone has a diameter of 1.4 mm and was encased in a brass tube with an outer diameter of 1.8 mm. Using a micromanipulator type M3301 (World Precision Instruments, Sarasota, FL, USA) attached to the vibration-reducing table, the hydrophone was centered and placed perpendicular and flush to the vestibular opening, completely sealing it. This allowed the hydrophone to lie in the opening with a good seal without entering the vestibule[12]. Jeltrate was used to fill the IAC and further seal the hydrophone in the vestibular opening. The hydrophone response was amplified by 60 dB using a SR-560 low noise amplifier (Stanford Research Systems, Sunnyvale, CA, USA).

The responses of the LDV and hydrophone were simultaneously collected three times; techniques mentioned in the previous section were used to derive V_s from the LDV response. Z_c was determined for each measurement from the ratio $P_v/(V_s \cdot A_{fp})$; the phase angle, $\angle Z_c$ was determined from the difference in phase between the outputs of the hydrophone and LDV. A_{fp} was determined from a calibrated digitized image of the footplate taken through the opening made in the vestibule. The average footplate area was 3.21 mm², with a standard deviation of 0.34 mm².

Using P_{ec} from the baseline measurements, the magnitude of GME was then determined from the ratio $|P_v|/|P_{ec}|$; the phase angle, $\angle$GME, was determined from the difference in phase between the outputs of the hydrophone and probe tube microphone. Measurements show that STF was the same before and after hydrophone insertion. For each ear, Z_c, STF and GME were derived using the mean of the three hydrophone and LDV measurements of P_v and V_s. The time required for the entire preparation and all measurements was less than eight hours for each temporal bone.

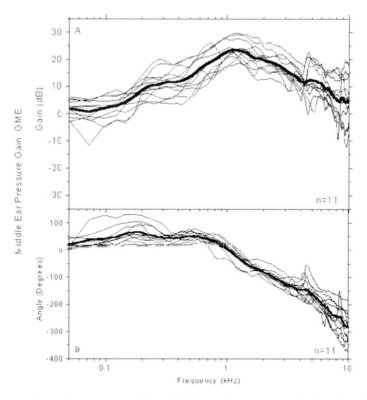

Fig. 2. Ear canal sound pressure to scala vestibuli sound pressure transfer function, GME, in 11 human temporal bone ears. Panel A shows the magnitude, panel B the phase angle. The curve for each ear represents the mean of three consecutive measurements of GME made within one hour of hydrophone insertion. Also shown is the mean magnitude and phase angle (thick line) of the 11 ears.

Results

Middle ear sound pressure gain

The ear canal sound pressure to vestibule sound pressure transfer function, GME, from 11 ears is shown in Figure 2. The mean GME magnitude has a maximum of 23.5 dB at 1.2 kHz, with a slope approximately 6 dB/octave from 0.1 to 1.2 kHz and around –6 dB/octave above 1.2 kHz. From 0.1-0.8 kHz, the mean GME phase angle is relatively flat with an average value of 48°. Above 0.8 kHz, the mean GME phase angle decreases with a slope of –87°/octave.

Stapes velocity transfer function

The ear canal sound pressure to stapes footplate velocity transfer function (STF) in the same 11 ears is shown in Figure 3. The mean STF magnitude has a maximum of 0.33 mm·s⁻¹/Pa at 1.0 kHz, with a mean slope of approximately 6 dB/octave from 0.1-1.0 kHz and around –7 dB/octave above 1.0 kHz. The mean STF phase angle is

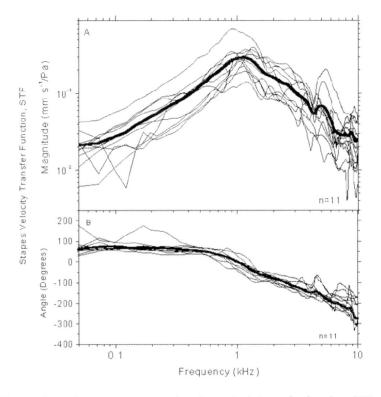

Fig. 3. Ear canal sound pressure to stapes footplate velocity transfer function, STF, in 11 human temporal bone ears. Panel A shows the magnitude, panel B the phase angle. The curve for each ear represents the mean of three consecutive measurements of STF. Also shown is the mean magnitude and phase (thick line) of the 11 ears.

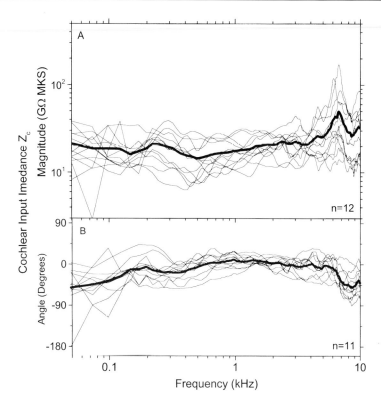

Fig. 4. Human cochlear input impedance (Z_c) in 12 human temporal bone ears. Panel A shows the magnitude, panel B the phase angle. The curve for each ear represents the mean of three consecutive measurements of vestibule pressure and stapes velocity made within one hour after hydrophone insertion. The mean magnitude and phase (thick line) of all ears is also shown. The phase from one ear was excluded because of a phase measurement error.

nearly the same as the mean GME phase angle, except for small differences below 0.2 kHz and above 5.0 kHz.

Cochlear input impedance

Figure 4 shows Z_c for each bone, including the mean. From 0.1-5.0 kHz, the mean Z_c magnitude is relatively flat, with a value of 21.1 GΩ. In the 0.5-5.0 kHz region, the Z_c phase angle is approximately 0° (±10°) and nearly flat, indicating Z_c is resistance dominated. At 0.1 kHz, the mean Z_c phase angle is –33° and increases to 0° at 0.5 kHz. The mean Z_c magnitude minimum is 13.4 acoustic GΩ MKS at 0.5 kHz, with a maximum of 49.9 GΩ at 6.7 kHz. Above 5.0 kHz, the mean Z_c magnitude increases with a peak at 6.7 kHz, and then decreases. Above 5.0 kHz, the mean phase angle of Z_c decreases 59°/octave to a minimum of –49° at 8.6 kHz, then increases to –40° at 10 kHz.

Effect of opening the scala vestibuli

STF was measured before and after inserting the hydrophone to assess the effect of opening the scala vestibuli. As shown in Figure 5, the average change in magnitude is about 1.0 dB, with a maximum of 3.7 dB at 5.7 kHz. The average change in phase angle is 5° with a maximum of 30° at 9.4 kHz. The effect of opening the scala vestibuli on STF measurement is small.

Effect of time on stapes velocity

In a temporal bone not used for cochlear impedance measurements, V_s was measured at 0.5, 1, 2, and 20 hours after preparation. The effect due to drying was less than 1.5 dB, and therefore, we conclude that V_s remained consistent over the measurement time of the experiments.

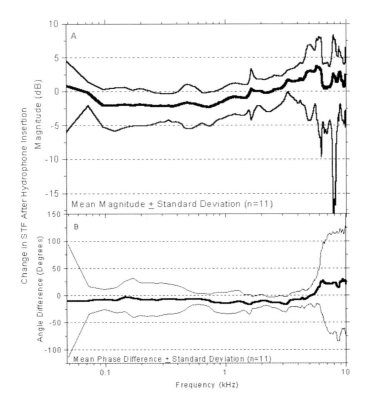

Fig. 5. The curves shown are the mean difference in STF after insertion of the hydrophone in 11 ears. Panel A shows the magnitude, panel B the phase angle. This comparison shows that hydrophone insertion has a negligible effect on stapes velocity, V_s.

Discussion

Previous measurements of middle ear pressure gain

In Figure 6, our mean GME is compared to the GME reported by others. There is relatively good agreement between our results and those obtained by Puria *et al.*[12], at most, disagreeing by 6 dB in magnitude and 40° in phase. However, there are differences in the shape of the curves. Puria *et al.* found a flat mean pressure gain of 20 dB between 0.5 and 2.0 kHz, decreasing to 18 dB at 4.0 kHz. From 0.1 Hz to 0.5 kHz, the magnitude increased by around 6 dB/octave, while above 4.0 kHz the magnitude rolled off by –8 dB/octave. In contrast, our data show a 23.5 dB peak gain at 1.2 kHz with a roll off of –6 dB/octave above this frequency; the gain is 20 dB at 2.0 kHz and 12 dB at 4.0 kHz. There is increased damping in their four ears compared with ours. Variations in method, primarily the absence of flush tubes in our preparation, may account for some of these differences. In addition, we studied a larger number of ears (11) so that individual variations tend to average out. The GME measurement by Hüttenbrink and Hudde[21] is overall greater than

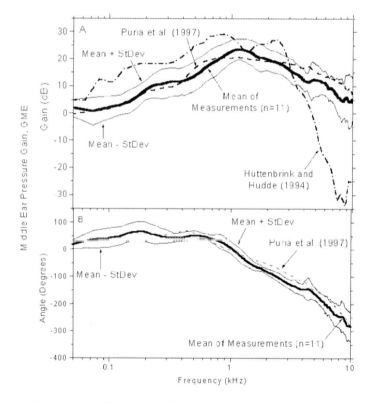

Fig. 6. Comparison of mean GME obtained in this study in 11 ears with mean GME reported by Puria *et al.*[12] in four ears and Hüttenbrink and Hudde[21] in one ear. Panel A shows magnitude, panel B the phase angle.

our mean result up to near 3.0 kHz, while above this frequency the gain rolls off precipitously. This may be due to air in the cochlea[12] or due to measurement artifact; only one ear was tested.

Previous measurements of stapes velocity

In Figure 7, we compare the mean STF obtained in this study with a previous STF measurement from our laboratory[11], and model calculations by Kringlebotn[22] based on temporal bone data obtained by Kringlebotn and Gundersen[2] using round window velocity as the output measure. In our previous measurements, peak gain was at 0.7 kHz rather than 1.0 kHz. The slopes above and below the resonant frequency of our previous measurements are essentially identical to the mean STF. However, because of the lower resonant frequency in the previous measurements, velocity magnitude at 0.5 kHz is about 5 dB greater, while above 1.0 kHz it is about 4 dB less, reaching a maximum difference of 7 dB at 4.4 kHz. No phase measurements were made in the 1994 experiments. In these previous measurements, a thin coat of oil was used on the TM to decrease any drying effects; this could add to the TM mass and decrease the resonant frequency. Comparing our current data with the

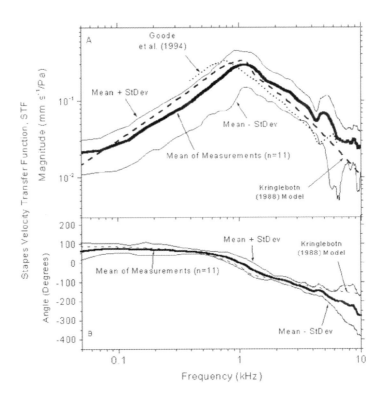

Fig. 7. Comparison of mean STF obtained in this study in 11 ears with the mean STF reported by Goode *et al.*[11] and the STF calculated by Kringlebotn[22]. No phase measurements were obtained in the earlier Goode study. Panel A shows magnitude, panel B phase angle.

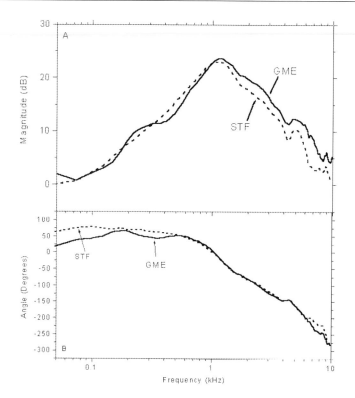

Fig. 8. Comparison of the mean GME and STF in the 11 ears. Panel A shows the magnitude, panel B the phase angle. The solid line represents GME and the dashed line represents STF. Zero dB for the STF curve was set at 2.1×10^{-2} mm·sec^{-1}/Pa at 0.05 kHz.

Kringlebotn model shows only small differences in magnitude and phase up to 4.0 kHz; the slopes are essentially identical. Above 4.0 kHz, there are increasing differences with rising frequency reaching a peak at 10 kHz where the magnitude differs by 7 dB and the phase angle by 90°.

Figure 8 shows the mean data of Figures 2 and 3 on one graph for comparison purposes. STF has been converted to magnitude in dB with 0 dB assumed to be 2.1×10^{-2} mm·sec^{-1}/Pa at 0.05 kHz. The METF magnitude curves are quite similar, separating slightly at higher frequencies. The METF phase is also similar but are slightly different at frequencies below about 0.5 kHz.

Previous measurements of cochlear input impedance

Prior to this report, only indirect estimations of Z_c have been reported. Figure 9 compares our measurement of Z_c to estimates made by Puria *et al.*[12], Merchant *et al.*[19] and a theoretical prediction by Zwislocki[20].

Puria *et al.*[12] measured vestibule pressure, but used stapes velocity from the Kringlebotn[22] model (Fig. 7, panel A) to estimate Z_c. Their mean magnitude and phase angle for Z_c is similar to ours for frequencies below 1 kHz. Above 1 kHz,

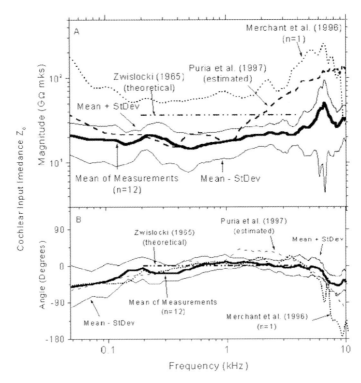

Fig. 9. Comparison of measured cochlear input impedance, Z_c, with previous estimates. Panel A shows magnitude, panel B phase. Merchant *et al.*[19] estimated Z_c for one ear by measuring the difference in stapes-cochlea acoustic input impedance after draining the cochlea. Puria *et al.*[12] estimated Z_c based on mean measured middle ear pressure gain and the Kringlebotn (1988) model calculation of STF. Zwislocki's[20] Z_c is based on theoretical parameters for cochlear input impedance.

their magnitude increases more rapidly than ours and is higher by a factor of four (12 dB) at 10 kHz. Between 1 and 10 kHz, their phase steadily decreases to below –90° at 10 kHz, whereas in the current phase measurements, $\angle Z_c$ is nearly constant at 0° to approximately 5 kHz. Above this frequency, $\angle Z_c$ decreases, levelling off near –45°.

Figures 6 and 7 provide an explanation for the differences between the present measurements of Z_c at higher frequencies and those reported by Puria *et al.*[12] Firstly, Figure 6 shows that, above 2 kHz, the Puria *et al.* GME magnitude is larger than the present measurements. Secondly, Figure 7 shows that above 1 kHz, the stapes velocity of Kringlebotn that Puria *et al.* used is lower in magnitude than our measurements. The combination of these differences leads Puria *et al.* to estimate a higher impedance magnitude, above 1.0 kHz, than we do from the present data. Similar arguments can be made for the differences in $\angle Z_c$. The primary reason why the $\angle Z_c$ estimated by Puria *et al.* continues to decrease is that the phase of the stapes velocity of Kringlebotn that Puria *et al.* used is greater than that found in the present experiments (Fig. 7, panel B).

Also shown in Figure 9 is an estimate of Z_c by Merchant *et al.*[19] from one ear. In that experiment, they first measured the acoustic input impedance of the stapes and cochlea, Z_{sc}, from the ratio of the sound pressure measured near the stapes head and the stapes head velocity. They then drained the cochlea and repeated the measurement. Z_c was calculated from the difference in Z_{sc} before and after draining the cochlea. The shapes of the Z_c curves are similar, however, the magnitude of Merchant *et al.* is higher than ours by as much as a factor of five. Their phase angle and the present measurements are in relative agreement up to 5 kHz, above which, theirs decreases rapidly to $-180°$ between 9 and 10 kHz. One possibility for the differences is that they measured stapes head velocity and we measured stapes footplate velocity. Also, we used intact middle ears and Merchant *et al.* used ears with the middle ear partially removed.

Model predictions by Zwislocki[20] for living humans predicts that Z_c has a magnitude of 35.2 acoustic $G\Omega$ and is purely resistive (0° phase) in the 0.2 to 4 kHz frequency range. The mean of our Z_c magnitude is about half as large as Zwislocki's, and the average difference from the mean phase angle is 4.7°, with a maximum difference of 17°. Zwislocki[15] contends that postmortem changes in the basilar membrane, observed in cats by Kohllöffel[23], decreases Z_c by a factor of two. Although our mean Z_c corroborates Zwislocki's contention, the question of postmortem changes in Z_c in the human is unanswerable at this time because of our inability to make the measurement in the living human ear.

Effect of stapes rocking motion on cochlear input impedance

Figure 10 shows that the peak in Z_c seen at 6.7 kHz correlates with a peak in the stapes footplate rocking ratio measured by Heiland *et al.*[14] The rocking ratio of the

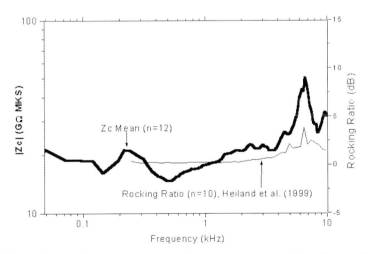

Fig. 10. Effect of stapes footplate rocking ratio on measurement of Z_c. The rocking ratio is defined as the maximum difference in displacement between the anterior and posterior footplate to displacement at the center of the stapes footplate. The peak in Z_c magnitude at 6.7 kHz is near the frequency of the peak in the rocking motion, and the two may be related.

Table 1. Definitions

P_{ec}	ear canal sound pressure at the surface of the tympanic membrane
V_s	stapes footplate velocity
A_{fp}	area of the stapes footplate
U_s	stapes footplate volume velocity, V_s times A_{fp}
P_v	scala vestibuli sound pressure near the stapes footplate
METF	middle ear sound transfer function
GME	middle ear sound pressure gain, ratio of P_v to P_{ec}
$\angle$GME	phase angle of middle ear sound pressure gain
STF	stapes velocity transfer function, ratio of V_s to P_{ec}
$\angle$STF	phase angle of stapes velocity transfer function
Z_c	acoustic input impedance of the cochlea
$\angle Z_c$	phase angle of acoustic input impedance of the cochlea

stapes is defined as the ratio of the maximum difference in displacement between the anterior and posterior sites of the footplate compared with displacement at the center of the footplate.

Conclusions

Figure 8 shows that METF measured by either GME or STF produces essentially the same curve when performed in the same ears. Therefore, either measure, if carefully performed, should provide equivalent METF results. Some differences exist between our GME data and that reported by others (Fig. 6). We suspect that the differences, which are not large, are due to the high standard deviations present in middle ear measurements in human temporal bones as well as differences in measurement methods[24]. The GME data presented in this paper are based on the largest number of human temporal bones reported to date, which should minimize the effect of individual variations in middle ear function. The GME magnitude curve has a band pass characteristic with a resonance at 1.2 kHz and around a 6 dB/octave slope from 0.1 to 1.2 kHz and a −7 dB/octave slope above this frequency.

The STF curves are similar to those reported by others using similar methods in intact ears[1,3,4,11,22]. Measures of middle ear acoustic function made by comparing stapes displacement before and after removal of the middle ear structures[6,8] produce a different result. Direct stimulation of the stapes with sound may produce a different type of vibration than in the intact middle ear. Studies where the cochlea has been drained in order to make the middle ear measurements are not considered reliable because of the lack of a cochlear load.

Direct measurement of Z_c, performed for the first time, reveals a flat, resistive cochlear input impedance of about 21.1 GΩ from 0.1-5.0 kHz. The impedance increases between 5.0 and 10.0 kHz with a maximum of 49.9 GΩ at 6.7 kHz. At higher frequencies above 5.0 kHz and at lower frequencies below 0.2 kHz, the phase angle becomes increasingly negative. The peak in Z_c at 6.7 kHz corresponds to a peak in the same frequency range as the stapes footplate rocking ratio[14]. This suggests that, in this frequency range, footplate motion is particularly complex and measurement of stapes velocity at one site, such as the center of the footplate, may not be adequate to determine the volume velocity. There may be another explanation, the presence of bubbles in the cochlea. Below 5.0 kHz, however, as seen in Figure 8, velocity measured at the center of the footplate is representative of footplate volume velocity, with only a small difference above 1.0 kHz.

While the mean data reported here provide us with a general scheme of how the human middle ear acoustically interacts with the cochlea, the relationship of Z_c and METF in individual ears is not as clear. Some temporal bones seem to function different than others, independent of quantitative differences. For example, since Z_c is flat and resistive at 0.5 to 5.0 kHz, P_v should be related to V_s, which should be related to the umbo velocity produced by a given TM. It would therefore be suspected that the highest METF would occur in ears with the highest umbo velocities. This is true in some but not all ears and needs further study.

Acknowledgments

This work was supported in part by grants from the VA (GDE 0010ARG) and the National Institute of Deafness & Other Communication Disorders of the NIH (DC03085).

References

1. Gundersen T: Prostheses in the Ossicular Chain. Baltimore, MD: University Park 1971
2. Kringlebotn M, Gundersen: 1985. Frequency characteristics of the middle ear. J Acoust Soc Am 77:159-164, 1985
3. Vlaming MSM, Feenstra L: Studies of the mechanics of the normal human middle ear. Clin Otolaryngol 11:353-363, 1986
4. Gyo K, Aritomo H, Goode RL: Measurement of the ossicular vibration ratio in human temporal bones by use of a video measuring system. Acta Otolaryngol (Stockh) 103:87-95, 1987
5. Brenkman CJ, Grote JJ, Rutten WL: Acoustic transfer characteristics in human middle ears studied by a SQUID magnetometer method. J Acoust Soc Am 82:1646-1654, 1987
6. Kurokawa H, Goode RL: Sound pressure gain produced by the human middle ear. Otolaryngol Head Neck Surg 113:349-355, 1995
7. Békésy G: Experiments in hearing, pp 745. New York, NY: McGraw-Hill 1960
8. Onchi Y: Mechanism of the middle ear. J Acoust Soc Am 33:794-805, 1961
9. Rubenstein M, Feldman B, Frei EH, Spria D: Measurement of stapedial-footplate displacements during transmission of sound through the middle ear. J Acoust Soc Am 40:1420-1426, 1964
10. Fishler H, Frei EH, Spira D: Dynamic response of middle-ear structures. J Acoust Soc Am 41:1220-1231, 1965
11. Goode RL, Killion M, Nakamura K, Nishihara S: New knowledge about the function of the

human middle ear: development of an improved analog model. Am J Otol 15:145-154, 1994

12. Puria S, Peake WT, Rosowski JJ: Sound-pressure measurements in the cochlea vestibule of human cadaver ears. J Acoust Soc Am 101:2754-2770, 1997

13. Dallos P: The Auditory Periphery: Biophysics and Physiology, pp 98-99. New York, NY: Academic Press 1973

14. Heiland KE, Goode RL, Asai M, Huber AM: A human temporal bone study of stapes footplate movement. Am J Otol 20:81-86, 1999

15. Zwislocki JJ: The role of the external and middle ear in sound transmission. In: Tower DB (ed) The Nervous System, Vol 3, Human Communication and its Disorders, pp 44-55. New York, NY: Raven Press 1975

16. Lynch TJ, Peake WT, Rosowski JJ: Measurements of the acoustic input impedance of cat ears: 10 Hz to 20 kHz. J Acoust Soc Am 96:2184-2209, 1994

17. Dancer A, Franke R: Intracochlear sound pressure measurements in guinea pigs. Hearing Res 2:191-205, 1980

18. Ruggero MA, Rich NC, Robles L, Shivapuja BG: Middle-ear response in the chinchilla and its relationship to mechanics at the base of the cochlea. J Acoust Soc Am 87:1612-1629, 1990

19. Merchant SN, Ravicz ME, Rosowski JJ: Acoustic input impedance of the stapes and cochlea in human temporal bones. Hearing Res 97:30-45, 1996

20. Zwislocki JJ: Analysis of some auditory characteristics. In: Luce E, Bush S, Galanter FE (eds) Handbook of Mathematical Physiology, pp 3-46. New York, NY: John Wiley 1965

21. Hüttenbrink KB, Hudde H: Untersuchungen zur Schalleitung durch das rekonstruierte Mittelohr mit einem Hydrophon. HNO 42:49-57, 1994

22. Kringlebotn M: Network model for the human middle ear. Scand Audiol 17:75-85, 1988

23. Kohllöffel LU: Studies of the distribution of cochlear potentials along the basilar membrane. Acta Otolaryngol (Stockh) Suppl 288:1-66, 1971

24. Goode RL, Nakamura K, Gyo K, Aritomo H: Comments on 'acoustic transfer characteristics in human middle ears studied by a SQUID magnetometer method'. J Acoust Soc Am 82:1646-1654, 1989

METHODOLOGY FOR LASER VIBROMETER STUDIES OF STAPES FOOTPLATE DISPLACEMENT

Eric W. Abel[1], Richard M. Lord[1], Robert P. Mills[2] and Zhigang Wang[1]

[1]*Medical Engineering Research Institute, University of Dundee, Dundee;*
[2]*Department of Otolaryngology, Lauriston Building, Royal Infirmary, Edinburgh, Scotland, UK*

Abstract

Most modern studies of stapes displacement use laser Doppler interferometry. However, there are some practical difficulties to be overcome if consistent results are to be obtained. The purpose of this study was to produce a reliable methodology for measuring stapes displacement *in vitro*, particularly for evaluation of ossicular prostheses and hearing implants

Reflectivity of the stapes footplate: Consistent optical reflection of the laser beam to the sensor has been improved by using retro-reflective paint instead of retro-reflective foil. Reflective foil was difficult to adhere to the footplate in a manner that gave stable results, so a retro-reflective paint was used. This method is similar to that of using glass micro-beads.

Surgical approach to the stapes: The internal meatal approach allows alignment of the beam along or close to the direction of vibration of the footplate, so cosine errors are small. It is a rapid, standard approach that does not need to disturb the middle ear cavity.

Other approaches restrict access to the beam, such that the vibration is measured at a large angle to the motion. This means that the actual level of vibration can be difficult to determine and there are problems in standardizing measurements when attempting to realign the temporal bone during multiple measurements on the same bone after, for example, inserting different types of prosthesis.

The methodology proposed is straightforward and gives reproducible results. It allows effective use of the time available for testing *in vitro* temporal bone specimens, while they remain viable.

Keywords: laser vibrometer, stapes displacement, stapes vibration measurement

Introduction

It is important for the middle ear researcher to be able to make reliable, repeatable measurements of ossicular displacement, when the middle ear is exposed to sound stimuli. A non-contact method that can be used on any of the moving

Address for correspondence: Eric W. Abel, PhD, Medical Engineering Research Institute, University of Dundee, Dundee, DD1 4HN, Scotland, UK

The Function and Mechanics of Normal, Diseased and Reconstructed Middle Ears, pp. 89–97
edited by J.J. Rosowski and S.N. Merchant
© *2000 Kugler Publications, The Hague, The Netherlands*

middle ear structures, tympanic membrane, ossicles and round window, is laser Doppler vibrometry. Laser vibrometry offers an accurate approach to measuring sound transmission through the ear. The methodology presented in this paper has been developed to investigate the performance of ossicular bone replacements and piezoelectric ossicular stimulators[1], by means of *in vitro* studies.

The magnitude of stapes vibration is of the order of 0.1 nm at the threshold of hearing[2]. A variety of instrumentation techniques have been attempted for measuring these low vibration magnitudes. Von Békésy[3] attempted microscopic observation using stroboscopic illumination and also succeeded in making measurements with a capacitive probe. The capacitive probe method was adopted by Møller[4] and was used by several researchers until the early 1980s. A problem with the capacitive probe method is that it loads the ossicles in a manner that may affect the transmission properties of the chain. A more promising technique used the Mössbauer effect, whereby a radioactive isotope was placed on the object under investigation[5-7]. The load that the source imposed could be minimized by using a very small particle. The Mössbauer technique suffers from certain drawbacks, especially the non-linear nature of its transduction characteristics and the long sampling times required due to the nature of the radiation[8].

A different approach was adopted by Khanna *et al.*[9] and used a Michelson interferometer for measurements in small biological structures. A laser is split into two beams, a reference beam and a 'measurement' beam. These are reflected back from a mirror and the target, respectively, and are recombined. The two beams interfere with each other, producing a series of bright bands, which can be used to measure the displacement of the target. Tonndorf and Khanna[10] applied this to middle ear measurements of tympanic membrane vibrations. A major advantage of laser velocimetry over the Mössbauer technique is its linearity over a wide dynamic range. Several other researchers have used the Michelson interferometer, but it has the disadvantage of its sensitivity to background noise, which is manifest as multiplicative noise in the measured signal.

Buunen and Vlaming[11] described the use of a laser Doppler velocity meter to measure tympanic membrane vibrations in cats. The laser Doppler vibrometer (LDV) measures the velocity of the target rather than displacement. Background noise appears as additive noise, which means that the measured signal-to-noise ratio will be high. It is now widely accepted that this technique is the best for laboratory study of ossicular vibrations. The LDV is readily available as laboratory equipment, with some commercial vibrometers being small enough to fit on the mounting bracket of an operating microscope. An example of a clinical application of the LDV is the work of Stasche *et al.*[12]

In 1996, Vogel *et al.* presented a comprehensive review of the opportunities and limitations of LDV studies of the middle ear[13]. One of the limitations is achieving a sufficient quantity of back-scattered light from the target. Biological tissues have a low reflectance[14] and therefore a reflective surface needs to be applied to the target. Different methods have been used to address this problem. Typically, a small reflective foil is attached to the target using petroleum jelly or capillary force[12,15,16]. However, the use of a reflective foil or sticker can give rise to problems from poor adhesion to the stapes, such that the vibration pattern of the foil may be different from that of the stapes. The reflected signal might not give a true representation of the ossicular vibration. The foil may change the properties of the surface on which it is placed; *e.g.*, it may change the elasticity of the tympanic membrane. One option that has become increasingly used and is to be recommended is the use of glass micro-beads, which are retro-reflective, *i.e.*, they reflect the light back to the direction of the source. The use of glass micro-beads has been reported by Nuttall *et al.*[17], who cover the appropriate optical ray theory adequately in their paper. Reflective beads have been used on tympanic membrane studies[18], inner ear studies[17], and for individual ossicular measurements[2]. The reflective beads are small and do not cause any significant loading effect. They can be attached by capillary action, or are bound in an adhesive that will hold it to the substrate.

Sound may be transmitted from the ear canal to the cochlea by the mechanisms of ossicular and acoustic coupling[19]. Acoustic coupling is negligible in normal ears, but has a significant role in diseased and reconstructed ears, where ossicular coupling has failed. An investigation of ossicular coupling via the mechanical chain can only be achieved by measuring stapes footplate displacements for known sound pressure stimuli.

The location of the target is dependent upon the aim and nature of the experiment. Many researchers have taken umbo displacement to be indicative of hearing function. One aspect of our research has been to compare the sound transmission performance of a prosthesis with that of the intact ossicular chain, so stapes displacement was measured. The laser target, as in many other studies, is therefore the stapes footplate.

Methods

The amplitude of stapes footplate velocity, representing the level of vibration transmitted through the ossicular chain, was measured by means of a commercial LDV (Polytec CLV 700-Head, 800-Laser and 1000-Controller). The vibrometer is suitable for measurement in the audio-frequency range.

The laser vibrometer and the temporal bone sample under investigation were both isolated from environmental vibration on an anti-vibration platform (isolation efficiency 90% @ 90 Hz). Air springs are very suitable for this purpose.

Temporal bone samples for the study were frozen immediately after extraction at the temperature of –20°C. They were allowed to thaw during preparation – typically 60-90 minutes. After this time, they were considered ready for use and would remain usable for up to six hours without deterioration of the os-sicular chain or dehydration of the ligaments, tendons or tympanic membrane[12,20].

Recent work has suggested that some changes may occur in temporal bone preparations that have been frozen, and that leaks within the inner ear may occur due to the expansion of the inner ear fluids[21]. The preparations used in this work had the cochlea removed and the vestibule drained, for access to the underside of the stapes footplate. Unless the annular ligament has been dam-aged, the effects of freezing the bone should not be evident. Puria *et al.* argue that the effects of freezing on the middle ear are small[22].

Initially, attempts were made to align the temporal bone sample in the path of the laser, such that the study could be made on the superior side of the stapes without disturbing the inner ear. The time required to make this alignment was assessed to be too large, as temporal bone experiments are limited to six hours[20]. The laser would also have to be directed at an angle to the direction of the vibration vector, so the true amplitude of the vibration would have to be calcu-lated using a cosine function. This would firstly result in a lower magnitude of signal, and secondly present problems in determining the angle between the laser beam and the stapes vibration vector.

The approach taken in this study of ossicular coupling meant that the co-chlea and perilymphatic fluid could be removed in order to assess the transmis-sion properties of the ossicles, compared with a prosthesis *in situ*. Exposing the stapes footplate via the internal auditory meatus proved to be the ideal ap-proach for this study, as displacement measurement of the stapes in the line of the velocity vector could be made. Alignment errors of up ten degrees from this line would result in vibration measurement errors of less than 2%. By using the internal auditory meatal approach to the underside of the stapes footplate, alignment time was significantly reduced and no correction to the measurement was re-quired. A separate investigation into the effect of removing the cochlea was undertaken, measuring stapes motion from the superior surface, before and af-ter the cochlea was drained.

For each experiment, the underside of the stapes footplate was exposed via the internal auditory meatus. The ear canal and tympanic membrane were left intact. A cortical mastoidectomy with a posterior tympanotomy exposed the ossicular chain. The prepared temporal bone was fixed in a holder by three clamps, the holder being mounted on tilt, rotation and translation micro posi-tioning stages. This enabled the sample to be maneuvered into the required position relative to the LDV. Figure 1 shows the experimental rig.

A comparison of retro-reflective foil (3M Scotchlite) and micro-beads was made. A small spot of retro-reflective paint (3M Scotchlite reflective liquid 7210, which contains glass micro-beads) was applied to the center of the stapes footplate using a pinhead. The mass of the paint spot was less than 0.5% that of the stapes, so its loading effect may be assumed to be negligible. The specimen was aligned in the optical path of the laser beam, which was then focused on the paint spot. The use of a Zeiss operating microscope aided this procedure.

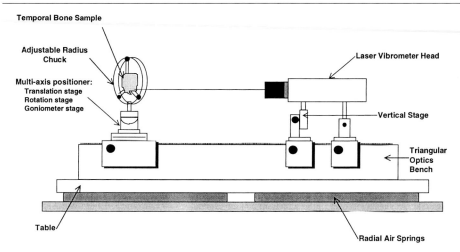

Fig. 1. Multi-axis positioning rig. The laser Doppler vibrometer was aligned with the temporal bone sample on an optics bench. The temporal bone was held in an adjustable radius chuck mounted on micro-adjusters allowing six degrees of freedom manipulation of the sample into the path of the laser beam.

To provide a method of introducing sound to the tympanic membrane, a 40-mm length of plastic tube, 4 mm in diameter, was attached to the ear canal using a rapid set epoxy resin. A side opening was made into the meatus, adjacent to the tympanic membrane and a 20-mm long, 2.2-mm diameter probe tube was adhered to the walls of the opening. This was attached to a microphone to allow the sound pressure level to be monitored at the tympanic membrane.

Pure-tone sound stimuli were applied to the eardrum in a closed field manner, using a 50-mm diameter transducer, attached to the acoustic tube via a conical flare. An arbitrary waveform generator (Thurlby Thandar Inst., TGA 1240) and an audio amplifier controlled the sound stimuli. A Knowles EK-3103 miniature microphone was calibrated for the 2.2-mm tube and acted as a probe microphone for monitoring the sound pressure level at the tympanic membrane. A 94-dB, 1-kHz tone was applied from a Brüel & Kjær 4230 calibrator to check the probe microphone arrangement.

The displacement characteristics of the ossicles were measured by applying a pure tone at frequencies between 125 Hz and 8 kHz. Pure tones rather than white noise were used to give a good signal-to-noise ratio. The vibrometer and microphone signals were acquired at a sampling rate of 30 kHz to a PC using an Eagle Technology PC30F data acquisition card. The laser signal was filtered using a band-pass filter of 0.08-10 kHz prior to acquisition. Measurement time for a complete characteristic was 20-25 minutes.

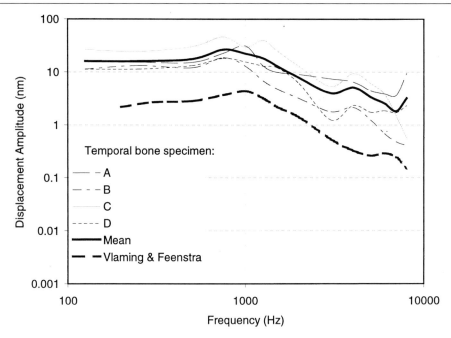

Fig. 2. Vibration characteristics of the stapes as a function of frequency at 80 dB SPL. Results from four temporal bone specimens (A-D) are shown with the arithmetic mean of all eight samples. The results of Vlaming and Feenstra[20] are plotted for comparison. Measured displacements are higher than those found in the normal middle ear due to removal of the cochlea.

Results

The stapes velocity responses to sound stimuli were measured in eight human temporal bones. Displacement amplitude was calculated by numerical integration of the velocity signal with respect to time.

Four plots of displacement response of the normal ossicular chain to a stimulation of 80 dB sound pressure level (SPL) are shown in Figure 2, illustrating the individuality of the ossicular chains, especially above 1 kHz. The plot of the arithmetic mean of all eight samples is also plotted, for clarity. Below 700 Hz, the displacement was flat, with amplitudes between 11 and 30 nm (mean of 19 nm). There are peaks and troughs in the spectrum above 1 kHz, which are different for the temporal bone samples. Above 1 kHz, the amplitude attenuation was approximately 12 dB/octave. This decrease in function shows a reduced transmission efficiency as frequency increases and may be attributed to the tympanic membrane 'breaking up' into less efficient vibrating areas[23].

The shape of the mean displacement plot is in good agreement with those reported by Vlaming and Feenstra[20], which are also represented in Figure 2. There is a discrepancy in magnitude of the displacements by between 10 and 20 dB. This may be attributed to the removal of the cochlea and the fact that Vlaming did not use a cosine correction on his measurements.

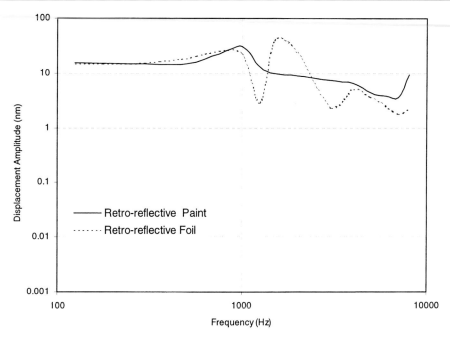

Fig. 3. Stapes footplate displacements measured using retro-reflective foil and retro-reflective tape, in human temporal bone, as a function of frequency at 80 dB SPL. The peaks measured in the response using the foil may be attributed to poor adhesion or altered ossicular characteristics.

Figure 3 shows the results of a comparison with retro-foil and with the retro-reflective paint. The same temporal bone was studied, the foil experiment being conducted prior to using paint. There are large peaks in the measured response above 1 kHz.

Discussion

Vlaming and Feenstra[20] were able to focus a laser vibrometer using a frontal approach to the stapes. This approach does not make it possible to focus the laser beam parallel with the direction of motion, and the angular deviation must be estimated if measurements of true displacement are to be made. It is technically difficult to make repeatable readings using their method, so an approach to the underside of the stapes footplate was used, which is much easier experimentally.

While the motion of the stapes is primarily piston-like at low frequencies, more detailed studies of the motion of the ossicular surfaces have shown the three-dimensional motion of the stapes. For example, Huber *et al.* found stapes motion to be piston-like at low frequencies, up to 1 kHz, with a small but identifiable additional rocking motion at higher frequencies[2]. The method presented in this paper does not require the application of a cosine correction to the displacement measurements, so our results are indicative of the one-dimensional stapes motion. The technique could be applied to measuring the motion at different locations across the stapes footplate, quantifying the ossicular motion in three-dimensions.

The internal auditory meatus was opened to expose the stapes footplate in order to gain access to the vibration vector of the stapes. This method required removal of the cochlea. The cochlea load is a result of the fluid acting to oppose motion of the stapes footplate. After removal of the cochlea fluid, there will still be some resistance to stapes motion due to the air behind the footplate, and so the cochlea does not vanish completely but is very small. Even so, results for the normal middle ear were found to be in agreement with those from previous middle ear studies[20]. The stapes exhibited a flat response at frequencies below 1 kHz with decreasing amplitude above 1 kHz, which is associated with transmission properties of the tympanic membrane. It was shown that the response to intensity, of the ossicular chain, over the frequencies (0.125-8 kHz) and intensities (80-100 dB) measured, was linear. Measurements in this study were considerably higher than the displacements measured by Vlaming and Feenstra. Some of this difference may be attributed to the fact that they did not make a cosine correction to the displacement values measured, but this would only account for between 1 and 2 dB. A more probable explanation is that there is another pathway for the stimulus to be driving the stapes footplate, and further investigations into mechanical coupling through the temporal bone sample are presently being undertaken.

A useful signal could not be achieved without the reflective coating. Using retro-reflective foil, resonances were recorded in the response above 1 kHz. This may have been due to the foil affecting the ossicular chain from loading, but it is more likely to be the measurement of the foil vibrating separately from the stapes. The use of reflective paint overcomes the practical difficulty of attaching tape and, maintaining a good attachment, avoids the possibility of obtaining erroneous recordings of vibration due to the tape vibrating separately from the stapes.

Acknowledgments

The authors acknowledge the support of the Scottish Hospital Endowments Research Trust, Edinburgh and Defeating Deafness, London.

References

1. Wang Z, Mills R, Abel E, Liu Y: A comparison of stapes vibration spectra in acoustic-eardrum stimulation and actuator-incus excitation. (Abstract). British Society of Audiology Short Papers Meeting on Experimental Studies of Hearing and Deafness, University of Essex, 21-22 Sept., 1999. Br J Audiol 34(2):119, 2000

2. Huber A, Asai M, Ball G, Goode R: Analysis of ossicular vibration in three dimensions. In: Hüttenbrink KB (ed) Proceedings of the International Workshop on Middle Ear Mechanics in Research and Otosurgery, Dresden, Germany, pp 82-87. 1996

3. Békésy G: Experiments in Hearing. New York, NY: McGraw-Hill 1960

4. Møller AR: Transfer function of the middle ear. J Acoust Soc Am 35:1526-1534, 1963

5. Hillman P, Schecter H, Rubenstein M: Applications of the Mössbauer technique to the measurement of small vibrations in the ear. Res Mod Phys 36:360, 1964

6. Johnstone BM, Boyle AJF: Basilar membrane vibrations examined with the Mössbauer technique. Science 158:389-390, 1967

7. Rhode WS: Observations of the vibration of the basilar membrane in squirrel monkey using the Mössbauer technique. J Acoust Soc Am 49:1218-1231, 1971

8. Ruggero MA, Rich NC: Application of a commercially-manufactured Doppler-shift laser velocimeter to the measurement of basilar-membrane vibration. Hearing Res 51:215-230, 1991

9. Khanna SM, Tonndorf J, Walcott WW: Laser interferometry for the measurement of submicroscopic displacement amplitudes and their phases in small biological structures. J Acoust Soc Am 44:1555-1565, 1968

10. Tonndorf J, Khanna SM: Submicroscopic displacement amplitudes of the tympanic membrane (cat) measured by laser interferometer. J Acoust Soc Am 44:1546-1554, 1968

11. Buunen TJF, Vlaming MSMG: Laser Doppler velocity meter applied to tympanic membrane vibrations in cat. J Acoust Soc Am 69:744-750, 1981

12. Stasche N, Foth HJ, Hormann K, Baker A, Hutloff C: Middle ear transmission disorders: tympanic membrane vibration analysis by laser-Doppler vibrometry. Acta Otolaryngol (Stockh) 114:59-63, 1994

13. Vogel U, Zahnert T, Hofmann G, Offergeld C, Hüttenbrink KB: Laser vibrometry of the middle ear: opportunities and limitations. In: Hüttenbrink KB (ed) Proceedings of the International Workshop on Middle Ear Mechanics in Research and Otosurgery, Dresden, Germany, pp 128-133. 1996

14. Khanna SM, Willemin JF, Ulfendahl M: Measurements of optical reflectivity in cells of the inner ear. Acta Otolaryngol (Stockh) Suppl 467:69-75, 1989

15. Goode RL, Ball G, Nishihara S: Measurement of umbo vibration in human subjects: method and possible clinical applications. Am J Otol 14(3):247-251, 1993

16. Nishihara S, Goode R: Measurement of tympanic membrane vibration in 99 human ears. In: Hüttenbrink KB (ed) Proceedings of the International Workshop on Middle Ear Mechanics in Research and Otosurgery, Dresden, Germany, pp 91-94. 1996

17. Nuttall AL, Dolan DF, Avinash G: Laser Doppler velocimetry of basilar membrane vibration. Hearing Res 51:203-214, 1991

18. Cohen YE, Rubin DM, Saunders JC. Middle ear development. I: Extra stapedius response in the neonatal chick. Hearing Res 58:1-8, 1992

19. Merchant SN, Ravicz ME, Voss SE, Peake WT, Rosowski JJ: Middle ear mechanics in normal, diseased and reconstructed ears. J Laryngol Otol 112:715-731, 1998

20. Vlaming MSMG, Feenstra L: Studies on the mechanics of the normal human middle ear. Clin Otolaryngol 11:353-363, 1986

21. Merchant SN, Ravicz ME, Rosowski JJ: Acoustic input impedance of the stapes and cochlea in human temporal bones. Hearing Res 97:30-45, 1996

22. Puria S, Peake WT, Rosowski JJ: Sound-pressure measurements in the cochlear vestibule of human cadavers. J Acoust Soc Am 101:2754-2770, 1997

23. Goode RL: The ideal middle ear prosthesis. In: Hüttenbrink KB (ed) Proceedings of the International Workshop on Middle Ear Mechanics in Research and Otosurgery, Dresden, Germany, pp 169-174. 1996

.

THE DISEASED MIDDLE EAR

OTITIS MEDIA AND MIDDLE EAR/INNER EAR INTERACTION

Including considerations of chronic silent otitis media

Hamid R. Djalilian[1] and Michael M. Paparella[1,2]

[1]Department of Otolaryngology, University of Minnesota; [2]Minnesota Ear, Head and Neck Clinic, Minneapolis, MN, USA

Background

Excluding viral upper respiratory infections, otitis media is the most common disease of childhood[1]. More than 15 million episodes of acute otitis media are treated annually in the USA[2]. In a study of children between birth and seven years old in Boston, more than 90% had had at least one episode of acute otitis media and 75% had experienced at least three episodes[3]. The cost of medical and surgical treatment of otitis media in children less than five years of age has been estimated to be approximately $5 billion dollars[4].

The etiology of otitis media appears to be multifactorial inheritance, *e.g.*, genetic factors that predispose to eustachian tubal dysfunction. There are several theories regarding the initiation of serous otitis media (SOM) and mucoid otitis media (MOM). In addition to eustachian tube obstruction and the *ex-vacuo* theory of Politzer[5], inflammation of the middle ear and eustachian tube epithelium has been implicated as a precipitating factor in the development of middle ear effusion. Another theory regarding the pathogenesis of middle ear effusion suggests that lymphatic or venous stasis in the eustachian tube and nasopharynx plays the most significant role. Other factors include, infection, and anatomical, patient, and environmental factors[6]. Infection includes both viral and bacterial types; while anatomical and pathophysiological factors pertain to eustachian tube dysfunction. Host factors include young age, impaired immunological status, presence of allergy, family history, male sex, and race. Of these factors, eustachian tube dysfunction may be one of the more important[6]. We have also found anatomical obstructive sites in the middle ear cleft to play a role in the etiology and pathogenesis of otitis media.

Address for correspondence: Michael M. Paparella, MD, Minnesota Ear, Head and Neck Clinic, Minneapolis, MN 55454-1449, USA

The Function and Mechanics of Normal, Diseased and Reconstructed Middle Ears, pp. 101–112
edited by J.J. Rosowski and S.N. Merchant
© *2000 Kugler Publications, The Hague, The Netherlands*

Classification and continuum

Paparella[7] described a classification system for otitis media and observed that certain forms can be interrelated and can occur in a continuum (Fig. 1). Serous otitis media (SOM), both acute and chronic, and mucoid otitis media (MOM), usually chronic, are clinically considered to be nonsuppurative middle ear inflammatory problems. SOM has somewhat more of a transudative effusion, while MOM is the result of active secretion by secretary cells, goblet cells, and subepithelial glands and therefore mucoid effusion. Purulent otitis media (POM) involves suppuration of the middle ear cleft with erythema and bulging of the tympanic membrane. Chronic otitis media (COM) refers to an inflammatory process within the middle ear cleft associated with irreversible tissue pathology. It may be active, with ongoing suppuration, or inactive, demonstrating sequelae of a previous infection[8]. Otitis media with effusion or SOM, along a continuum, can lead to intractable pathological conditions or to COM. These findings may be undetected or undetectable. These slowly evolving pathological changes can ensue behind an intact tympanic membrane[9]. In 1980, we proposed the existence of 'silent otitis media'. This is defined by histological evidence of some form of otitis media without any clinical abnormality in the tympanic membrane[10]. Many intractable changes in the middle ear, and thus in the inner ear, can occur behind an intact tympanic membrane, referred to as chronic silent otitis media. This is differentiated from COM and chronic mastoiditis which, as the literature defines, requires a tympanic membrane perforation and otorrhea.

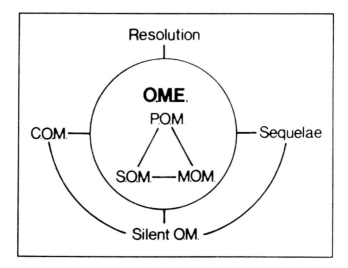

Fig. 1. Classification and continuum of otitis media.

Chronic silent otitis media

Chronic silent otitis media, which may or may not manifest clinically, is more prevalent than suspected. In one study of 333 temporal bones with pathological changes of COM, only 36 had clinical symptoms suggestive of otitis media. Only 19% had as associated tympanic membrane perforation[10]. Chronic silent otitis media may follow as a continuum from otitis media with effusion (OME). Since symptoms may be silent or subtle, they receive no treatment, which leads to perpetuation of the disease and the risk for complications. This is especially the case in young children who cannot communicate the subtle changes, such as hearing loss, vertigo, tinnitus, or clumsiness, that may occur in the setting of silent otitis media with inner ear involvement. Studies of 12 pediatric temporal bones with *Haemophilus influenza* meningitis that appeared clinically to arise from silent otitis media, have shown evidence of extensive otitis media pathology including, inflammatory cells in the region of the round window[11]. This points to the potentially serious role of middle ear/inner ear interaction in the presence of silent otitis media.

Middle ear/inner ear interaction

The classical labyrinthine extracranial and intracranial complications of otitis media have been well documented. However, the quiet development of sensorineural hearing loss (SNHL), which can develop as a concomitant or sequela of otitis media, has not been fully appreciated or understood. In certain patients, toxins from otitis media are thought to be transported across the round window membrane. This first leads to end organ dysfunction of the silent basal turn, and ultimately to involvement of lower frequencies readily recognized through audiological testing[12].

Vertigo is perhaps the most difficult symptom to identify in children. Descriptions of vertigo in children are generally reserved for older children or adolescents, whereas young children may be described as being only clumsy. In a study of pediatric vertigo, otitis media was the most common cause, identified in five of 34 patients with vertigo[13]. Objective testing of children with middle ear effusions has demonstrated spontaneous nystagmus in 36% and positional nystagmus in 23% of 97 children with otitis media with effusions[14]. Findings on electronystagmography returned to normal following insertion of tympanostomy tubes. In a related study, 85% of patients became symptom free after the insertion of ventilation tubes[15]. Pathologically, tympanogenic labyrinthitis may develop by spread from the middle ear via the round window, resulting in SNHL and vertigo[16]. Enzymatic erosion by cholesteatoma over the horizontal semicircular canal may also result in vestibular symptoms[17].

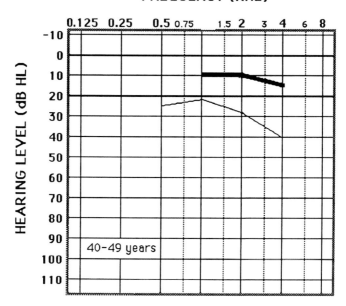

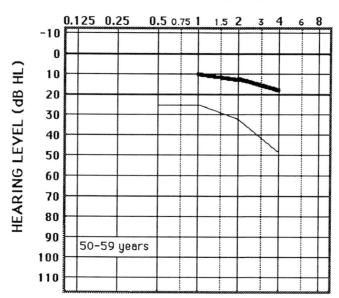

Fig. 2. Decade audiograms compared with normative data. The difference between the thin line and the bold line indicates aggregate sensorineural hearing losses due to otitis media for each decade. (Adapted from Paparella et al.[12] by courtesy of the Publisher.)

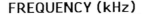

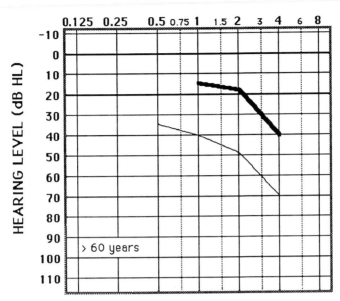

Fig. 2. Continued.

Audiology

Perhaps the most distressing finding in the setting of otitis media (silent or otherwise) is the presence of SNHL. This SNHL is usually secondary to changes in the basal turn of the cochlea, and thus in the highest frequencies[17]. There have been few references to this problem in the literature. We studied 279 patients with COM[18]. In these patients, mean bone conduction audiograms were compared regarding characteristics of otorrhea, duration of disease, and extent of pathology. In patients with unilateral disease, a cochlear deficit was frequently seen on comparison with the normal control ear. An increased incidence of SNHL in otitis media was seen in patients in all decades, in comparison with normative decade data taking into account presbycusic factors (Fig. 2), and typically high frequency cochlear dysfunctions were noted. Other studies including Moore and Best[19] and Arnold *et al.*[20] have also described SNHL as a component of otitis media. We also found that extended high frequency auditory function in POM, SOM, MOM, and COM is compromised[12] (Fig. 3).

In a study of chinchillas at our laboratory, inoculation of their middle ears with 7-F *Streptococcus pneumoniae* resulted in a 13-36 dB SNHL three to four days after otitis media was first detected. The SNHL persisted for several weeks after inoculation[21]. In a series of 76 patients with perilymphatic fistulas, 76% had an antecedent history of otitis media with effusion[22]. When the route of communication to the inner ear was grafted, only 10% had additional hearing

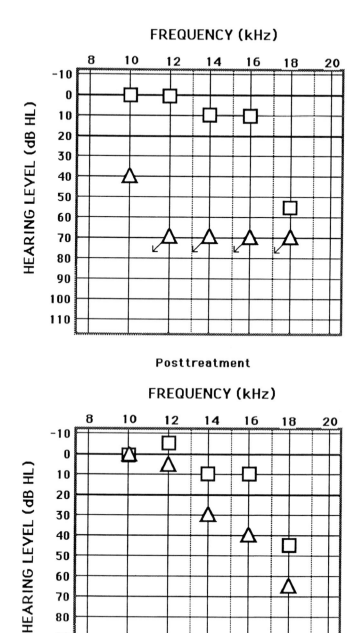

Fig. 3. Extended high frequency audiometry in a patient with purulent otitis media pre- and posttreatment, demonstrating temporary threshold shift in extended high frequencies in purulent otitis media. (Adapted from Paparella *et al.*[12] by courtesy of the Publisher.)

loss. Animal models have shown that the round window appears to be the route of entry. In another study from our laboratory, chinchillas underwent grafting of the round window, and were compared with a control group; all were inoculated with *S. pneumoniae*. In animals without round window grafts, bacteria were identified in all cochlear turns, and neural damage was evident[23]. In addition, because bacteria were not observed in the stapedial ligament, investigators believed that the only route of bacterial entry was via the round window[17].

Histopathology

Clinical and pathological features of suppurative labyrinthitis including tympanogenic, meningogenic, and hematogenic types, have been described[12]. The pathology of suppurative labyrinthitis can be divided into the acute suppurative stage, fibrous stage, and ossification stage[24]. In 1972, Paparella *et al.*[25] described the pathology and clinical features of patients with tympanogenic suppurative labyrinthitis and complete cochlear deafness. Of interest was the fact that these patients demonstrated minimal or no tympanic membrane findings and minimal or no vestibular symptoms or findings. We studied 75 human temporal bones with otitis media and subtle cochlear changes. Significant pathological findings were serofibrinous precipitates and inflammatory cells in the perilymph of the scala tympani of the basal turn (Fig. 4). Abnormal or missing hair cells localized to the lower basal turn were seen occasionally in certain cases[12]. The histopathological correlate for temporary threshold shift (TTS) appears to be serous (toxic) labyrinthitis predominantly in the basal turn, which can lead to permanent threshold shift (PTS) involving first the basal turn (high frequencies) and later all frequencies with permanent damage to cellular elements.

A recent study[26] used histopathology, immunostaining and immunohistochemistry to study cochlear changes in *S. pneumoniae* otitis media in mice. Immunohistochemistry showed the presence of fibrinogen in the cochlea, especially in the lower portion of the spiral ligament and in the spiral limbus. This finding was not found on histopathological studies of the tissues. There was decreased immunostaining for connexin 26 in the spiral ligament, accompanied by marked fibrinogen staining. Immunostaining for sodium-potassium-adenosine triphosphatase in the stria vascularis and in the type II fibrocytes of the spiral ligament showed that these two areas were not affected. The authors concluded that the presence of fibrinogen in the cochlea suggests disruption of the blood-labyrinth barrier caused by the middle ear inflammation. They supposed that changes in connexin 26 staining could suggest that the spiral ligament may be among the regions responsible for the cochlear malfunction[26].

Sometimes, a patient may have a flat SNHL in the presence of COM. We postulate endolymphatic hydrops related to otitis media in such cases[27]. In those cases, histological evidence of both otitis media and hydrops, including apical hydrops, were found. Studies indicate a strong correlation between histopathological findings in the middle and inner ear and audiometric and other inner ear problems.

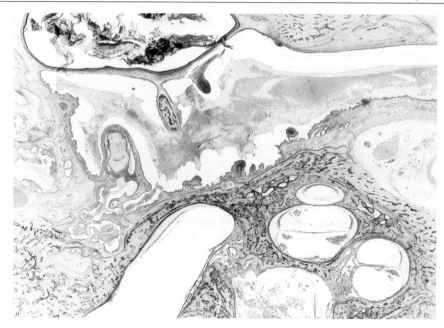

Fig. 4. Histopathology of tympanogenic labyrinthitis showing the serofibrinous precipitates and inflammatory cells in all turns of the cochlea.

Round window morphology and pathology

We performed a study on the pathogenesis of otitis media[28]. We found that the form that otitis media takes relied mostly on relative activity of the subepithelial space, which is contiguous with the round window membrane and the epithelium. A study of the pathology of COM found that granulation tissue was found more commonly than cholesteatoma; and sequelae of otitis media tended to occur more commonly secondary to granulation tissue than to cholesteatoma[8].

Round window and anatomical studies in otitis media have shown many changes. Gross changes consisted of dilation of the vessels within the fibrous layer, thickening of the membrane, infiltration of inflammatory cells, marked metaplasia, hyperplasia or cystic changes (Fig. 5). These changes were more prevalent in POM than in SOM[25]. A few studies have found that cytological changes in the round window were comparable to those in the mucoperiostium of the middle ear. A study by Schachern *et al.*[23] demonstrated that *Streptococcus pneumoniae* type 7F passed through an intact, normal round window membrane to enter the inner ear[29]. The absence of bacteria within the stapedial ligament or in the inner ears of the grafted round window membrane, proved that the round window membrane was the only portal of entry. The bacteria then entered the scala media through the Schuknecht's channels and along the myelinated nerve fibers[23]. The round window membrane has been found to be infiltrated with inflammatory cells in 9% of temporal bones with COM[8]. In 18% of cases, the round window membrane was convex and fixed by contrac-

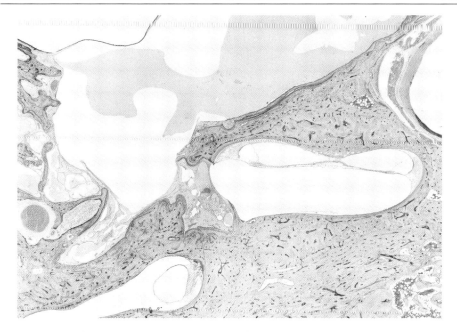

Fig. 5. Round window membrane changes in otitis media, demonstrating granulation tissue, inflammatory cells, and hyperplasia in the round window niche.

ture of mature fibrous granulation tissue. The most common change in the round window membrane seen in COM is its thickening to an average of twice its former thickness, primarily due to collagen in the subepithelial space. This may provide the round window membrane a better protective function in cases of COM.

Round window diffusion studies

The anatomy and location of the round window niche are ideally suited to a dependent accumulation of pus in cases of otitis media, especially POM. The membrane is approximately 0.065 mm thick, and the niche, which varies considerably, is approximately 1 mm deep and 2 mm in diameter. Many studies have been carried out in which various drugs and other agents have been placed in the middle ear, whereupon they readily passed through the round window and are recovered in the perilymph. Under normal conditions, low molecular-weight molecules, such as sodium, iodide ions and horseradish peroxidase (MW = 45,000 Da), can easily cross the round window membrane[30]. On the other hand, albumin (MW = 70,000 Da) does not traverse the round window membrane under normal conditions[30]. The permeability of the round window niche to tritiated albumin has been demonstrated in cat ears with experimentally induced acute POM, compared to normal membranes. Thus, the membrane of the round window may be more permeable in cases of POM[31]. A study by Ikeda[32] confirmed this finding, when increased round window membrane permeability was found in the setting of inflammation caused by staphylococcal or *Escherichia coli* exotoxins. Various studies have shown that various exotoxins, such as Staphylococcus[33] and Pseudomonas exotoxins[34], and endotoxins from *Haemophilus influenzae*[35] and *E. coli*[36], can cross the round window membrane.

Frank invasion of pus cells through the membrane of the round window membrane in cases of POM has been described. The subepithelial space shows a great deal of acute inflammatory response and edema in such cases. Diapedesis of occasional leukocytes through the membrane of the round window and collections of such leukocytes in the scala tympani have been seen in chronic suppurative otitis media. Serofibrinous precipitates are much more commonly seen in POM than in COM in case studies of human temporal bones. Granulomatous, fibrotic, and cystic changes in the membrane can be seen in human temporal bone studies of cases with COM[25]. As demonstrated by a study in our laboratory, the membrane of the round window thickens to an average of twice its former thickness in human cases of COM, primarily due to collagen in the subepithelial space. Such a change may provide the membrane of the round window a better protective function in certain cases of COM than in POM.

Conclusions

Silent otitis media, defined as intractable pathology beneath an intact tympanic membrane, is more prevalent than commonly believed. Interaction between the middle ear and inner ear occurs commonly in the presence of silent chronic otitis media, especially purulent acute or chronic otitis media, which can lead to irreversible damage in the inner ear and in particular the basal turn of the cochlea. The most common route of spread of middle ear enzymes and inflammatory elements into the inner ear occurs through the permeable round window membrane. The labyrinthine changes usually manifest themselves as hearing loss, especially in the high frequencies, tinnitus, and vertigo. The clinician must be aware of chronic silent otitis media and pathology associated with the symptoms it can cause in the middle ear as well as in the inner ear.

Acknowledgments

Supported by National Institutes of Deafness and Communicative Disorders Grants P50DC03093, RO1DC03433, and The International Hearing Foundation.

References

1. Jung TTK, Hanson JB: Classification of otitis media and surgical principles. Otolaryngol Clin N Am 32(3):369-383, 1999

2. Stool SE, Field MJ: The impact of otitis media. Pediatr Infect Dis J 8:11, 1989

3. Teele DW, Klein JO, Rosner B. Epidemiology of otitis media during the first seven years of life in children in greater Boston: a prospective, cohort study. J Infect Dis 160:83, 1989

4. Gates GA: Cost-effectiveness considerations in otitis media treatment. Otolaryngol Head Neck Surg 114:525, 1996

5. Politzer A: Textbook of the Disease of the Ear and Adjacent Organs. Philadelphia, PA: Lea's Son 1883

6. Bluestone CD: Anatomy, physiology, and pathophysiology of the eustachian tube. In: Lalwani AK and Grundfast KM (eds) Pediatric Otology and Neurotology, pp 11-28. Philadelphia, PA: Lippincott Raven 1998

7. Paparella MM: Middle ear effusions: definitions and terminology. Ann Otol Rhinol Laryngol 85 (Suppl 25):8-11, 1976

8. Meyerhoff WL, Paparella MM, Kim CS: Pathology of chronic otitis media. Ann Otol Rhinol Laryngol 87:749-760, 1978

9. Paparella MM, Goycoolea M, Bassiouni M, Koutroupas S: Silent otitis media: clinical applications. Laryngoscope 96(9):978-985, 1986

10. Paparella MM, Meyerhoff WL, Goycoolea MV: Silent otitis media. Laryngoscope 90:1089-1098, 1980

11. Djeric DR, Schachern PA, Paparella MM, Jaramillo M, Haruna S, Bassioni M: Otitis media (silent): a potential cause of childhood meningitis. Laryngoscope 104(11):1453-1460, 1994

12 Paparella MM: Insidious labyrinthine changes in otitis media. Acta Otolaryngol (Stockh) 92:513-520, 1981

13. Bower CM, Cotton RT: The spectrum of vertigo in children. Arch Otolaryngol Head Neck Surg 121:91-95, 1995

14. Golz A, Westerman T, Gilbert LM et al: Effect of middle ear effusion on the vestibular labyrinth. J Laryngol Otol 105:987-989, 1991

15. Grace ARH, Pfleidrer AG: Dysequilibrium and otitis media with effusion: what is the association? J Laryngol Otol 104:682-684, 1990

16. Paparella MM, Schachern PA, Yoon TH: Survey of interactions between middle ear and inner ear. Acta Otolaryngol (Stockh) Suppl 457:9-24, 1988

17. Vambutas A, Paparella MM: Tympanoplasty: prudent considerations of silent otitis media and interactions of middle ear and inner ear. Otolaryngol Clin N Am 32(3):505-512, 1999

18. Paparella MM, Brady DR, Hoel R: Sensori-neural hearing loss in chronic otitis media and mastoiditis. Trans Am Acad Ophthalmol Otolaryngol, 74:108-115, 1970

19. Moore DC, Best GF: A sensorineural component in chronic otitis media. Laryngoscope 90(8/1):1360-1366, 1980

20. Arnold WJ, Nitze R, Ilberg CH, Gazer M; Qualitative Untersuchungen der Verbindungswege der Subarachnoidalrames mit dem lymphatischen System des Kipfes und des Malscs. Acta Otolaryngol (Stockh) 74:411, 1972

21. Morizono T, Giebink GSL: Sensorineural hearing loss in experimental purulent otitis media due to Streptococcus pneumoniae. Arch Otolaryngol 111(12):794-798, 1985

22. Bluestone CS: Otitis media and congenital perilymphatic fistula as a cause of sensorineural hearing loss in children. Pediatr Infect Dis 7(Suppl):141-145, 1988

23. Schachern PA, Paparella MM, Hybertson R, Sano S, Duvall AJ 3rd: Bacterial tympanogenic labyrinthitis, meningitis, and sensorineural damage. Arch Otolaryngol Head Neck Surg 118(1):53-57, 1992

24. Paparella MM, Sugiura S: The pathology of suppurative labyrinthitis. Ann Otol Rhinol Laryngol 76(3):554-586, 1967

25. Paparella MM, Oda M, Hiraide F, Brady D: Pathology of sensorineural hearing loss in otitis media. Ann Otol Rhinol Laryngol 81:632-647, 1972

26. Ichimiya I, Suzuki M, Hirano T, Mogi G: The influence of pneumococcal otitis media on the cochlear lateral wall. Hearing Res 131(1/2):128-134, 1999

27. Paparella MM, Goycoolea MV, Meyerhoff WL, Shea D: Endolymphatic hydrops and otitis media. Laryngoscope 89(1):43-58, 1979
28. Paparella MM, Kim CS, Goycoolea MV, Giebink S: Pathogenesis of otitis media. Ann Otol Rhinol Laryngol 86(4/1):481-492, 1977
29. Bhaya MH, Morizono T, Schachem PA, Paparella MM: Tympanogenic labyrinthitis and meningitis. Am J Otolaryngol 13(6):386-389, 1992
30. Hellström S, Eriksson PO, Yoon YJ, Johansson U: Interactions between the middle ear and the inner ear: bacterial products. Ann NY Acad Sci 830:110-119, 1997
31. Goycoolea M, Paparella MM, Goldberg B: Permeability of the round window membrane in otitis media. Arch Otolaryngol 106:430-433, 1980
32. Ikeda K: Changes of the permeability of round window membrane in otitis media. Arch Otolaryngol 114:895, 1988
33. Goycoolea M, Paparella MM, Goldberg B, Schlievert PM, Carpenter A: Permeability of the middle ear to staphylococca pyrogenic exotoxin in otitis media. Int J Pediatr Otorhinolaryngol 1:301-308, 1980
34. Lundman L, Santi PA, Morizono T, Harada T, Juhn SK, Bagger-Sjoback D: Inner ear damage and passage through the round window membrane of pseudomonas aeruginosa exotoxin A in a chinchilla model. Ann Otol Rhinol Laryngol 101:437-444, 1992
35. Lundman L, Juhn SK, Bagger-Sjoback D, Svanborg C: Permeability of the normal round window membrane to Haemophilus influenzae type B endotoxin. Acto Otolaryngol (Stockh) 112:524-529, 1992
36. Spandow O, Anniko M, Hellstrom S: Inner ear disturbances following inoculation of endotoxin into the middle ear. Acta Otolaryngol (Stockh) 107:90-96, 1989

HISTOPATHOLOGY OF OTITIS MEDIA WITH AN INTACT TYMPANIC MEMBRANE

Chiaki Suzuki and Iwao Ohtani

Department of Otolaryngology, Fukushima Medical University School of Medicine, Fukushima, Japan

Abstract

Otitis media frequently occurs behind a genuinely intact tympanic membrane, but cannot be routinely observed via otomicroscopy. Therefore, from 186 autopsy subjects, the authors examined 310 temporal bones with genuinely intact tympanic membranes in order to examine pathological conditions in the middle ear histopathologically. Ninety-eight temporal bones (31.6%) had middle ear pathology, with no significant difference being found in the incidence of inflammatory changes in each middle ear site. The phase of otitis media in all bones was subacute and/or chronic. Serous effusion was most frequently revealed. Mastoid air cells showed comparatively good pneumatization. Given these results, the authors suggest that it is important to account for the possibility of inflammation in the tympanic cavity, even if the tympanic membrane appears normal. Furthermore, clinicians should account for the possibility of otitis media in patients with a comparatively well-pneumatized mastoid.

Keywords: otitis media, intact tympanic membrane, human temporal bone

Introduction

Otitis media is one of the most common infectious diseases. Recurrence and/or the development of otitis media with effusion can occur even if the condition of the tympanic membrane has returned to normal. One of the reasons for inflammation existing in the tympanic cavity was thought to be that its presence cannot be observed through the tympanic membrane, and therefore it was not treated.

In 1980, Paparella *et al.*[1] introduced the concept of silent, insidious otitis media, a pathological condition behind an intact tympanic membrane. Furthermore, Jaisinghani *et al.*[2] stated that a normal tympanic membrane does not exclude the possibility of middle ear pathology, and Costa *et al.*[3] reported that considerable pathological changes were found to exist behind a non-perforated

Address for correspondence: Chiaki Suzuki, MD, Department of Otolaryngology, Fukushima Medical University School of Medicine, 1 Hikarigaoka Fukushima-shi, 960-1247, Japan

The Function and Mechanics of Normal, Diseased and Reconstructed Middle Ears, pp. 113–121
edited by J.J. Rosowski and S.N. Merchant
© 2000 Kugler Publications, The Hague, The Netherlands

tympanic membrane. However, the non-perforated tympanic membrane in his report showed pathological changes such as retraction and myringosclerosis. Today, otomicroscopy is routinely used to observe the tympanic membrane, and reveals pathological changes in the tympanic membrane in detail, including perforation, vessel dilatation, hemorrhage, myringosclerosis, and retraction. Therefore, we report here the histopathological findings of middle ear inflammation in the presence of a genuinely non-pathological tympanic membrane.

Material and methods

From the collection of 1200 human temporal bones at Fukushima Medical University, we selected 310 temporal bones from 186 autopsy subjects with genuinely intact tympanic membranes, in order to examine pathological conditions in the middle ear histopathologically. Temporal bones which showed not only perforation, but also any additional swelling, vessel dilatation, calcification or infiltration of inflammatory cells in the tympanic membrane, were excluded as pathological findings. Moreover, temporal bones from infants and patients with systemic diseases such as leukemia and lymphoma were excluded.

The temporal bones had been removed during autopsy at our university, fixed in Heidenhain-SuSa solution and/or 10% formaldehyde, decalcified in 5% trichloroacetic acid solution, dehydrated in graded solutions of alcohol, and embedded in celloidin. Each section was cut horizontally at a thickness of 25 µm. Every tenth section was stained with hematoxylin and eosin, and then examined under light microscopy.

Pathological findings within the middle ear included the presence of leukocytic infiltration, edematous swelling of the submucosa, vessel dilatation, hemorrhage, round cell infiltration, extensive fibrosis, proliferation of the mucous membrane, increased gland formation, granulation tissue, cholesterol granuloma, cholesteatoma, and tympanosclerosis in the middle ear. These findings were classified according to anatomical location: supratubal recess, scutum, Prussak's space, pars flaccida, epitympanum, mastoid antrum, mastoid cells, eustachian tube, oval window niche, facial recess, promontory, tympanic sinus, and round window niche. The definition and classification of otitis media was made according to Senturia et al.'s criteria[4]. The phase of otitis media was classified into three groups: acute, subacute, and chronic, that is to say, in the acute state there are extensive leukocytic infiltrations and edematous swelling of the submucosa, whereas in chronic inflammation there are more round cell infiltration, extensive fibrosis, proliferation of the mucous membrane, and increased gland formation. The subacute state was defined as the interval phase between the end of the acute phase and the beginning of the chronic process. Effusion was classified as serous, mucoid, purulent, and no effusion. Furthermore, the development of pneumatization in the mastoid air cells was classified into four groups: well, moderate, poor, and sclerotic.

Results

The photomicrographs in Figures 1a-c show typical subacute otitis media behind a normal intact tympanic membrane. However, the facial recess and/or epitympanum show infiltration of inflammatory cells with serous effusion. Figures 2a-c also show typical chronic otitis media behind an intact tympanic membrane. Granulation and inflammatory cells with mucous effusion are present in the tympanic sinus, round window niche and/or epitympanum.

Of the 310 temporal bones with genuinely intact tympanic membranes, 98 (31.6%) had middle ear pathology. The presence of inflammation at each site in the middle ear cleft ranged from 17.1-27.6% (Fig. 3). No significant difference in the incidence of inflammatory changes at each site, with the exception of the promontory, was revealed. The phase of otitis media in all bones was subacute and/or chronic, with no acute incidence.

Effusion incident rates in the tympanic cavity are shown in Figure 4. Serous effusion occurred most frequently, and was found in 70 (72.2%) temporal bones. Mucoid effusion was found in three (3.1%), purulent in three (3.1%) and no effusion in 21 (21.6%) temporal bones, respectively.

The development of pneumatization in mastoid air cells is shown in Figure 5. The incidence of well and/or moderately pneumatized temporal bones was 88 (90.7%) and of poor and/or sclerotic temporal bones 10% or less. Overall, mastoid cells had comparatively good pneumatization.

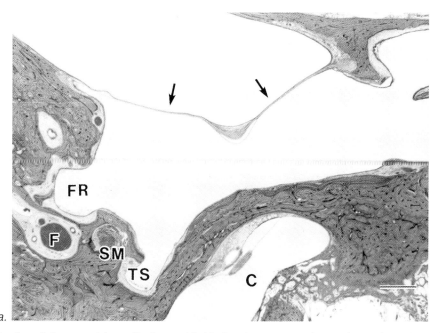

a.

Fig. 1. a. Subacute otitis media detected behind an intact tympanic membrane (arrow). Facial recess (FR) and/or tympanic sinus (TS) show infiltration of inflammatory cells. Bar: 1.0 mm; C: cochlea; F: facial nerve; SM: stapedial muscle.

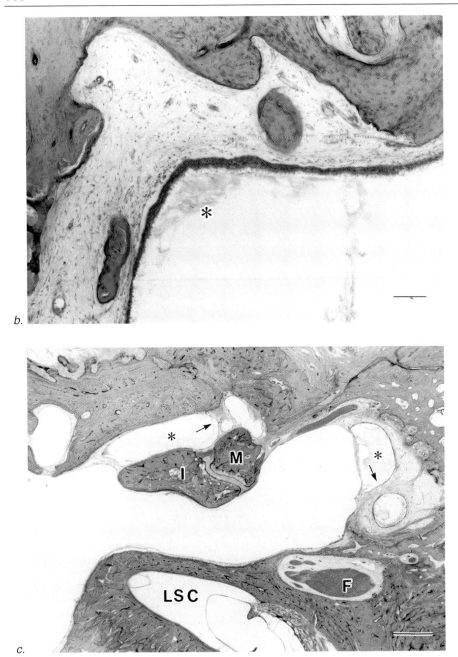

Fig. 1. b. High magnification of facial recess. Round cell infiltration was found in subepithelial tissue. Bar: 0.1 mm; effusion (*). *c.* Epitympanum also shows infiltration of inflammatory cells (arrow) and effusion (*). Bar: 1.0 mm; M: malleus; I: incus; F: facial nerve; LSC: lateral semi-circular canal.

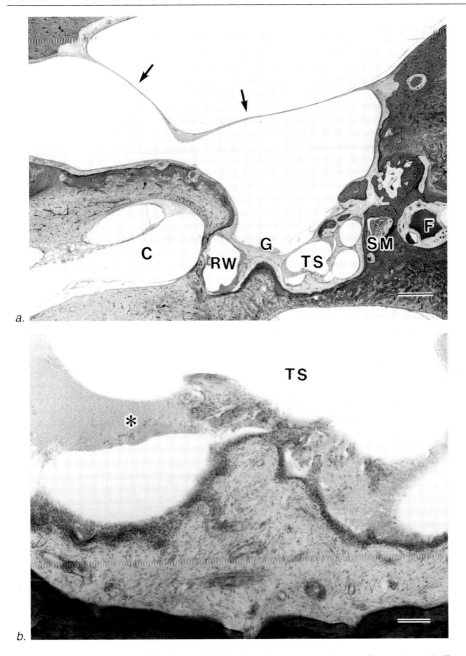

Fig. 2. a. Chronic otitis media detected behind an intact tympanic membrane (arrow). Tympanic sinus and/or the round window niche (RWN) show granulation (G) and inflammatory cells. Bar: 1.0 mm; C: cochlea; F: facial nerve; SM: stapedial muscle; TS: tympanic sinus. *b.* High magnification of tympanic sinus (TS) reveals granulation and round cells infiltration and/or serous effusion (*). Bar: 0.1 mm.

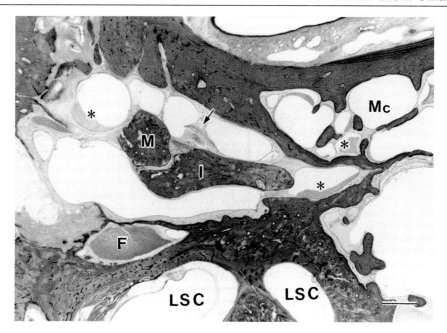

Fig. 2. c. Epitympanum also shows granulation (arrow) and/or infiltration of inflammatory cells and effusion. Bar: 1.0 mm; M: malleus; I: incus; F: facial nerve; LSC: lateral semicircular canal; Mc: mastoid cells; effusion (*).

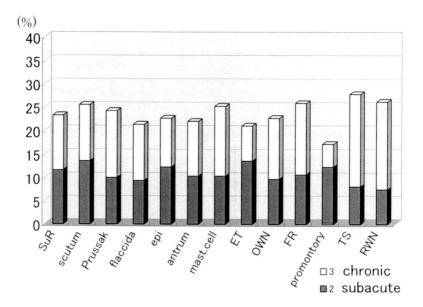

Fig. 3. Incidence of inflammation at each middle ear cleft site. SuR: supratubal recess; Prussak: Prussak's space; flaccida: pars flaccida; epi: epitympanum; mast. cell: mastoid cells; ET: Eustachian tube; OWN: oval window niche; FR: facial recess; TS: tympanic sinus; RWN: round window niche.

Effusion type of tympanic cavity

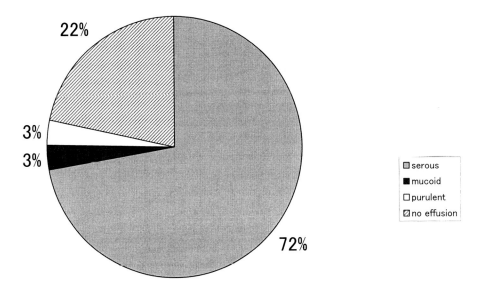

Fig. 4. Incidence of each type of effusion in the tympanic cavity.

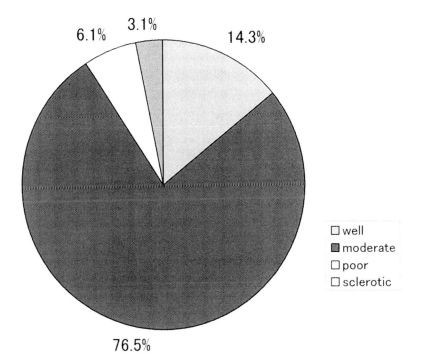

Fig. 5. Development of pneumatization in mastoid air cells.

Discussion

Paparella et al.[1] reported a low (19.5%) histopathological incidence of tympanic membrane perforation in temporal bones associated with other manifestations of chronic otitis media. Costa et al.[3] stated that chronic otitis media associated with an intact tympanic membrane was more common than that with a perforated membrane. This study's results (incident rate 31.6%), support the finding that a normal tympanic membrane can be associated with inflammation in the tympanic cavity. Therefore, it is important for clinicians to attend to the otitis media, even if the tympanic membrane appears normal.

Meyerhoff et al.[5] reported the localization of chronic otitis media in temporal bones. They indicated that the most common sites for chronic inflammation in the middle ear cleft were the epitympanic cavity, mastoid air cells, and round window niche. Furthermore, Takahara and Sando[6] reported that different degrees of inflammation in chronic otitis media existed in different portions of the middle ear cleft, and that inflammatory changes existing in the mesotympanum were more severe than in other parts of the middle ear. However, in cases with a genuinely intact tympanic membrane, there were neither special sites nor common sites of inflammation in the middle ear cleft. These findings indicate that inflammation behind a genuinely intact tympanic membrane may occur at any middle ear cleft sites.

In this study, it is conceivable that middle ear inflammation behind a normal tympanic membrane was mild, when we consider the phase of inflammation and/or effusion. This could account for patients with a normal tympanic membrane presenting with no clinical symptoms such as otalgia, otorrhea and/or fever. Thus, an inflammatory lesion behind an intact tympanic membrane might become a focus for persistent otitis media in patients with poor general health.

In this study, cases of silent otitis media had comparatively good pneumatization. However, it remains unclear whether this is a necessary requirement for silent otitis media, but, at the very least, our results show that we have to be cognizant of the inflammation in the tympanic cavity behind an intact tympanic membrane in well-pneumatized mastoid cases.

Conclusions

Given our results, we propose, firstly, that it is important to account for the possibility of inflammation in the tympanic cavity, even if the tympanic membrane appears normal and, secondly, that clinicians should be cognizant of the silent otitis media in patients with a comparatively well-pneumatized mastoid. Furthermore, we suggest that the inflammatory lesion behind an intact tympanic membrane might become a focus of persistent otitis media in patients with poor general health.

Acknowledgments

Appreciation is expressed to Mrs. Etsuko Sato and Mr. Akihiko Sato for their assistance in this study.

References

1. Paparella MM, Shea D, Meyerhoff WL, Goycoolea MV: Silent otitis media. Laryngoscope 90:1089-1098, 1980
2. Jaisinghani VJ, Paparella MM, Schachern PA, Le CT: Tympanic membrane/middle ear pathologic correlates in chronic otitis media. Laryngoscope 109:712-716, 1999
3. Costa SS, Paparella MM, Schachern PA, Yoon TH, Kimberley BP: Temporal bone histopathology in chronically infected ears with intact and perforated tympanic membranes. Laryngoscope 102:1229-1236, 1992
4. Senturia BH, Bluestone CD, Klein JO, Lim DJ, Paradise JL: Report of the AD HOC committee on definition and classification of otitis media and otitis media with effusion. Ann Otol Rhinol Laryngol 89(Suppl 68):3-4, 1980
5. Meyerhoff WL, Kim CS, Paparella MM: Pathology of chronic otitis media. Ann Otol Rhinol Laryngol 87:749-760, 1978
6. Takahara T, Sando I: The common site for otitis media in human temporal bones: a quantitative histopathological study. Auris Nasus Larynx 12(Suppl 1):173-176, 1985

DETECTING FIBRONECTIN AND LAMININ IN THE SERUM AND MIDDLE EAR EFFUSIONS WITH SECRETORY OTITIS MEDIA

Clinical significance

Qiuju Wang, Deliang Huang and Weiyan Young

Department of Otolaryngology, Chinese PLA General Hospital, Beijing, China

Abstract

The etiology and pathogenesis of middle ear effusions (MEE) and adhesions are not fully understood. Previous studies have shown that high levels of expression of cytokines, cell adhesion molecules, plasmins and fibronectin fragments in MEE are directly related to the recurrence of middle ear effusions and the formation of middle ear adhesions. Fibronectin (FN) and laminin (LN) are components of the extracellular matrix (ECM) and ligands of integrins. The authors determined the levels of FN and LN in MEE using enzyme-linked immunosorbentasssay (ELISA) and radioimmunoassay (RIA) methods. The aim of the study was to understand the roles of FN and LN in MEE.

Levels of FN and LN in MEE were significantly higher than those in serum of both patients and controls ($p<0.005$ and $p<0.02$, respectively). However, serum levels of FN and LN in patients with MEE were not significantly different from those in the controls ($p>0.05$). The mean values of FN and LN were different among different cytological types of MEE. The authors believe that the increased levels of FN and LN in MEE are the result of local changes. The significance of FN and LN, as well as their source and their role in the formation of MEE, effusions will be discussed.

Introduction

The etiology and pathogenesis of middle ear effusions (MEE) and adhesions are not fully understood, although multiple theories exist. Among these theories are eustachian tube dysfunction with failure to ventilate the middle ear cleft, allergic reactions, and local immune dysfunction associated with persistence of pathogenic bacteria or bacterial components. Recently, studies also showed that high levels of expression of cytokines, cell adhesion molecules,

Address for correspondence: Qiuju Wang, MD, Department of Otolaryngology, Chinese PLA General Hospital, 28 FuXing Road, Beijing, China 100853

The Function and Mechanics of Normal, Diseased and Reconstructed Middle Ears, pp. 123–128
edited by J.J. Rosowski and S.N. Merchant
© 2000 Kugler Publications, The Hague, The Netherlands

plasmins and fibronectin fragments in MEE are directly related to recurrent middle ear effusions and the formation of middle ear adhesions[1-5]. Our laboratory has focused on the role of components of the extracellular matrix (ECM), fibronectin (FN) and laminin (LN), in the early stages of secretory otitis media. FN and LN are both high-molecular-weight glycoproteins. FN can increase cellular adhesion activity, affect cell migration and differentiation, and take part in cytoskeleton reconstruction and cellular formation[6]. LN plays an important role in inflammation reaction, immune response, tissue fibrosis and tumor metastasis[7]. Previous studies on various diseases, including atherosclerosis, pulmonary fibrosis and glomerulosclerosis, have revealed the diverse biological activities of FN and LN in different situations[8]. However, little is known about the significance of FN and LN in MEE. Our hypothesis is that FN and LN are present in MEE, play a significant role in the pathological changes, and may determine the resolution or persistence of MEE. In this study, we used enzyme-linked immunosorbentassay (ELISA) and radioimmunoassay (RIA) systems to detect significant quantities of FN and LN in MEE from adults with secretory otitis media. Our results are presented and interpreted in the context of our clinical data, and in the context of the important roles of FN and LN in various diseases studied previously.

Material and methods

Samples of MEE were obtained from 19 ears that had undergone routine myringotomy and collection of exudate from the middle ear cavity. At the same time, 1.0 ml venous blood was also obtained from these patients. Their average age was 44.5 years. The mean course was 20.1 days. Sera were obtained from ten voluntary blood donors (control group). Their average age was 35.5 years.

MEE were classified into two types according to the gross appearance: serous (thin fluid, $n=13$); mucoid (thick fluid, $n=6$). Samples of MEE were centrifuged at 3000 rpm for ten minutes; supernatants were then collected for later assays. The residuals (subnatants) were stained with May-Giemsa and were examined during the cytological studies. For cytological investigation, MEE were classified into four types, according to the method of Palva[9]: neutrophil dominant (N); monocyte (M); neutrophil and lymphocyte mixed (NL); few-cell (FC). All supernatants were stored at $-80°C$ until used.

FN was assayed by ELISA. The first antibody was mouse-anti-human FN antibody (Zhong Shan Biology Company); the second was rabbit-anti-human FN antibody (Hua Mei Biology Company); the third was horseradish peroxidase labelled (HRP) goat-anti-rabbit IgG (Zhong Shan Biology Company). The results were read from an auto-enzyme-labelled-reader instrument (Model 2550 EIA Reader, Japan).

LN was assayed with commercially-available laminin radioimmunoassay kits (Second Military Medical University Navy Medicine Institute, Shanghai).

All experimental data were expressed as mean ± standard error. The differences between groups were compared using *t* tests.

Results

Diagnosis by gross examination of 19 samples of MEE showed 13 ears with serous type (68.4%) and six ears with mucoid type (31.6%). Cytological examinations performed on 19 samples revealed the following: N type in eight ears (42.1%); NL type seven ears (36.8%); FC type four ears (21.1%); no samples showed M type.

Levels of FN and LN in MEE and serum

Levels of FN
With ELISA assay, significant levels of FN (absorbency) were detected in MEE. The mean and standard error levels of FN (absorbency) in MME, in patients' and controls' sera, respectively, were as follows: 0.786 ± 0.123, 0.507 ± 0.033, 0.502 ± 0.026 (Fig. 1). Absorbency of FN in MEE was significantly higher than those in sera collected from the patients and from normal healthy controls ($p<0.005$). The levels of FN in patients' sera were higher than those in controls, but there was no significant difference ($p>0.5$).

Levels of LN
Using RIA kits, significant levels of LN (ng/ml) were also detected in MEE. Mean and standard error levels of LN in MEE, patients' sera and controls' sera were, respectively: 116.88 ± 13.02, 100.09 ± 5.85 and 97.33 ± 9.56 ng/ml (Fig. 2). The mean levels of LN in MEE were significantly different from those

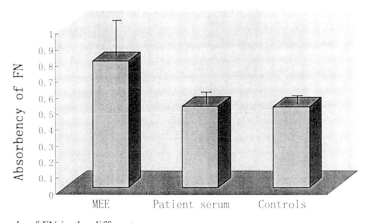

Fig. 1. Levels of FN in the different groups.

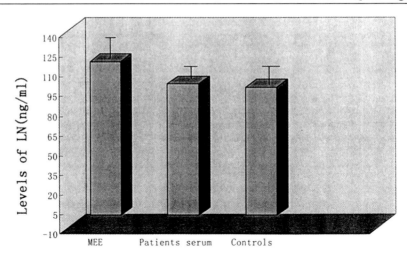

Fig. 2. Levels of LN in the different groups.

in sera collected from patients and normal healthy controls ($p<0.02$ and $p<0.05$, respectively). Although the mean levels of LN in patients' sera was higher than those in controls, there was no significant difference ($p>0.5$).

Levels of FN and LN in different types of MEE
Table 1 lists the mean and standard errors of FN and LN in different types of MEE. Levels of FN and LN were not found to be correlated with type of effusion (serous or mucoid) ($p>0.2$).

Levels of FN and LN in MEE of different cytological types
The mean levels of FN were highest in the NL type (Table 2). The mean levels

Table 1.

MEE type	Absorbency value of FN (M±SE)	Level of LN (ng/ml) (M±SE)
Serous type	0.819±0.194	113.48±11.98
Mucoid type	0.726±0.049	126.23±59.66

Table 2.

Cytological type	Cases	Absorbency value of FN (M±SE)	Level of LN (ng/ml) (M±SE)
N type	8	0.717±0.092	123.93±60.01
NL type	7	0.879±0.124	106.16±21.54
FC type	4	0.806±0.356	119.35±22.24

of LN were highest in the N type. However, the differences in FN and LN between the various types were not significant (*p*>0.2).

Discussion

The main new finding in this study was the successful detection of FN and LN, suggesting that an active response produced by inflammatory cells was going on in the middle ear cleft. The results also suggest that FN and LN take part in the response activity in the early stages of MEE. The levels of FN and LN in MEE were much higher than those in sera from patients and controls. This result may imply that the increase of FN and LN in MEE was a result of local changes. Salonen *et al.*[5] found that, in the early stages of MEE, the basement membrane of the mucosa is disrupted very early in a middle ear inflammatory reaction, as extravasated polymorphonuclear cells cross the basement membrane during infiltration of the middle ear cavity. The basement membranes underlying the epithelial cells include several components, such as fibronectin and heparan sulfate proteoglycan, involved in the maintenance of tissue integrity. Therefore, the source of FN in MEE may come from the destruction of basement membranes that induce FN degradation to the middle ear cavity. On the other hand, the source of FN may be the result of the proliferated active fibroblasts secreting FN in the cavity. LN has previously been shown to be present in high levels in inflammation reactions, immune responses, and tissue fibrosis processes[7]. Therefore, the detection of high levels of FN and LN in MEE suggests an ongoing inflammatory state that has the potential for mucosal changes, bone erosion, and hearing loss.

In our study, we failed to find a correlation between levels of FN and LN and type of effusion (serous or mucoid). Neither could we correlate FN/LN levels to the cytological type of effusion. Clearly, the study of glycoproteins in human ear pathology is difficult, with many variables being uncontrollable. Thus, we hope to develop and validate an animal model to simulate the middle ear cleft of a human, and to study the components ECM FN and LN, as they relate to the development and persistence of MEE.

Taken together, our data suggest that FN and LN may play a role in the pathogenic process of MEE, especially in the early stages.

References

1. Bikhazi PBS, Ryan AF: Expression of Immunoregulatory cytokines during acute and chronic middle ear immune response. Laryngoscope 105:629-634, 1995
2. Johnson MD et al: Murine model of otitis media with effusion: immunohistochemical demonstration of IL-1α antigen expression. Laryngoscope 104:1143-1149, 1994
3. Himi T et al: Quantitative analysis of soluble cell adhesion molecules in otitis media with effusion. Acta Otolaryngol (Stockh) 114:285-288, 1994

4. Johnson MD, Fitzgerald TE, Leonard G: Cytokines in experimental otitis media with effusion. Laryngoscope 104:191-196, 1994
5. Salonen EM et al: Plasmin and fibronectin degradation in chronic secretory otitis media. Arch Otolaryngol Head Neck Surg 115:48-53, 1989
6. Kosmehl H, Berndt A, Katenkamp D: Molecular variants of fibronectin and laminin: structure, physiological occurrence and histopathological aspects. Virchows Arch 429(6):311-322, 1996
7. Von der Mark K: Laminin and its receptor. Biochim Biophys Acta 17/823(2):147-160, 1985
8. Barnes JL, Torres ES, Mitchell RJ et al: Expression of alternatively spliced fibronectin variants during remodeling in proliferative glomerulonephritis. Am J Pathol 147(5):1361-1371, 1995
9. Palva T: Lymphocyte in middle ear effusions. Ann Otol Rhinol Laryngol 89(Suppl 68):143-146, 1980

CLICK-EVOKED OTOACOUSTIC EMISSION STIMULUS WAVEFORM AS AN INDICATOR OF MIDDLE EAR PATHOLOGY IN NEONATES

P.J.A. de Jager[1,2], P. Brienesse[1*], P. van Dijk[1] and L.J.C. Anteunis[1]

[1]Department of Otorhinolaryngology, Head and Neck Surgery, University Hospital Maastricht, Maastricht; [2]Hoensbroeck Audiological Centre, Hoensbroek, The Netherlands

Abstract

In a retrospective study of 57 neonates (114 ears), whose ears exhibited click-evoked otoacoustic emissions (CEOAEs) in at least one of two trials, the shape of the click response in the individual trials was found to be related to the presence or absence of emissions. Since all ears had passed the screening at least once and there were no other indications for sensorineural hearing loss, the authors assumed that the absence of an emission was due to either middle ear pathology or outer ear obstruction. The stimulus waveform was described by a damped sinusoid, with a natural frequency f_n and a damping coefficient δ. The natural frequency and the damping coefficient correlated with the presence or absence of CEOAE. It proved to be convenient to describe the stimulus waveform with the ratio of the natural frequency and the damping coefficient f_n/δ. A value smaller than 14 kHz indicated middle ear pathology. Sensitivity was 78%, specificity 94%, the positive predictive value was 54% and the negative predictive value 98%.

Keywords: click-evoked otoacoustic emissions, neonate, middle ear, acoustic impedance, otitis media

Introduction

During click-evoked emission (CEOAE) testing, the sound pressure measured in the ear canal results from a combination of the short-latency interaction of the earphone stimulus with the passive properties of the middle and inner ear, as well as the longer-latency emitted sound produced by active processes within

*Present affiliation: The Dutch Foundation for the Deaf and Hearing Impaired Child, Amsterdam, The Netherlands

Address for correspondence: P.J.A. de Jager, MSc, Department of Otorhinolaryngology & Head and Neck Surgery, Division of Audiology, University Hospital Maastricht, P. Debeyelaan 25, P.O. Box 5800, 6202 AZ Maastricht, The Netherlands

The Function and Mechanics of Normal, Diseased and Reconstructed Middle Ears, pp. 129–133
edited by J.J. Rosowski and S.N. Merchant
© 2000 Kugler Publications, The Hague, The Netherlands

the inner ear. A reasonable approximation is that the shape of the first few msec of the click 'stimulus' is determined by the mechanical properties of the middle ear and the earphone output. Kok et al.[1] noted that, for CEOAEs, a higher than usual stimulus level indicates a higher reflectance of the middle ear, and that fluid in the middle ear is a plausible cause of this higher reflectance. Therefore, we expect the stimulus waveform parameters to be correlated with the presence of CEOAEs.

This study aimed to correlate the presence of otoacoustic emissions in term neonates to the stimulus waveform.

Subjects and methods

CEOAEs were recorded in the ears of 57 neonates (114 ears) in two trials. During the first trial, the neonates were aged 6.0 ($\pm$2.2) days, during the second trial they were 35.6 ($\pm$4.4) days. All neonates were healthy term babies and not at risk for sensorineural hearing loss. All ears showed an emission at least once. Therefore, the absence of CEOAEs was assumed to be indicative of middle ear pathology. All measurements were performed with the ILO88 Otoacoustic Emission Analyser (Otodynamics, London, UK).

An emission was considered 'present' when the signal-to-noise ratio was 3 dB or more. In the cases where emissions were absent, only those observations with a noise estimate of less than 10 dB SPL were included. Others were classified as 'failed attempts' due to the high noise floor.

The stimulus waveform p(t) was described in the time domain by a damped oscillation, and characterized by a natural frequency f_n and a damping coefficient δ[2,3]:

$$p(t) = \exp(-2\pi f_n \delta t)\sin(2\pi f_n \sqrt{(1-\delta^2)}t)$$

The ratio $S = f_n/\delta$ proved to be suitable for describing the stimulus waveform with one single figure. The parameters f_n, δ and S related to the measurements with emissions 'present' were compared to those related to the measurements with emissions 'absent'.

Results

The results were as presented in Table 1. In the first trial, we found significant differences in the damping δ and ratio S between the emission present and emission absent groups. In the second trial, significant differences were found in all three parameters. When the right and left ears were analyzed separately, the significance remained the same for the right ear. For the left ear, no significant differences were found during the first trial, while all differences were significant during

Table 1. Stimulus waveform parameters

		n		δ	f_n (kHz)	S (kHz)
First trial	emission present	102	(90%)	0.18±0.08*	4.0±0.6	26.0±8.5*
	emission absent	7	(6%)	0.28±0.07*	3.8±0.3	14.9±6.0*
	failed attempt	5	(4%)	–	–	–
Second trial	emission present	88	(77%)	0.15±0.06*	4.1±0.3*	32.0±17.5*
	emission absent	11	(10%)	0.33±0.11*	3.1±0.5*	10.5±4.3*
	failed attempt	15	(13%)	–	–	–

*Significant differences between means with and without emissions (significant if $p<0.05$, independent samples t-test); n: number of ears

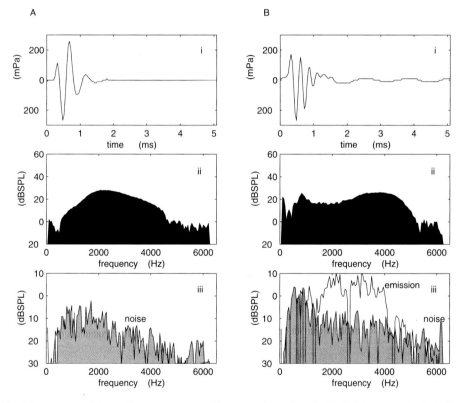

Fig. 1. Responses of the auditory system to a click, as registered by the ILO88 Otoacoustic Emission Analyser (OtoDynamics, London, UK). Both cases A and B represent the same ear (left). A was recorded during the first trial, B during the second trial. In case A, CEOAEs were absent in the ear, as can be seen in the emission spectrum A.iii, where the grey spectral area is a measure of the noise floor. In case B, emissions were present. Here, B.iii represents the corresponding emission spectrum. A.i and B.i show the time domain registrations of the click response immediately after offering the click. A.ii and B.ii show the spectra of these click responses. It can be seen that, in case A, the click response has a lower resonance frequency than in case B. Corresponding values for the damping δ, resonance frequency f_n, and ratio S for case A, were 0.33, 2482, and 7613 Hz, respectively. For case B, these values were 0.13, 3756, and 28892 Hz, respectively. This is in agreement with the general findings.

the second trial. If we assume that the absence of a CEOAE is indicative of a conductive hearing loss, a ratio S of less than 14 kHz describes 78% of the ears with no emissions (a sensitivity score of 78%), with a specificity of 94%, a positive predictive value of 54%, and a negative predictive value of 98%. Two examples of recorded stimulus waveforms and the corresponding CEOAEs are given in Figure 1.

Discussion

Middle ear pathology can block CEOAEs[4-7]. As a result, while screening neonates for hearing impairments using CEOAEs, the absence of CEOAEs may reflect both a conductive and a sensorineural hearing loss. Consequently, it is not possible to determine the nature of the hearing loss on the grounds of absent CEOAEs. This is unfortunate because a conductive loss requires a different treatment from a sensorineural loss.

The use of the standard test to detect middle ear pathology – single frequency tympanometry – is controversial in neonates. The proposed technique uses a broadband stimulus (click). It might also be possible to detect changes in the impedance of the middle ear or the ear canal with reflectance techniques[8,9] or with multifrequency impedance measurements[10]. However, the advantage of our technique is that substantial impedance changes and the presence of CEOAEs can both be detected in a single measurement.

Our subjects were not at risk for cochlear damage. We therefore assumed that middle ear pathology or outer ear obstruction was responsible for failing the CEOAE test. Our results showed that the stimulus waveform parameters correlate with the presence of CEOAEs. Therefore, the waveform can be indicative of middle ear pathology in neonates.

Acknowledgment

Neonate data were provided by the Dutch Foundation for the Deaf and Hearing Impaired Child, Amsterdam, The Netherlands.

References

1. Kok MR et al: Click-evoked oto-acoustic emissions in 1036 ears of healthy newborns. Audiology 32:213-224, 1993
2. Jerger J: Handbook of Clinical Impedance Audiometry, pp 10-16. American Electromedics Corporation, Acton, USA 1975
3. Oppenheim AV, Willsky AS, Young IT: Signals and Systems, 1st edn, pp 243-250. London: Prentice-Hall Int 1983
4. Amedee RG: The effects of chronic otitis media with effusion on the measurement of transiently evoked otoacoustic emissions. Laryngoscope 105:589-595, 1995
5. Engdahl B, Arnesen AR, Mair IWS: Otoacoustic emissions in the first year of life. Scand Audiol 23:195-200, 1994

6. Sutton GJ, Gleadle P, Rowe SJ; Tympanometry and otoacoustic emissions in a cohort of special care neonates. Br J Audiol 30:9-17, 1996

7. Chang KW et al: External and middle ear status related to evoked otoacoustic emission in neonates. Arch Otolaryngol Head Neck Surg 119:276-282, 1993

8. Keefe DH et al: Ear-canal impedance and reflection coefficient in human infants and adults. J Acoust Soc Am 94:2617-2638, 1993

9. Bollag U, Bollag-Albrecht E, Braun-Fahrlander C: The use of acoustic reflectometry in the study of middle ear effusion in children suffering from acute otitis media, upper respiratory tract infection and in healthy children. Eur J Pediatr 155:1027-1030, 1996

10. Holte L, Margolis RH, Cavanaugh RM: Developmental changes in multifrequency tympanograms. Audiology 30:1-24, 1991

MIDDLE-EAR MECHANICS IN THE DISEASED EAR

MECHANISMS OF SOUND CONDUCTION IN NORMAL AND DISEASED EARS

John J. Rosowski

Eaton-Peabody Laboratory and Department of Otolaryngology, Massachusetts Eye and Ear Infirmary, Boston; Department of Otology and Laryngology, Harvard Medical School, Boston; Speech and Hearing Sciences Program, Harvard – MIT, Division of Health Sciences and Technology, Cambridge, MA, USA

Abstract

This paper reviews the four basic processes of sound conduction from the environment to the inner ear: *1.* sound collection by the head, body and external ear; *2.* sound transformation by the tympanic membrane (TM) and ossicles of the middle ear; *3.* direct-acoustic stimulation of the inner ear by sound in the middle ear cavity; and *4.* stimulation of the inner ear by sound that is conducted by the whole body. These four processes are combined into three sound-conduction routes, where one route results from the combination of the external ear and TM and ossicular processes, the second route results from the combination of the external ear and the direct-acoustic processes, and the third route is the whole-body process that also depends on the normal operation of the external and middle ear structures. The contribution of the three routes to normal hearing is discussed, as well as how these routes are differentially affected by pathologies. It is concluded that, in the normal ear, sound conduction via the external ear and TM-ossicular system dominates sound conduction via the other routes. However, in cases of severe TM and ossicular pathology, the acoustic and whole-body routes can dominate sound conduction and thereby limit the magnitude of conductive hearing losses to generally less than 60 dB HL.

Keywords: external ear, middle ear, conductive hearing loss

Sound conduction to the inner ear in normal cars

The structures involved in the conduction of sound from the environment into the auditory inner ear include the structures of the external and middle ear, as

Address for correspondence: John J. Rosowski, PhD, Eaton-Peabody Laboratory, Massachusetts Eye and Ear Infirmary, 243 Charles Street, Boston, MA 02114, USA. *email:* jjr@epl.meei.harvard.edu

The Function and Mechanics of Normal, Diseased and Reconstructed Middle Ears, pp. 137–145
edited by J.J. Rosowski and S.N. Merchant
© *2000 Kugler Publications, The Hague, The Netherlands*

well as the structures of the head and body. These structures can be combined into four different sound conducting processes.

Sound collection by the head, body and external ear

The first process important to the conduction of sound to the cochlea is sound collection from the environment. In the case of air-conducted sound, the structures of the head and body act together with the peripheral parts of the external ear to diffract and scatter sound (Fig. 1A), leading to a sound pressure at the entrance to the external ear, P_{EX}, which can be greater or less than the sound pressure in the absence of the head and body, P_{FF}. Conduction through the ear canal results in a further transformation to the sound pressure at the tympanic membrane (TM), P_{TM}.

The relative magnitudes of P_{EX} and P_{FF} depend on the direction of the sound source relative to the head. Low-frequency sounds (f<300 Hz) are little affected by the directional processes, but mid- and high-frequency sounds directed towards the ear are amplified by 'back-scattering' from the head, body, pinna, and concha. Mid- and high-frequency sounds directed towards the opposite side of the head are reduced in magnitude by the head shadow (Fig. 1B). The transformation from P_{EX} to P_{TM} is independent of direction, but can be greatly affected by variations in the middle ear load on the external ear.

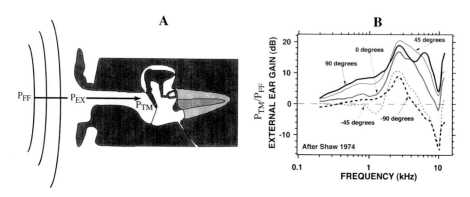

Fig. 1. Sound collection by the head, body and external ear. *A.* A uniform plane wave of free-field sound pressure, P_{FF}, interacts with the head, body and external ear to produce a directionally dependent sound pressure, P_{EX}, at the entrance to the ear canal. The resultant sound wave in the ear canal is transformed to the sound pressure at the TM, P_{TM}, in a manner that depends on the canal geometry and the acoustic impedance of the middle ear load on the ear canal. *B.* The transformation of sound by the head, body and external ear for sound sources at different azimuthal positions on the horizontal plane. The abscissa is sound frequency; the ordinate is the magnitude of the sound pressure gain in dB produced by the sound collection process. The parameter for the different curves is the azimuth of the sound source relative to the ear under study. A 90° azimuth is that of a sound source pointing at the ear of interest. A 0° azimuth describes a sound source on the sagittal midline pointing at the face. A –90° azimuth describes a sound source directed at the ear on the opposite side of the head. After Shaw[1].

Middle ear sound conduction: the tympanic membrane and the ossicles

The second sound-conduction process is the transformation of ear canal sound pressure, P_{TM}, to a sound pressure produced by the TM and ossicles on the oval window (the entrance to the inner ear). We call the output pressure the stapes pressure, P_S, since it results from the application of an ossicularly derived force over the area of the stapes footplate (Fig. 2A). Because of the middle ear transformer mechanism[2,3], the magnitude of the stapes pressures in humans is of the order of 25 dB greater than the magnitude of the pressure in the ear canal (Fig. 2B). The transformer mechanism is mostly explained by the larger area of the TM relative to the area of the stapes footplate. Though dependent on a simple area ratio, the middle ear pressure gain is limited by the mechanics of the middle ear structure in a frequency-dependent manner, such that the gain depends on sound frequency, with the largest gains near 1-2 kHz and smaller gains at higher and lower frequencies.

Middle ear sound conduction: direct acoustic stimulation of the cochlear windows

The inner ear is known to respond to the difference between the sound pressures at the oval and round windows[5,6]. The middle ear ossicular process makes use of this sensitivity to differential pressure by applying its output to the oval window only, but there is another mechanism through which the middle ear can stimulate the inner ear. As the TM is set in motion by sound pressure in the ear canal, it produces a change in the air volume in the middle ear, and a resultant sound pressure within the air spaces that directly stimulates the cochlear windows[7] (Fig. 3A). If the sound pressure produced by this mechanism were the same at the two cochlear windows ($P_{OW} = P_{RW}$), their difference would be zero and this mechanism would not

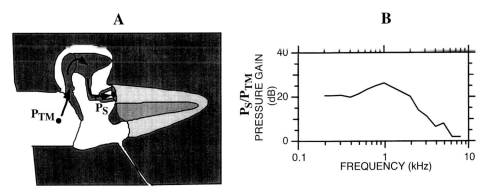

A **B**

P_{TM} P_S

P_S/P_{TM} PRESSURE GAIN (dB)

40

20

0

0.1 1 10
FREQUENCY (kHz)

Fig. 2. The ossicular mechanism of middle ear sound conduction. *A.* Sound pressure in the ear canal, P_{TM}, pushes on the TM, creating a force on the ossicles. The resultant force pushes on the stapes with its broad flat footplate and produces a sound pressure, P_S, in the oval window. *B.* The gain in sound pressure produced by the TM and ossicles as measured by Kurokawa and Goode[4].

A   **B**

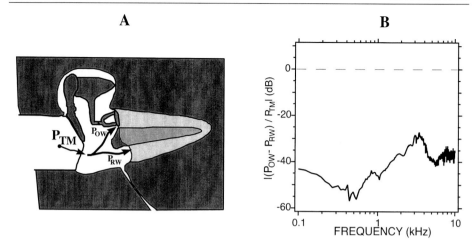

Fig. 3. Direct acoustic stimulation of the inner ear. *A.* The sound pressure in the ear canal produces motion of the TM and results in sound pressures in the middle ear space just opposite the oval, P_{OW}, and round windows, P_{RW}, into the cochlea. *B.* Because the two windows are only separated from each other by a small fraction of a wavelength, the window sound pressures P_{OW} and P_{RW} are nearly equal in magnitude and phase, and the magnitude of their difference is small (–25 to –55 dB) compared to the sound pressure in the ear canal.

stimulate the inner ear. However, even small differences in the magnitude or phase of the sound pressures (P_{OW} P_{RW}) outside the two windows can effectively stimulate the inner ear (Fig. 3B).

Sound conduction to the inner ear via the whole body

Environmental sound can also reach the inner ear by producing vibrations of the body, which are then conducted to the inner ear by bones and muscle. This is a more general process than audiological 'bone conduction' where a vibrator acts only on the mastoid portion of the skull. The processes involved in whole-body sound conduction are not easily separable from the external and middle ear mechanisms[8]. *1.* Sound-induced vibrations of the body's bones and muscles compress the walls of the external and middle ear, producing sound pressures which are then conducted to the inner ear via the normal middle ear mechanism. *2.* These vibrations can also produce relative motions of the head and ossicles that mimic normal ossicular transduction of sound. *3.* These vibrations produce compressions of the inner ear fluid compartments that result in the vibration of the inner ear lymphs.

Estimates of the magnitude of the sound conducted by the whole-body mechanism come from several sources, including measurements of the hearing loss introduced by pathologies such as external ear atresia that close off the external ear to sound, thereby reducing the influence of air-borne sound, and measurements of the hearing loss introduced by hearing protection devices (Fig. 4B). These measurements suggest that the whole-body route can provide a stimulus to the inner ear, which is 50-60 dB smaller than when the external ear is open to air-borne sound.

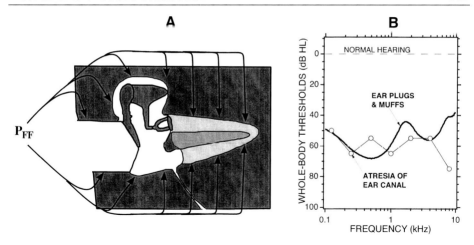

Fig. 4. Whole body sound conduction. *A.* Sound-induced vibrations of the whole body and head can generate sound pressures via compressions of the ear canal and middle ear walls, cause relative motions of the ossicles and inner ear, and also directly compress the inner ear. *B.* Measurements of the magnitude of these effects from measurements of the hearing loss when the ear canal is closed off by a pathological atresia plate[9] or by hearing protectors[10].

The three routes of sound conduction in the normal ear

The two middle ear processes described above both depend on sound gathering by the external ear, so that we combine the four processes into three routes of sound conduction: *1.* The *ossicular route* is defined by the combination of the external ear and ossicular processes. *2.* The *direct acoustic route* is defined by the combination of the external ear and the middle ear's direct acoustic process. *3.* The *whole-body route* is determined by the whole-body sound conduction process. Figure 5 shows an estimate of the relative magnitude of the sound conducted by these three routes in the normal ear. Clearly, normal sound conduction is dominated by the ossicular route, which conducts 30-60 dB more sound to the inner than the other routes. The comparison of the direct acoustic and whole-body routes suggests that they are of roughly similar magnitude in the normal ear.

A complication in the comparison of Figure 5 is that both of the estimates of the whole-body route are measured under conditions that maximize the *occlusion effect*. Occluding the ear canal has long been known to increase the sensation produced by bone-conduction vibrators, and we suspect that the measurements illustrated in Figures 4B and 5 actually overestimate the whole-body route contribution by about 10 dB at frequencies below 2 kHz[8].

Effects of pathology on the three routes of sound conduction

Each of the three sound-conduction routes can be affected by middle ear pathology. Any ossicular pathology will interfere with the ossicular route, while ossicular

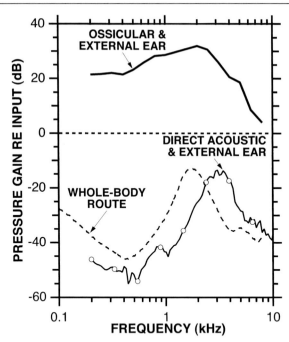

Fig. 5. Estimates of the magnitude of sound conduction via the three routes in the normal ear. The estimate of the *ossicular route* (plain solid line) is calculated from the middle ear gain measured by Kurakowa and Goode[4] and the external ear gain defined by Shaw[1] for a sound source positioned at 0° azimuth on the horizontal plane. The *direct acoustic route* conduction is estimated from the measurements of Voss[11] combined with the ear-canal gain of Shaw[1]. The *whole-body route* conduction is estimated from Zwislocki's[10] measurements of the hearing loss produced by ear protectors, where the dB difference between the *whole-body* and *ossicular* routes equals the hearing loss measured by Zwislocki.

interruptions may increase the acoustic route conduction[7], and ossicular fixations will reduce acoustic route conduction by interfering with the motion of the stapes. The effect of ossicular pathologies on the whole-body route is unclear, in that changes in the ossicular mobility will alter the 'ossicular inertial' component of whole-body conduction[8], and also affect the direct compressions of the inner ear capsule. The 'Carhart notch' observed in audiological bone conduction suggests that the final result of stapes fixation is to reduce conduction by the whole-body route. (A more clinically oriented discussion of the effects of selected pathologies is presented in Merchant *et al.*[12].)

Middle ear fluid will also have different effects: it will clearly reduce the sound conduction by the ossicular route, but will also serve to increase the sound pressure within the middle ear cavity, and could conceivably increase sound conduction by the direct-acoustic route. Fluid's effect on the whole-body route is unclear, but more likely than not, middle ear fluid will act to limit the motion of the stapes and round window and will decrease the contribution of the inner ear compression mechanism to whole-body sound conduction.

Perforations of the TM are one pathology whose effects on the different routes are better understood. Figure 6 illustrates the effects of perforations on the three processes involved in the ossicular and direct acoustic routes. Figure 6A contains model estimates of the effect of TM perforations on the external ear gain. The model is that of Rosowski[3], and the effect of the perforation is estimated by replacing the normal middle ear input impedance that terminates the external ear of the model, with the middle ear input impedance measured by Voss[11] in temporal bones with a 5-mm diameter perforation. The figure shows that the model of the normal ear has some similarities to the data, and also that perforating the TM should have serious effects on the frequency dependence of external ear gain, including introducing minima in the gain. Figures 6B and C illustrate measurements made by Voss[11] of the changes in ossicular sound transfer produced by TM perforations (quantified by measurements of stapes velocity) and on the direct acoustic stimulus (quantified by taking the difference of sound pressures measured at the oval and round window). TM perforations introduce large decreases in ossicularly-coupled sound at low frequencies, with smaller changes at higher frequencies. On the other hand, the 5-mm TM perforation leads to a 20-dB increase in middle ear sound pressure and the window pressure difference, $P_{OW} - P_{RW}$, at many frequencies. The effects of perforations on the whole-body route are not known; however, it seems unlikely that perforations will increase sound conduction through the whole-body route.

Figure 7 shows a comparison of the three sound conduction routes with a 5-mm diameter TM perforation. Conduction by the ossicular route still dominates at middle and high frequencies, but is decreased at low frequencies to the point where it is smaller than the sound conducted by the other two routes. The increased sound conducted by the direct acoustic route is now larger than ossicular route sound conduction at frequencies of less than 300 Hz and, therefore, the acoustic route should act to limit the low-frequency hearing loss produced by a TM perforation[11].

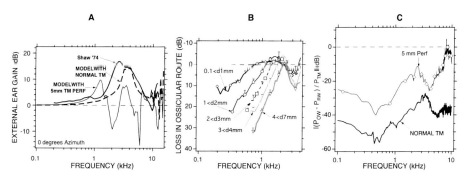

Fig. 6. Measurements and model estimates of the effect of TM perforations on external and middle ear function. *A.* Comparison of measurements of the external ear gain for a sound source of 0° azimuth (from Shaw[1]) with model estimates of the gain with a normal TM[3] and after replacing the TM impedance with that of a TM with a 5-mm perforation[11]. *B.* Measurements of the loss in middle ear sound transfer produced by TM perforations of different diameters[11]. *C.* Measurements of the window pressure difference relative to ear-canal sound pressure in temporal bones with normal TMs and with a 5-mm diameter perforation[11].

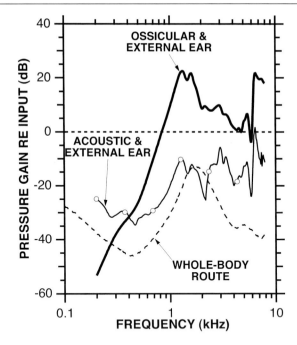

Fig. 7. Comparisons of sound conduction by the three routes after a TM perforation of 5 mm in diameter. The ossicular and direct acoustic routes have been adjusted by the data from Figure 6.

The sound conducted by the whole-body route is of the same magnitude as acoustic route conducted sound in the middle frequencies and smaller at lower and higher frequencies. (Again, we have assumed that the whole-body route is unaltered by the perforation, but since a TM perforation should interfere with conduction of the sound produced by compressions of the ear canal and middle ear walls, there is reason to suspect that whole-body sound conduction would be reduced somewhat after TM perforations and could really be lower than the direct acoustic sound conduction at all frequencies.) Peake *et al.*[7] have analyzed audiograms after total perforations of the TM and have argued that, in these cases, the direct acoustic route can explain residual hearing.

Conclusions

We argue that sound conduction to the inner ear can occur by way of three routes: *1.* The *ossicular route*, defined by the combination of external ear sound gathering function and the transduction of ear canal sound pressure into sound pressures acting on the stapes by the TM and ossicular chain. *2.* The *direct acoustic route*, defined by the combination of the external ear sound gathering function and the generation of a window-pressure difference ($P_{OW} - P_{RW}$) from sound in the ear canal. *3.* The *whole-body route*, sound that reaches the inner ear by way of vibrations of the muscle and bones of the head and body. We also argue that the ossicular route dominates sound conduction in the normal ear, but that pathologies can lead to dominance of the other sound conducting routes, such that those other routes can limit the hearing loss produced by pathologies. This limiting function has been best described in cases of TM perforation[11] and in cases of total ossicular disarticulation[7]. Better understanding of the interaction of these routes in pathological ears will depend on improvements in our knowledge of the effect of pathology on the three routes, especially the whole-body route.

References

1. Shaw EAG: The external ear. In: Keidel WD, Neff WD (eds) Handbook of Sensory Physiology. Vol V/1: Auditory System, pp 455-490. New York, NY: Springer-Verlag 1974
2. Wever EG, Lawrence M: Physiological Acoustics. Princeton, NJ: Princeton Univ Press 1954
3. Rosowski JJ: Models of external and middle ear function. In: Hawkins H, McMullen T, Popper A, Fay R (eds) The Springer Handbook of Auditory Research. Vol 6: Auditory Computation, pp 15-61. New York, NY: Springer-Verlag 1996
4. Kurokawa H, Goode RL: Sound pressure gain produced by the human middle ear. Am J Otol 113:349-355, 1995
5. Wever EG, Lawrence M: The acoustic pathway to the cochlea. J Acoust Soc Am 22:460-467, 1950
6. Voss SE, Rosowski JJ, Peake WT: Is the pressure difference between the oval and round windows the effective acoustic stimulus for the cochlea? J Acoust Soc Am 100(3):1602-1616, 1996
7. Peake WT, Rosowski JJ, Lynch TJ III: Middle ear transmission: acoustic vs. ossicular coupling in cat and human. Hearing Res 57:245-268, 1992
8. Tonndorf J: Bone conduction. In: Tobias JV (ed) Foundations of Auditory Theory, Vol 2, pp 197-237. New York, NY: Academic Press 1972
9. Gill NW: Congenital atresia of the ear: a review of the surgical findings in 83 cases. J Laryngol Otol 83:551-587, 1969
10. Zwislocki J: In search of the bone-conduction threshold in a free sound field. J Acoust Soc Am 29(7):795-804, 1957
11. Voss SE: Effects of tympanic-membrane perforations on middle ear sound transmission: measurements, mechanisms and models. PhD Thesis, Massachusetts Institute of Technology 1998
12. Merchant SN, Ravicz ME, Voss SE, Peake WT, Rosowski JJ: Middle ear mechanics in normal, diseased and reconstructed ears. J Laryngol Otol 112:715-731, 1998

ON THE FINE STRUCTURE OF MULTIFREQUENCY TYMPANOGRAMS

Evidence for multiple middle ear resonances

Thomas Hocke[1], Joachim Pethe[1], Albrecht Eiber[2], Ulrich Vorwerk[3] and Hellmut von Specht[1]

[1]*Abteilung für Experimentelle Audiology und Medizinische Physik Otto-von-Guericke-Universität Magdeburg, Magdeburg;* [2]*Institut B für Mechanik, Universität Stuttgart, Stuttgart;* [3]*St. Salvator Krankenhaus, HNO-Klinik, Halberstadt, Germany*

Abstract

This paper concerns the evaluation of resonances in multifrequency tympanograms. Multifrequency tympanograms (MFT) of 20 normal hearing subjects were recorded. The frequency range of the tympanometric measurements was extended to 6 kHz with a resolution of 15 Hz. In the pattern of the recorded multifrequency tympanograms, several resonances can be detected. This investigation evaluated all the resonances in the tympanometric fine structure, not just the so-called main ossicular resonance. It is shown that a reproducible fine structure can be found in the MFTs of normal hearing subjects. A procedure for the evaluation of this fine structure was derived from the authors' own measurements and experimental findings in the literature. The existence of this fine structure may explain the great inter-subject variability in middle ear resonance described in the literature.

Keywords: multifrequency tympanometry, middle ear, resonance, fine structure

Introduction

In conventional tympanometry, the admittance Y is measured as a function of the static ear canal pressure with the fixed frequency of 220 Hz[1]. This measurement gives insufficient information about the condition of the middle ear, in patients with confirmed middle ear pathology normal conventional tympanograms can be recorded[2]. More detailed information is available if the tympanometric

Address for correspondence: Thomas Hocke, MD, Abteilung für Experimentelle Audiology und Medizinische Physik, Otto-von-Guericke-Universität Magdeburg, Leipziger Strasse 44, 39120 Magdeburg, Germany. *email:* thomas.hocke@medizin.uni-magdeburg.de

The Function and Mechanics of Normal, Diseased and Reconstructed Middle Ears, pp. 147–155
edited by J.J. Rosowski and S.N. Merchant
© *2000 Kugler Publications, The Hague, The Netherlands*

measurements are performed with several probe frequencies[3-6], the so-called multifrequency tympanogram (MFT).

MFT measurements made over a broad frequency range with fine frequency resolution yield complex MFT patterns with an observable fine structure[7].

As well as the determination of the so-called main resonance frequency in MFT patterns[4], several curve parameters (tympanometric width, peak pressure and gradient) can be analyzed[8,9].

False assessment of the condition of the middle ear cannot be excluded if the main ossicles' resonance, which may be defined by different criteria[10-12], is evaluated. The present paper focuses on the description and classification of the resonance fine structure[7] in MFT patterns. An improved evaluation is performed utilizing an enhanced recording technique[13] and a comparison of our own experimental findings with results in the literature[12,14].

Methods

The MFTs of 20 normal hearing subjects (ten females and ten males with ages ranging from 20-42 years) were recorded. The subjects were examined otoscopically before measurement. MFTs of both ears were recorded with an experimental MFT system. In four subjects, recordings were limited to one side due to ear canal irritations. The MFT system was calibrated using hard-walled cavities with volumes ranging from 0.4-2.0 cm^3. Pressure p was varied manually between –300 and +220 daPa with a step size of $\Delta p \approx 20$ daPa between –100 and +100 daPa, and otherwise $\Delta p \approx 40$ daPa. Phase noise (equations 1 and 2), containing all stimulation frequencies simultaneously with randomized phases ϕ_k, was used as a stimulus

$$x(t_n) = \sum_{k=l}^{m} A_k(\omega_k) \cdot \sin(\omega_k t_n + \phi_k), \tag{1}$$

$$\omega_k = \frac{2\pi k}{N \cdot \Delta t} \quad \text{with} \quad k=l, l+1, ..., m-1, m. \tag{2}$$

With l=14 and m=393, the frequency resolution of the MFT recording was 15 Hz in the frequency range from 0.2-6.0 kHz. For averaging, the stimulus was presented cyclically (length of one stimulus cycle was 65 msec), requiring a recording time at a distinct static pressure of about two seconds. In practise, the recording time for the whole MFT varied from five to ten minutes. The stimulus level was kept below 30 dB HL. The coefficients $A_k(\omega_k)$ in equation (1) were used to equalize the frequency response of the loudspeaker.

Results and discussion

The MFT of a normal hearing subject is shown in Figure 1. In this MFT pattern, the maximum of the real part of the admittance, Re(Y) at 4.5 kHz with p from –300 to +220 daPa, is due to the first ear canal resonance. The frequency of the first ear canal resonance differs considerably in the individual measurements. The pattern of this MFT below 4 kHz is due to the dynamic behavior of the middle ear. The resonances of the middle ear apparatus appear like ridges or hills in a map of a landscape. Variations in the MFT parameter with frequency and static pressure distinguish different types of middle ear resonances by their dependence on pressure and frequency: some resonances have their maximum amplitude at the tympanometric peak pressure p^*, others have their maximum amplitude at pressure $p \neq p^*$. Resonances can also be distinguished with maxima at a certain pressure $p \neq p^*$, *e.g.*, in Figure 1 at p ≈ +80 daPa (with f ≈ 1.6 kHz) and resonances where the amplitude increases with greater $\Delta p = |p^* - p|$ up to the edges of the measured pressure-frequency plane, *e.g.*, in Figure 1 at p ≈ +220 daPa (with f ≈ 3.0 kHz).

In this paper, the evaluation of MFT patterns is focused on the resonances with maximum amplitude at a frequency between 3.0 and 4.0 kHz with p = –300 or +220 daPa, as well as on the fine structure below 1.5 kHz (resonances with their maximum amplitude at p^*).

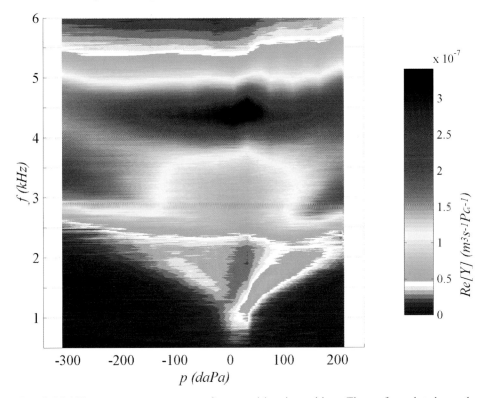

Fig. 1. Multifrequency tympanogram of a normal-hearing subject. The surface plot shows the real part of the admittance, Re(Y), as a function of frequency and ear canal pressure.

For an undamped simple spring-mass system, the resonance frequency is defined as the frequency with zero susceptance. Considering the middle ear apparatus to be a complex system of coupled oscillators and problems with compensating for the ear canal volume[10], this resonance definition is not applicable. A resonance involves an increased excursion of certain parts of the middle ear, and therefore leads to an increased conductance. Theoretically, these conductance maxima do not exactly match the resonance frequencies of an oscillating system, but are very near the resonance frequencies in terms of the frequency resolution used in our measurements. For this reason, we practicably define the resonance frequency as the frequency with the conductance that has a local maximum or a shoulder. A shoulder is an increased conductance with another resonance being present (*e.g.*, s2 at 850 Hz in Fig. 2). A local maximum or shoulder was defined only if it occurred in at least two adjacent measurements of Re(Y) at different static pressures (*see* also Fig. 2B).

Figure 2A shows Re(Y) of three subjects at their individual p*, and illustrates some of the problems in evaluating the MFT pattern. For subject s1, the maximum at 960 Hz dominates the pattern. This maximum has a frequency that would match the main ossicles' resonance described in the literature[11]. But in the case of subjects s2 and s3, evaluation becomes more complicated. In the Re(Y) curve of s2, several maxima occur at 640, 980, and 1100 Hz, and a shoulder occurs at 850 Hz. For s3, a very dominating maximum is found at 820 Hz and a local maximum at 630 Hz. Our working hypothesis at this stage is that each local maximum or shoulder is due

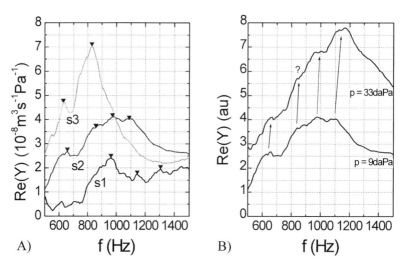

Fig. 2. (A) Real part of the admittance, Re(Y), as a function of frequency in three normal-hearing subjects with the pressure equal to the tympanometric peak pressure. Local maxima and shoulders are indicated by down triangle symbols. The tympanometric peak pressure p* is the pressure at which, in the classical 220 Hz tympanogram, the admittance is at its maximum. (B) Two adjacent Re(Y) curves for subject s2 in Figure 2A. The curves illustrate the determination of resonances, utilizing the similarity of adjacent Re(Y) curves in the MFT. The arrows indicate the shift of resonances due the static pressure change.

to a certain mode of vibration with a certain resonance frequency of the middle ear apparatus and furthermore that, in a measurement, different maxima due to different modes of vibration dominate the MFT pattern[14]. Figure 2B shows the Re(Y) of subject s1 at the tympanic peak pressure, and its adjacent curve. The maxima and shoulders marked in Figure 2A are shifted slightly towards higher frequencies, due to the varied static pressure. The shoulder (question mark) in the Re(Y) curve with p = 20 daPa at about 850 Hz is not absolutely certain, but is confirmed in the curve at p = 0 daPa and *vice versa*.

In Figure 3, the distribution of all local maxima from all subjects is shown. The evaluation procedure for an MFT pattern was derived by means of Figure 3. This distribution has several peaks which, in the frequency range below 1.2 kHz, coincide with some of the peaks found by Valvik *et al.*[12], indicated by star symbols in Figure 3. The coincidence is quite convincing for the three lower frequency peaks. The increased deviation of the 1100 Hz peaks between Valvik *et al.*'s[12] and our results may be due to the different methods. The meaning of Figure 3 is not only the coincidence in frequency, but also more that there are at least four peaks in both distributions, indicating a certain scheme of appearance. This coincidence supports our hypothesis that there are multiple modes of middle ear vibration and that different modes in different ears may be identified to be the ossicles' 'main resonances'. The individual situation, and probably the particular measurement conditions, may influence which of the resonances is the dominating one and thus considered to be the main resonance in previously published papers[10-12]. Gender, age, and postural effects[12,15-17] have been demonstrated to have no sufficient effect on the distribution pattern[12]. One useful interpretation of Figure 3 is, that if the maxima of both distributions coincide, in the corresponding frequency range, reproducible resonances should be expected between individuals. The coincidence provides a basis for defining classes of resonances in the MFT pattern (fine structure).

Evaluating the recorded MFTs and sorting out the maxima with reference to these classes yields distributions such as those presented in Figure 4. The classes were labelled with respect to the frequency range they occur in, *e.g.*, f^{1000} means that a resonance of this class is likely to be detected at around 1000 Hz. If a resonance was determined at the boundaries of the classes, the classification was made by considering the other resonances in the same MFT. Assuming that a resonance was determined at 720 Hz, it might belong to the 650 Hz class as well as to the 800 Hz class. But if another resonance was detected at 600 Hz in this MFT ('occupying' the place in the 650 Hz class), the 720 Hz resonance was assigned to the 800 Hz class. No more than one local maximum is classified to each resonance class per MFT. For five of the 110 classified by us, there were no other nearby resonances and the maximum/shoulder was assigned to the class of the closest frequency. Empty classes were also observed in the case of very flat MFT patterns in the frequency range from 500-1200 Hz.

The basic content of Figure 4 is that, in the frequency range from 500-1200 Hz, four different modes of vibration are detectable. Each of them may dominate the

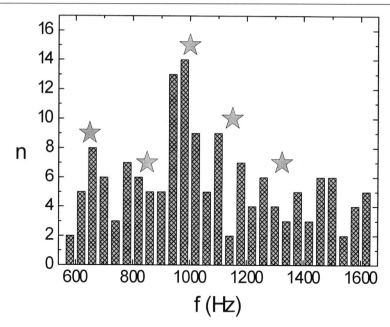

Fig. 3. Overall distribution of local maxima/shoulders in the MFT pattern. The star symbols indicate maxima of the distribution of the main ossicles' resonance (100 normal hearing subjects), as found by Valvik *et al.*[12].

MFT pattern. This interpretation of Figures 3 and 4 is also supported by other experimental findings and theoretical considerations[14].

Figure 5 shows a distribution for the two resonances that are reliably detectable in the higher frequency range. The maximum amplitude of these resonances can be found at the edges of the measured pressure-frequency plane, p = −300 daPa with f ≈ 3.5 kHz and p = +200 daPa with f ≈ 3.2 kHz. This characteristic makes these two resonances easy to detect in the MFT pattern. If the lowest ear canal resonance covers the frequency range of these resonances, they were evaluated as not detectable because an exact determination of the resonance frequency was not possible.

Table 1 summarizes some characteristics of the resonances described in this paper. There is a gap of ≈2 kHz between the lower four classes of resonances (f^{650}, f^{800}, f^{1000} and f^{1100}) and the two upper classes (f^{3200} and f^{3500}). This does not indicate that no resonances exist in this frequency range. But the authors are not presently in a position to determine reliable criteria in order to classify the fine structure in this gap. Either there was no coincidence between our results and the literature, or we could not derive a reliable scheme based on our results in normal hearing subjects. This should be the focus of future investigations in large groups of subjects.

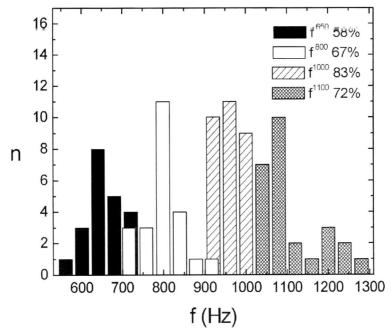

Fig. 4. The stacked column plot shows the distribution of resonances in the MFT pattern. The resonance frequencies were determined at the tympanometric peak pressure. The percentage values next to the class name of the resonances indicate the detectability.

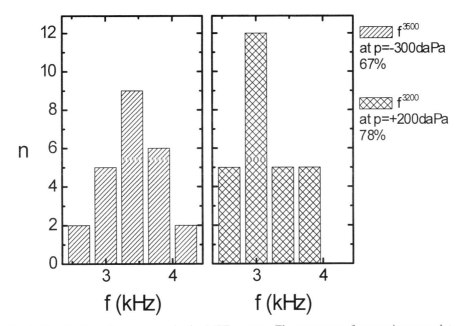

Fig. 5. Distribution of resonances in the MFT pattern. The resonance frequencies were determined at p = –300 or +200 daPa. The percentage values given next to the class name of the resonances indicate the detectability.

Table 1. Detectability, mean value, and standard deviation of the resonance frequencies evaluated

Resonance class	Detectability (%)	Resonance frequency (Hz) (mean value ± standard deviation)
f^{650} at p = p*	58	660 ± 39
f^{800} at p = p*	67	798 ± 52
f^{1000} at p = p*	83	963 ± 29
f^{1100} at p = p*	72	1110 ± 72
f^{3500} at p = −300 daPa	67	3380 ± 475
f^{3200} at p = +200 daPa	78	3224 ± 405

Conclusions

A fine structure can be found in the MFT pattern of normal-hearing subjects. In contrast to other publications, four classes of resonances were evaluated in the frequency range below 1.2 kHz. In the frequency range above 1.2 kHz, two resonances were found to be reproducible. By considering these results, the great variability in the main ossicles' resonance described in literature can be explained. The concept of the main ossicles' resonance in MFT patterns should be revised.

References

1. Terkildsen K, Thomson KA: The influence of pressure variations on the impedance of the human ear drum. J Laryngol Otol 73:409-418, 1959
2. Margolis RH: Tympanometry in infants. In: Harford ER (ed) Impedance Screening for Middle Ear Disease, pp 41-57. New York, NY: Grune and Stratton 1979
3. Lidén G, Harford E, Hallén O: Tympanometry for the diagnosis of ossicular disruption. Arch Otolaryngol 99:23-29, 1974
4. Colletti V: Methodologic observations on tympanometry with regard to the probe tone frequency. Acta Otolaryngol (Stockh) 80:54-60, 1975
5. Vanhuyse V, Creten W, Van Camp K: On the W-notching of tympanograms. Scand Audiol 4:45-50, 1975
6. Margolis RH, Van Camp KJ, Wilson RH, Creten WL: Multifrequency tympanometry in normal ears. Audiology 24:44-53, 1985
7. Hocke T, Eiber A, Pethe J, Von Specht H, Vorwerk U, Begall K: Zur Feinstruktur von Multifrequenztympanogrammen bei normaler Mittelohrfunktion. Z Audiol 1:38-43, 1998
8. Koebsell KA, Margolis RH: Tympanometric gradient measured from normal preschool children. Audiology 25:149-157, 1986
9. Margolis RH, Hunter LL, Giebink GS: Tympanometric evaluation of middle ear function in children with otitis media. Ann Otol Rhinol Laryngol 103:34-38, 1994
10. Shanks JE, Wilson RH, Cambron NK: Multiple Frequency Tympanometry: effects of ear canal volume compensation on static acoustic admittance and estimates of middle ear resonance. J Speech Hearing Res 36:178-185, 1993
11. Colletti V, Fiorino FG, Sittoni V, Policante Z: Mechanics of the middle ear in otosclerosis and stapedoplasty. Acta Otolaryngol (Stockh) 113:637-641, 1993

12. Valvik BR, Johnsen M, Laukli E: Multifrequency tympanometry. Audiology 33:245-253, 1994
13. Hocke T, Eiber A, Vorwerk U, Pethe J, Mühler R, Von Specht H, Begall K: Multifrequency tympanometry: results in normal hearing subjects. Audiology (in press)
14. Eiber A, Freitag H-G, Hocke T: On the relationship between multifrequency tympanogram pattern and the dynamic behavior of the middle ear. This volume
15. Holte L: Aging effects in multifrequency tympanometry. Ear Hear 17:12-18, 1996
16. Margolis RH, Goycoolea H: Multifrequency in normal adults. Ear Hear 14:408-413, 1993
17. Meredith R, West JA, Osborne D: No postural effects on middle ear resonance. Br J Audiol 29:255-258, 1995

ON THE RELATIONSHIP BETWEEN MULTIFREQUENCY TYMPANOMETRY PATTERNS AND THE DYNAMIC BEHAVIOR OF THE MIDDLE EAR

Albrecht Eiber[1], Hans-Georg Freitag[1] and Thomas Hocke[2]

[1]Institute B of Mechanics, University of Stuttgart; [2]Department of Experimental Audiology and Medical Physics, Otto-von-Guericke-University, Magdeburg, Germany

Abstract

Multifrequency tympanograms (MFT) show frequency and pressure dependent peaks (fine structure) representing the dynamic behavior of the middle ear structures and the tympanic membrane. The association of behavior and structure should allow detection of pathological changes from the MFT patterns. The classical MFT procedure was enhanced to include frequencies up to 6 kHz with a resolution of 15 Hz and was applied to cadaver specimens and living subjects. The opinion that the MFT describe only one 'main resonance' is misleading because at least three different resonances have been found around 1 kHz. The authors hypothesize that each of these resonances is related to a natural frequency associated with a particular vibration mode, as can be shown by evaluating the equations of motion. This statement was tested with the aid of so-called local MFTs constructed from measurements of the velocity of distinct points on the eardrum and ossicular chain on cadaver specimens using laser Doppler velocimetry. In addition, simulations using a mathematical model of the middle ear structure support these findings. The results support the idea that differences in the fine structure of the MFT are useful for distinguishing different middle ear pathologies.

Keywords: multifrequency tympanometry, fine structure, mechanical models, nonlinear behavior

Introduction

In the last few years, multifrequency tympanometry (MFT) has become a useful diagnostic tool. However, the interpretation of the measured results is neither easy nor clear. Because of the restricted frequency range and poor frequency resolution of the standard MFT technique, much valuable information

Address for correspondence: Dr.-Ing. Albrecht Eiber, Institute B of Mechanics, Pfaffenwaldring 9, 70550 Stuttgart, Germany. email: ae@mechb.uni-stuttgart.de

The Function and Mechanics of Normal, Diseased and Reconstructed Middle Ears, pp. 157–166
edited by J.J. Rosowski and S.N. Merchant
© 2000 Kugler Publications, The Hague, The Netherlands

remains hidden. Moreover, we believe that the definition of one main middle ear resonance[1,2] leads to misinterpretation. We suggest that the fine structure of various resonances within the MFT is diagnostic and can be explained on the basis of mechanical considerations. This paper describes investigations of mathematical models and measurements of temporal bones which test the relationship between MFT fine structures and middle ear dynamics.

Dynamic behavior of the middle ear

A steady-state sound pressure wave acting on the eardrum causes a very complex vibration pattern. The vibrating eardrum transmits forces to the ossicular chain, bringing it in motion. This process is highly frequency-dependent due to the dynamic behavior of the middle ear structure, which can be modelled as a dynamic system of coupled mechanical vibrators[3].

Generally, a dynamic system with f degrees of freedom has f eigenvalues associated with f eigenvectors. In an undamped system, the eigenvalues correspond to the natural frequencies and the eigenvectors correspond to the natural modes. For these modes, all elements of the system vibrate in phase or counter phase. (The general solution is a superposition of the modes.)

Lightly damped systems show damped natural modes similar to undamped ones, but there are phase shifts between the individual elements. Undamped systems under harmonical excitation show strict resonance if the excitation is identical to a natural frequency. As a consequence, there is an infinite system response at least in one of its coordinates.

The frequency response in damped systems shows resonance phenomena with large but finite amplitudes if the excitation frequency is near the natural frequencies of the undamped system. The corresponding forms of vibration strongly depend on the point where the excitation is applied, on its direction as well as on the internal dynamics, i.e., on the coupling between the individual degrees of freedom. On the other hand, a peak in the frequency response of a certain point of the system due to a certain excitation can generally be considered a resonance phenomena or resonance in the system.

In Figure 1, the velocity of the piston-like motion v_S of the stapes footplate is sketched to show the frequency-dependent behavior. The solid curve results from measurements on a temporal bone preparation with the cochlea removed by reason of a reduced number of parameters and better access to the stapes footplate. The dashed line represents the calculated response, obtained from simulations with a mathematical model. The model with 25 degrees of freedom consists of the three ossicles viscoelastically hinged in the tympanum by various ligaments. Simplified vibrators representing the air in the outer ear canal and the eardrum are included; these were derived from detailed finite element models[3], whereby the air in the middle ear spaces is not included. Due to the use of a standard set of parameters which had not been adapted to the indi-

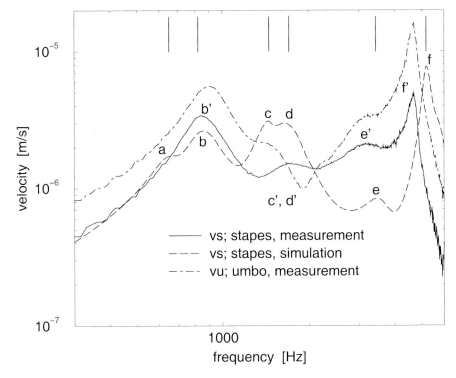

Fig. 1. Velocity of the simulated and measured piston-like motion of the stapes footplate and measured inward-outward velocity of the umbo due to a sound excitation of 60 dB SPL.

vidual temporal bone, there are some quantitative differences between the measured and the calculated frequency response.

Several peaks between 600 Hz and 4 kHz can be seen due to natural frequencies of the eardrum and the middle ear. The natural frequencies of the simulation model are indicated by tics at the abscissa. These correspond to the peaks 'a' to 'f' in the simulated frequency response. The ensemble of peaks 'a' to 'e' is referred to as 'fine structure'. The peak 'f' between 4 and 5 kHz is due to the first resonance of the ear canal closed by the probe. Qualitatively, the structure of the peaks 'b'' to 'f'' in the measured response is similar to the simulated behavior.

At the other end of the ossicular chain, at the manubrium and at the eardrum, the fine structure shown above is also observable, see velocity v_U in Figure 1.

The peaks in Figure 1 are due to the natural frequencies of the middle ear structure, eardrum and ear canal, represented by the coupled three-dimensional mechanical system. Considering the masses as given, the natural *frequencies* are determined by the stiffness coefficients of the eardrum, ligaments, incudo-stapedial joint and annular ring, and the *amplitudes* of the velocities v_S and v_U in the resonance peaks are determined by the corresponding damping coefficients.

It should be mentioned that each element in the structure influences several natural frequencies, depending on its sensitivity, and as a corollary, a distinct natural frequency is governed by several elements of the model.

Stiffening of the compliant elements can occur due to pathological effects, such as calcification processes. Because of the progressive nonlinear mechanical behavior of the compliant elements within the tympanic membrane, joints, ligaments and annular ring, stiffening occurs due to a pretension applied by a static pressure in the ear canal[4].

Multifrequency tympanometry

In tympanometry, the stiffening effect of the middle ear structure is caused by applying a static pressure p in the ear canal. Using a multifrequency excitation, the fine structure in the dynamic behavior or resonance characteristics can also be seen in MFTs[5].

Global tympanograms (MFT)

The admittance Y is calculated from the pressure p_{EC} measured in the ear canal with a microphone, $Y = Y(p_{EC})$. This acoustic pressure depends on the motion of all surface points on the eardrum. These motions are influenced by the dynamic behavior of the whole middle ear structure expressed by its natural frequencies. In the MFT, not all of the resonance frequencies are clearly distinct. This is because not all of the natural frequencies cause distinct peaks in the umbo's and eardrum's motion. Furthermore, a complex averaging over these motions is carried out in the MFT.

Dealing with higher frequencies, the dynamic behavior of the air column between microphone and eardrum, as well as the geometrical shape of the ear canal and the eardrum, has to be considered.

A deeper insight into the fine structure is given by considering the admittance of the particular points without averaging. This leads to 'local MFTs'.

Local tympanograms (LMFT)

Using laser Doppler vibrometry (Polytec OFV 303 with controller OFV 3001), it is possible to measure the velocity of a single point of the eardrum. This was carried out under the same conditions as multifrequency tympanometry, varying the static pressure and the excitation frequency. The mechanical admittance is proportional to the velocity and can be calculated taking the excitation into account.

Graphic representation of tympanograms

The signal considered, *e.g.*, admittance or velocity, as a function of static pressure p and excitation frequency is converted into a color scale and plotted like the map of a landscape, where the resonance peaks can be seen as ridges or hills (Fig. 2). Sections in the vertical axis show the resonances (fine structure) in the frequency behavior. Sections in the horizontal axis show the traditional MFT plots at constant frequency. The increasing resonance frequencies at increasing absolute pressure values represent the nonlinear behavior of the springs in the form of shifted natural frequencies. As examples in Figure 2, the cuts for p = 0 and p = 100 daPa, as well as for three frequencies, are shown on the left side and at the bottom of the LMFT plot.

Simulations

The mathematical model[3] is based on mechanical analogies and includes a representation of the stimulus and recording probe at the entrance to the ear canal. Nonlinear behavior of the viscoelastic elements was also considered. The nonlinear stiffening effect due to static pressure p is modelled to be symmetric for positive or negative pressure. Figure 2 shows a simulated LMFT based on the umbo's velocity $v_U(t)$ because the velocity corresponds to the admittance.

Generally, the frequency response at a certain point of the system to a harmonical excitation is also harmonical, and can be described as amplitude of the response signal and the phase angle between excitation and response, or as the complex transfer function with its real and imaginary part containing both amplitude and phase information. In this paper, we were interested in the dynamic behavior of the middle ear evaluating the velocity of various points on the eardrum, and therefore we only utilized the amplitude information of the response function. Figure 2 shows the amplitude of v_U simulated for various pressures p with an increment of $\Delta p = 20$ daPa, the increment in the excitation frequency is $\Delta f = 15$ Hz.

Similar behavior can be seen in the simulated LMFT of a point P in the posterior inferior part of the eardrum in Figure 3. Both LMFT patterns contain information on the dynamic behavior of the entire middle ear since all elements of the system are coupled. However, each of the middle ear vibration modes contributes differently to the motion of the different points. In the LMFT of the umbo, the modes with major contributions from the ossicular chain are clearly distinct, and the LMFT of point P contains more information about the motion of the eardrum. The LMFTs at both locations are dominated by an ear canal resonance of around 5.2 kHz.

For p = 0, there are several peaks in umbo velocity magnitude (Fig. 2) near 0.65, 0.87, 1.7, and 2.6 kHz, which are interpreted as middle ear resonances. The lowest one is probably the contribution of the pars flaccida, while the others are due to the eardrum and ossicular chain. The frequency shift for variations in p can clearly be seen following the ridges.

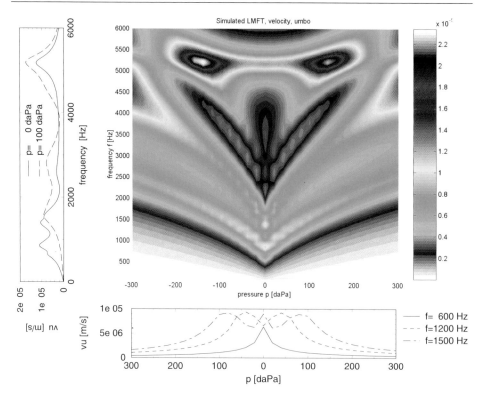

Fig. 2. Simulated local multifrequency tympanogram (LMFT) of the umbo. Left: constant pressure; bottom: constant frequency.

In the case of otosclerosis, the ossicular chain, and in particular the annular ligament, is stiffened. Consequently, those resonance peaks dominantly governed by the stiffness of the annular ring are shifted to higher values. In Figure 4, a beginning otosclerosis is considered. The LMFT pattern of the umbo looks different compared to the normal case in Figure 2. In particular, the resonance peaks between 1 and 3 kHz are shifted to higher values.

Measurements

We performed measurements of tympanic membrane velocities in temporal bones, checking for the effects described above. The external ear canal was removed from the temporal bones near to the annulus fibrosus, and replaced by a transparent adapter that allowed a view of the eardrum by laser. Loudspeaker and microphone were placed in a probe which was glued at the entrance of the adapter. This adapter had a relatively large air volume, leading to a natural frequency of the air column at around 4500 Hz. A multisinusoidal stimulus consisting of 400 components in the frequency range between 15 Hz and 6 kHz, with a resolution of 15 Hz, was used; the increment in static pressure between –100 and +100 daPa was $\Delta p = 20$ daPa,

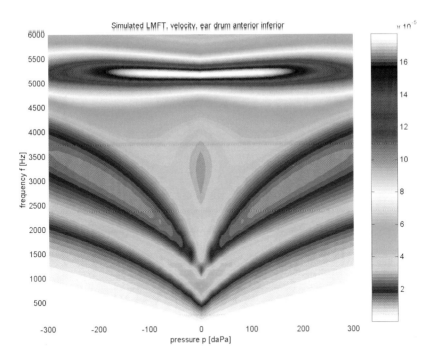

Fig. 3. Simulated local multifrequency tympanogram (LMFT) of a point on the eardrum in the inferior region.

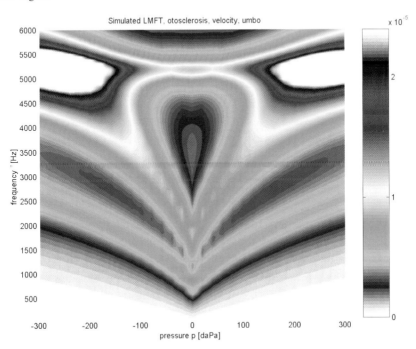

Fig. 4. Simulated local multifrequency tympanogram (LMFT) of the umbo of a beginning otosclerosis.

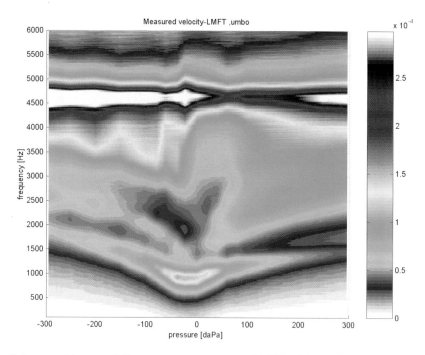

Fig. 5. Measured local multifrequency tympanogram (LMFT) of the umbo.

otherwise it was Δp = 50 daPa. For clinical use of the apparatus on living subjects, the air volume between the eardrum and probe is smaller, and the natural frequencies of the ear canal occur at higher values. Therefore, the frequency range up to 6 kHz can be used for diagnosis.

The main information about the ossicular chain can be gained from the motion of the umbo. The measured velocity normalized to 60 dB SPL in Figure 1 shows the fine structure with various resonances for p = 0 and, in Figure 5, the velocity depending on the static pressure forms the LMFT. Except in the frequency range between 2 and 4 kHz, it is quite symmetrical with respect to p, indicating that the ossicular chain exhibits relatively similar behavior for positive and negative static pressures. The values of the resonance frequencies are minimal at pressure p* = –20 daPa. In the case of closed middle ear cavities, such a p* may indicate a negative pressure in the tympanum. In our experiments, the cavity was open and therefore p* was due to pretension in the middle ear structure.

The LMFT of the pars flaccida is plotted in Figure 6, showing considerable motion around 650 Hz. For positive pressure, that the structure of MFT is not distinct may be due to the unfavorable angle of view of the laser. The obvious peaks detected in Figures 5 (umbo) and 6 (pars flaccida) show a different stiffening effect due to the increased static pressure, in particular the lowest peak.

Here an advantage of MFT becomes obvious: the frequency response measured at different static pressures leads to a coherent set of results. Missing measurement

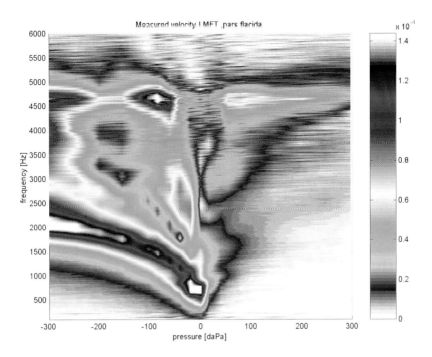

Fig. 6. Measured local multifrequency tympanogram (LMFT) of the pars flaccida.

values in some response functions can be interpolated from the adjacent ones.

It should be mentioned that, in the clinical use of MFT, the pressure in the ear canal is measured, not the velocity of points on the eardrum. Partially to compensate for the influence of the air column in the ear canal, the acoustic admittance with its real and imaginary part is used to represent the tympanograms[6]. It can be shown that the maxima of the real part of the acoustic admittance are near the resonance frequencies of the system.

Conclusions

Due to the complex mechanical structure of the middle ear, there are several resonance phenomena in the frequency range up to 6 kHz. The frequencies and amplitudes of these resonances are determined by the mechanical parameters of the system. Changes in the resonance behavior of the system are due to changes in the parameter values caused by specific diseases in the middle ear. Therefore, changes in dynamic behavior can be used to estimate mechanical middle ear parameters. In some cases, a relationship to a specific disease is obvious from the fine structure in the MFT.

Otosclerosis in the annular ring or partial malleus head fixation lead to an increased stiffness that shifts the natural frequencies to higher values. The insertion of an implant or a cholesteatoma lead to an increased mass shifting the natural frequencies to lower values. Both effects may occur simultaneously.

The amplitude in the resonance peaks is governed by the damping, but the individual assignment to the distinct parameters and the detection of the corresponding disease is difficult.

For practical use, the tympanograms from the MFT procedure are a superposition of the dynamic behavior of the air column and of all points on the eardrum simultaneously. In the motion of the eardrum, some dynamic effects of the ossicular chain are visible, and the tympanograms are useful for diagnosis.

A more distinct insight into the fine structure of the resonance behavior of the middle ear is given by measuring the motion of particular points of the eardrum and the manubrium, and by plotting the LMFTs. In particular, it was shown that the resonance peaks in the fine structure have a distinct physical meaning and must be interpreted separately. Restriction to the dominant one only as the 'main resonance' may lead to misinterpretation. The existence of the fine structure has clearly been shown by MFTs from clinical practice and statistical evaluation[7], by measurements of temporal bones and the evaluation of the resulting LMFTs and MFTs, as well as by simulations with a mathematical model, comparing calculated LMFTs and MFTs with measured ones.

References

1. Coletti V, Fiorino FG, Sittoni V, Policante Z: Mechanics of the middle ear in otosclerosis and stapedoplasty. Acta Otolaryngol (Stockh) 113:637-641, 1993
2. Valvik BR, Johnsen M, Laukli E: Multifrequency tympanometry. Audiology 33:245-253, 1994
3. Eiber A, Freitag HG: Description of sound transfer through the middle ear. In: Gonçalves PB et al (eds) Applied Mechanics in The Americas, Vol 6, pp 49-52. Rio de Janeiro: Brazilian Society of Mechanical Sciences 1999
4. Price R, Kalb J: Insights into hazard from intense impulses from a mathematical model of the ear. J Acoust Soc Am 90:219-227, 1991
5. Hocke T, Eiber A, Vorwerk U, Pethe J, Mühler R, Von Specht H, Begall K: Multifrequency tympanometry: results in normal hearing subjects. Audiology (in press)
6. Hocke T, Pethe J, Eiber A, Vorwerk U, Von Specht H: On the fine structure of multifrequency tympanograms: evidence for multiple middle-ear resonances. This volume
7. Vorwerk U, Eiber A, Hocke T, Begall K: The diseased middle ear: effects on the fine structure of multifrequency tympanogram patterns: a clinical view. This volume

THE DISEASED MIDDLE EAR: EFFECTS ON THE FINE STRUCTURE OF MULTIFREQUENCY TYMPANOGRAM PATTERNS

A clinical view

Ulrich Vorwerk[1], Albrecht Eiber[2], Thomas Hocke[3] and Klaus Begall[1]

[1]Department of Oto-, Rhino-, Laryngology, St. Salvator Hospital, Halberstadt; [2]Institute B of Mechanics, University of Stuttgart, Stuttgart; [3]Department of Experimental Audiology and Medical Physics, Otto-von-Guericke-University, Magdeburg, Germany

Abstract

The influence of pathophysiological changes of the middle ear apparatus on the fine structure of multifrequency tympanogram (MFT) patterns was investigated. MFT patterns of 12 patients with otosclerosis before and after stapedoplasty were recorded and compared with those of 32 normal hearing ears. It was shown that an evaluation of the fine structure of MFT patterns can provide additional information about the condition of the middle ear apparatus. It is also shown that a statement about the condition of the middle ear has to be based on detailed considerations involving the fine structure of MFT patterns in normal hearing subjects. The reasons for the particular characteristics of the fine structure in the MFT patterns of pathological middle ears are given. Individual evaluation of MFT patterns can be a presurgical help for the middle ear surgeon.

Keywords: middle ear, multifrequency tympanometry, fine structure, MFT patterns, otosclerosis, stapedoplasty

Introduction

Conventional tympanometry uses one or two sound probe frequencies and is of limited value in assessing middle ear function[1]. A more successful technique is multifrequency tympanometry (MFT). Most MFT apparatus operates with probe frequency in the range of 226-2000 Hz. We believe that precise examination of the middle ear requires the use of probe-tone frequencies above 2 kHz. The

Address for correspondence: Dr. med. Ulrich Vorwerk, HNO-Klinik, St.-Salvator Krankenhaus, Gleimstrasse 5, 38820 Halberstadt, Germany. *email:* vorwerk@hno.salvator-kh.de

The Function and Mechanics of Normal, Diseased and Reconstructed Middle Ears, pp. 167–176
edited by J.J. Rosowski and S.N. Merchant
© 2000 Kugler Publications, The Hague, The Netherlands

MFT apparatus described by Hocke *et al.*[2], which extends the frequency range beyond 2 kHz, was used in the present study. The expansion of the frequency range and the resolution in the frequency and pressure areas has increased the potential utility of MFTs in recent years. Classical tympanometry only provides the clinician with an overall picture of middle ear impedance, rather than the detailed knowledge of middle ear mechanics that is potentially available in multifrequency tympanograms[3,4]. Uncertainties in the interpretation of multifrequency tympanograms is the reason why they are not commonly applied clinically[5,6].

Otosclerosis serves as a suitable model for the pathological middle ear, since the well-documented pathology associated with the disease facilitates the interpretation of the results. In addition, the extent of the disease can be surgically assessed during stapedoplasty. The otosclerosis-induced stiffening of the ossicles, in particular the annular ring ligament, is expected to cause an increase in the frequency of resonance in MFTs. A companion paper details the existence of multiple resonances in the fine structure of the MFT[7]. The present study demonstrates that the fine structure of MFT patterns is altered by middle ear pathology.

Another pathology with well-defined effects is fixation of the malleus head. MFTs from ears with both diseases were compared with those of patients whose ears and hearing were normal.

Material and methods

The MFTs of 32 ears of normal subjects aged between 20 and 45 years served as controls[8]. Five males and seven females, aged from 35-56 years, with otosclerosis were also examined. The MFTs were recorded one day prior to, and six to eight weeks after, stapedoplastic surgery. Similar recordings were carried out on six patients with fixation of the malleus head. The multifrequency tympanometer (MFT 2370) used was constructed by us[2] and consisted of the following components: measuring probe, programmable stimulator, microphone amplifier, technique to generate (pump), and measure (pressure difference sensor) pressure, a PC with analogue/digital converter (IPR; Braunschweig). The probe-tip contained a measuring microphone (Type EK 3133, Knowles) as well as a miniature loud speaker (Type ED1932, Knowles), and was shaped to enable it to connect with the auditory canal. The difference between the pressure in the auditory canal and the atmosphere was measured, and will be referred to as static pressure. The stimulator and pre-amplifier were controlled by computer. Pressure was controlled manually. The system was calibrated in hardwall cavities, ranging in volume from 0.8-2.0 ml. The admittance $Y = Y(p,f)$ was measured for 96 frequencies in the range of 220 Hz to 6 kHz. The static pressure was varied between -300 and $+200$ daPa. The measurement sequence was initiated by setting the ear canal pressure to $p = -300$ daPa. After measurement of admittance as a function of frequency, the static pressure was changed in steps of 50 daPa up to +200 daPa. The measurement of pressure between –100 and +100 daPa was conducted in steps of 25 daPa. Analysis of the data was carried out using the program package MATLAB (version 5.1, The Mathworks, Inc.). The real parts of the admittance between the measured points were interpolated linearly. Representing these values in a color scale, as described by Hocke et al.[9] (this volume), the resonances can be depicted as local maxima. These local maxima appear as ridges or hill lines in a landscape map and show the dependence of resonance frequencies on static pressure[7]. Such ridges are generally U-shaped in the static-pressure versus frequency plane (e.g., Fig. 2).

The measurement at one static pressure lasts approximately ten seconds. A complete MFT examination requires approximately five to ten minutes.

Results

Hocke et al.[8,9] describe the detectability and frequency range of individual resonances for normal subjects. The MFTs of 12 patients with otosclerosis and 32 normal hearing subjects were analyzed according to the methodology described. The results of both study groups are shown in Table 1 and plotted in Figure 1. A classification of resonance frequencies, taking the statistical exploration of measurement results and the characteristic vibrational behavior, is given in Hocke et al.[9] (this volume) and is used here. MFTs of the otosclerotic patients show a significantly higher frequency in four resonance areas compared to the control subjects. As expected, this is due to increased stiffness in the annular ligament. The average frequency shift for these four ranges is 254.5 Hz. The vibration qualities of the middle ear change after stapedoplasty. A resonance peak was

Table 1. Detectability, mean value, and standard deviation of the evaluated resonance frequencies

| | | Resonance | | | | |
		f_{650}	f_{800}	f_{1000}	f_{1750}	f_{3200}
Normal hearing group	detectability	62%	69%	88%	34%	78%
(reference group)	resonance frequency (Hz)	656	798	963	1728	3192
(n=32)	mean value					
	± standard deviation	±38	±54	±29	±326	±405
Otosclerosis	detectability	0%	25%	100%	16%	66%
preoperatively	resonance frequency (Hz)	-	873	1396	2000	3430
(n=12)	mean value					
	±standard deviation		±95	±194	±0	±469
Otosclerosis	detectability	0%	100%	89%	22%	0%
postoperatively	resonance frequency (Hz)	-	744	1150	1500	-
(n=9)	mean value					
	±standard deviation		±125	±269	±0	

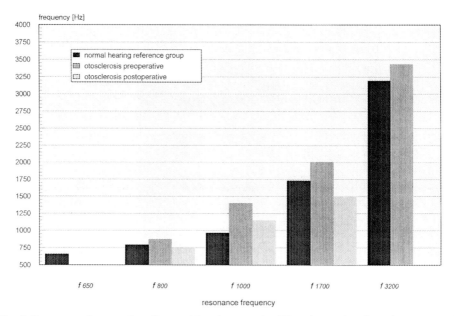

Fig. 1. Resonance frequencies of normal hearing ears (*n*=32) and otosclerotic patients pre- and postoperatively (*n*=12, *n*=9, respectively).

not obvious above 2000 Hz. We hypothesize that the postoperative decrease of the resonance frequencies is explained by a reduction of stiffness in the ossicular chain of otosclerosis patients because the annular ligament is no longer involved.

The morphological changes caused by the operation varied in a broad range. Hence, it seems advisable to interpret the MFT pattern not statistically, but rather at an individual level. We will now proceed to discuss the MFTs of two otosclerotic patients, one postoperative MFT after stapedoplasty and one patient with malleus head fixation. To compare with MFTs of normal hearing subjects see the paper of Hocke *et al.*[9] (this volume).

In Figures 2 to 4, the surface plot of the MFTs shows the admittance's real part, *Re(Y)*, as a function of frequency and ear canal pressure.

Case 1 (Fig. 2)

This patient, aged 33 years, was suffering from otosclerosis in the left ear, with no obvious eardrum defects. The case history did not reveal any infections, but the patient had suffered from increasing deafness over the years. The audiogram revealed an air-bone gap of 40-60 dB with 20 dB bone conduction. The other ear showed normal hearing. Stapedoplasty under local anesthesia showed that the stapes was completely fixed. The footplate was greatly altered due to otosclerosis and was very thick in the frontal aspect. The stapes could not be moved, in contrast to the malleus and incus. A well-structured MFT pattern

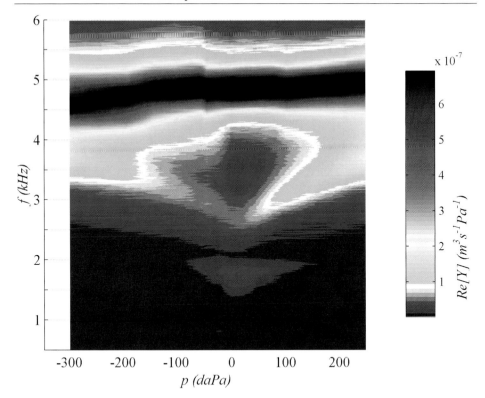

Fig. 2. (Case 1): MFT of an otosclerotic ear.

was seen from 1 kHz with a resonance of the auditory canal due to the residual volume at approximately 5 kHz. The U-shape is significantly narrower compared to normal subjects, suggesting a stronger dependence on static pressure. Resonances near f_{650} and f_{800} are not apparent and other natural frequencies are shifted to the higher values. The fine structure of the MFTs is generally not as distinct as in the case of normal subjects.

Case 2 (Fig. 3)

This patient, aged 52 years, was suffering from otosclerosis in the left ear, with no obvious eardrum defects. The case history did not reveal any infections, but the patient had suffered from increasing deafness for many years. The audiogram revealed an air-bone gap of 30-70 dB with 50 dB bone conduction. The left ear had been operated on two years previously for otosclerosis. Stapedoplasty under local anesthesia showed that the stapes was completely fixed, but that the malleus and incus were mobile. A well-structured MFT pattern was seen from 1 kHz with a resonance of the auditory canal residual volume at approximately 5 kHz. The U-shaped configuration is significantly narrower compared to normal subjects. The f_{650} and f_{800} resonances are apparent, but are slightly shifted

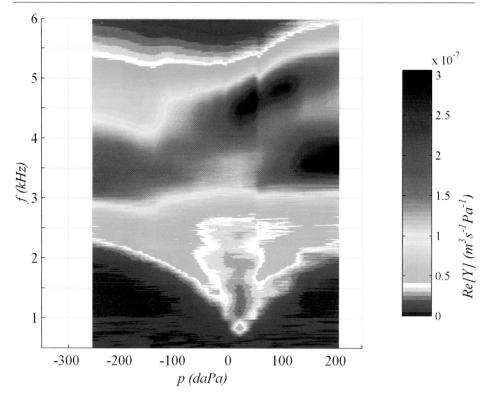

Fig. 3. (Case 2): MFT of an otosclerotic ear.

to the higher frequencies. The resulting resonances are clearly asymmetrical and non-linear. This example is not characteristic of the typical findings seen in otosclerosis in that, here, we find a well-structured MFT in the lower frequency range. However, knowledge of the fine structure and high pressure resolution permits a description of the MFT pattern.

Case 3 (Fig. 4)

This patient, aged 38 years, was suffering from otosclerosis in the right ear, with no obvious eardrum defects. The case history did not reveal any infections, but the patient had suffered from increasing deafness over the years. The audiogram revealed an air-bone gap of 60 dB with 20 dB bone conduction. The left ear had been operated on for otosclerosis three years previously. Stapedoplasty under local anesthesia showed that the stapes was completely fixed. The footplate was greatly altered due to otosclerosis and was very thick in the frontal aspect, and the malleus was fixed due to scar formation. This resulted in limited mobility of the malleus and incus. There was a distinctly structured MFT pattern. The representative resonances show distinct asymmetry and non-linearity. The U-shaped configuration is not as obvious in the other patients. with the excep-

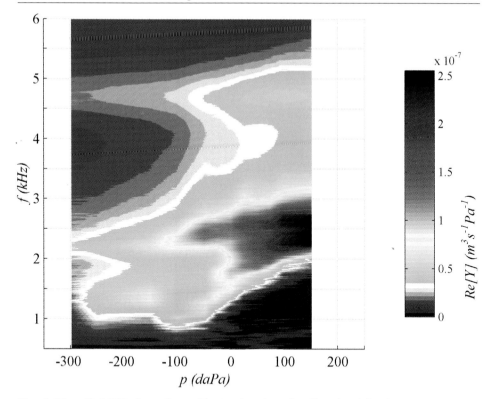

Fig. 4. (Case 3): MFT of a patient with otosclerosis and malleus head fixation.

tion of f_{650}, the other resonances are present, but shifted to higher frequency ranges. The fine structure of the MFTs is as indistinct as in normal cases. This is also not a typical example of findings seen in otosclerotic patients. The asymmetric MFT pattern is even more distinct in this case, due to the malleus head fixation. However, knowledge of the fine structure and sufficient pressure resolution permits a description of the MFT pattern.

Case 4 (Fig. 5)

This patient, aged 54 years, was suffering from otosclerosis in the right ear, with no obvious eardrum defects. The case history did not reveal any infections, but the patient had suffered from increasing deafness over the years. The audiogram revealed an air-bone gap of 70-80 dB with 30-50 dB bone conduction before stapedoplasty. This ear had been operated on two years previously for otosclerosis. Stapedoplasty under local anesthesia showed that the stapes was completely fixed, but that the malleus and incus were mobile. Six weeks after stapedoplasty, we found an audiogram with an air-bone gap of from 10-15 dB with 20-50 dB bone conduction. A non-well-structured MFT pattern was seen from 1 kHz with a resonance of the auditory canal residual volume at approximately 5-6 kHz. The U-shaped configuration is only obvious in the

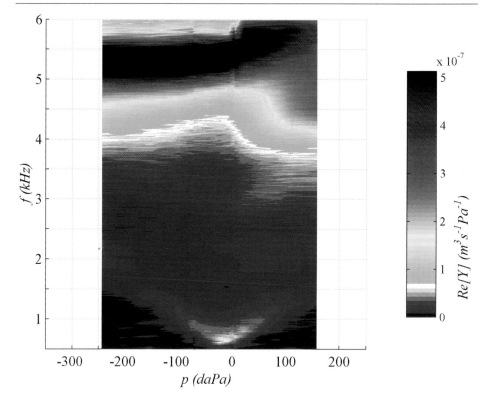

Fig. 5. (Case 4): MFT of a patient after stapedoplasty.

1 kHz frequency region. So we found a structured MFT in the lower frequency range. The higher natural frequencies were not apparent. This example is characteristic of the typical findings seen in postoperative patients.

Discussion

The appearance of numerous resonance maxima in the MFT can be explained by the mechanics of the eardrum: ossicle apparatus, which corresponds to a complex system of coupled oscillators[10,11]. Therefore, the number of resonances within the eardrum and ossicle chain corresponds to the various degrees of freedom of the system. The numerical nomenclature suggested by Hocke *et al.*[2] in 1998 has been used until now. However, recent studies using mechanical simulation and laser measurements have shown that not all resonances can be clearly identified in pathological middle-ear conditions. There is no common nomenclature for MFTs in the literature[12-14]. The present study aims to designate frequency ranges to the corresponding resonance maximum. It turns out that the recording and analysis of the 'main resonance' only can lead to a false interpretation of the results (Valvik *et al.*[15]). The fine structure found in normal subjects also requires a detailed description of all individual resonances in the pathological situation. This means that a correspondingly high pressure and frequency resolution is needed. Unfortunately, this is not possible when using commercially-available equipment. Also, the frequency range of the probe should be extendible beyond 2 kHz, since an altered function of the stapes leads to MFT alterations in the higher frequency ranges. An additional aspect is the reduction of the residual volume between the tip of the probe and the ear-drum[16-18]. This involves the dead space around the probe in addition to the remaining volume in the auditory canal. With a small residual volume, it is possible to elevate this limit to approximately 5-6 kHz. This enables detection of MFT fine structure below this frequency. The special construction of the probe utilized has made this possible.

Otosclerosis is an appropriate model for studying a pathological middle ear, since the pathology is relatively uniform and restricted. Exact definition and description of the disease is possible during the operation (stapedoplasty), which enables conclusions derived from changes in the MFT to be compared with the normal situation. The mass bondage in the area of the annular ligament leads to stiffening of the middle ear structure. This results in an increase in the resonance frequencies[17-22]. It has been shown that, if only the main resonance detected from the MFT is considered, this resonance shift cannot be correctly ascertained. If all resonance maxima are considered, it is possible to detect the expected shifts of resonance peaks, in particular of that around at 1.5 kHz. In their examinations, Eiber et al.[7] describe comparative laser measurements on temporal bones. They have shown that changes in the ossicular chain, especially in the region of the stapes, in particular influences the frequency range above 1.5 kHz. The resonance maximum of the eardrum is found at approximately 1 kHz. Stapedoplasty enables the removal of the suprastructures of the stapes, which can be replaced by a prosthesis. In our measurements, we found that the loss of stapes is reflected in the loss of higher resonance frequencies. A resonance in the range above 2.5 kHz was no longer evident. The prosthesis alters the middle ear structure and subsequently the oscillation of this system, leading to a postoperative reduction in the f_{800}, f_{1000} and f_{1700} resonances. This phenomenon has seldom been described by other authors. The altered MFT pattern in the lower frequency range is attributed to the altered ossicle mobility, but it also depends on the difference in resonance behavior of the individual components of the eardrum, which becomes more strongly effective. In general, for patients with middle ear pathology, the systemization of MFT patterns is even more limited than that in normal subjects. This is also true in the case of additional functional disorders, such as connective tissue fixation of the malleus head. Strong asymmetry and non-linearity is evident in the frequency-pressure behavior of these patients. The altered pattern, rather than the resonance frequency itself, is of importance. Indications from the MFT regarding the expected middle ear pathology could be helpful to the surgeon.

References

1. Terkildsen K, Thomsen K: The influence of pressure variations on the impedance of the human eardrum. J Laryngol Otol 73:409-418, 1959
2. Hocke T, Eiber A, Pethe J, Von Specht H, Vorwerk U, Begall K: Zur Feinstruktur von Multifrequenztympanogrammen bei normaler Mittelohrfunktion. Z Audiol 1:38-43, 1998
3. Hunter L, Margolis R: Effects of tympanic membrane abnormalities on auditory function. J Am Acad Audiol 8:431-446, 1997
4. Colletti V: Methodologic observations on tympanometry with regard to the probe tone frequency. Acta Otolaryngol (Stockh) 80:54-60, 1975
5. Margolis RH: Tympanometry in infants. In: Harford ER (ed) Impedance Screening for Middle Ear Disease, pp 41-57. New York, NY: Grune and Stratton 1979
6. Hudde H: Mittelohrdiagnostik durch Impedanzmessung. Audiol Akustik 2:40-58, 1992
7. Eiber A, Freitag HG, Hocke T: On the relationship between MFT patterns and the dynamic behavior of the middle ear. (this volume)
8. Hocke T, Eiber A, Vorwerk U, Pethe A, Mühler R, Von Specht H, Begall K: Multifrequency tympanometry: results in normal hearing subjects. Audiology 1999 (submitted for publication)
9. Hocke T, Pethe J, Eiber A, Vorwerk U, Von Specht H: On the fine structure of multifrequency tympanograms: evidence for multiple middle-ear resonances. (this volume)
10. Eiber A: Mechanical modelling and dynamical investigation of middle ear. In: Hüttenbrink KB (ed) Middle Ear Mechanics in Research and Otosurgery, Dresden: University Press Dresden, pp 61-66. 1997
11. Wada H, Koike T, Kobayashi T: Three-dimensional finite-element method (FEM) analysis. In: Hüttenbrink KB (ed) Middle Ear Mechanics in Research and Otosurgery, Dresden: University Press Dresden, pp 76-81, 1997
12. Colletti V: Tympanometry from 200 to 2000 Hz probe tone. Audiology 15:106-119, 1976
13. Margolis RH, Goycoolea H: Multifrequency tympanometry in normal adults. Ear Hear 14:408-413, 1993
14. Margolis R, Saly G: Wideband reflectance tympanometry in normal adults. J Acoust Soc Am 106:265-280, 1999
15. Valvik BR, Johnsen M, Laukli E: Multifrequency tympanometry. Audiology 33:245-253, 1994
16. Shanks JE, Wilson RH, Cambron NK: Multiple frequency tympanometry: effects of ear canal volume compensation on static acoustic admittance and estimates of middle ear resonance. J Speech Hear Res 36:178-185, 1993
17. Hudde H: Eardrum impedance and drum coupling region. In: Hüttenbrink KB (ed) Middle Ear Mechanics in Research and Otosurgery, Dresden: University Press Dresden, pp 48-55. 1997
18. Hanks WD, Mortensen BA: Multifrequency tympanometry: effects of ear canal volume compensation on middle ear resonance. J Am Acad Audiol 8:53-58, 1997
19. Vorwerk U, Neumann U, Begall K: Der Einsatz eines Multifrequenztympanometers zur Bestimmung der Mittelohrresonanz. Freiburg: University Press Freiburg, (Abstract) 1997
20. Neumann U, Vorwerk U, Begall K: Multifrequenztympanometrie und Mittelohrresonanz bei gesunden und pathologischen Ohren. Freiburg: University Press Freiburg, (Abstract) 1997
21. Coletti V, Fiorino F, Sittoni V, Policante Z: Mechanics of the middle ear in otosclerosis and stapedoplasty. Acta Otolaryngol (Stockh) 113:637-641, 1993
22. Shahnaz N, Polka L: Standard and multifrequency tympanometry in normal and otosclerotic ears. Ear Hear 18:326-341, 1997

EXPERIMENTAL INVESTIGATIONS OF OSSICULAR JOINT ANKYLOSIS

Christian F.E. Offergeld[1,2], Karl-Bernd Hüttenbrink[1,2], Thomas Zahnert[1,2] and Gert Hofmann[2]

[1]Department of Otorhinolaryngology, Head and Neck Surgery; [2]Middle Ear Laboratory, Dresden Medical School, University of Dresden, Dresden, Germany

Abstract

The normal ossicular chain contains two joints (incudo-malleal and incudo-stapedial joint). While these joints are functionally fixed during acoustic sound transfer, they perform gliding movements during atmospheric pressure changes. In the classical concept of middle ear function, it is assumed that these gliding motions protect the internal ear from exceeding atmospheric pressure loads. In cases of fixed ossicular joints (ankylosis), this natural protection mechanism is missing. Possible consequences for the internal ear have not been investigated precisely up to now, since clinical diagnosis of ossicular joint ankylosis is difficult.

The purpose of this experimental study was to discover the effect of artificially fixed ossicular joints on the middle ear transfer function during altered atmospheric pressure changes in the external auditory meatus. The suitability of this method for detection of ossicular joint ankylosis was investigated using a combination of atmospheric pressure changes and sound stimulation.

Experiments were performed using ten fresh temporal bone specimens. Acoustic transfer characteristics were determined by laser Doppler vibrometry (LDV) of the stapes footplate during atmospheric pressure changes in the external auditory meatus. Measurements of the normal middle ear were repeated in all specimens after artificial fixation of the ossicular joints using cyanoacrylate glue. The transfer function of the ankylosed middle ear demonstrated a more emphasized decrease in the middle frequency range compared to the normal middle ear during pressure changes of up to 10 kPa. Due to the fact that these magnitude differences were only in the range of 5-10 dB, it is unlikely that this effect will be useful clinically.

Keywords: ossicular joints, transfer characteristics, middle ear, displacement, annular ligament, pressure, ankylosis, internal ear disorders

Address for correspondence: Christian F.E. Offergeld, MD, Department of Otorhinolaryngology, Head and Neck Surgery, Dresden Medical School, University of Dresden, University Hospital 'Carl Gustav Carus', Fetscherstrasse 74, 01307 Dresden, Germany. email: Offi@rcs.urz.tu-dresden.de

The Function and Mechanics of Normal, Diseased and Reconstructed Middle Ears, pp. 177–186
edited by J.J. Rosowski and S.N. Merchant
© 2000 Kugler Publications, The Hague, The Netherlands

Introduction

The normal middle ear is designed with a mechanical protection system against high static and dynamic pressure influences[1,2]. The gliding of the incudo-malleal joint, *e.g.*, during the valsalva maneuver, leads to decoupling of the ossicular chain. Due to this mechanism, the ossicles serve as a cushion in order to protect the internal ear against exceeding tympanic membrane displacement. The un-impeded gliding in the ossicular joints is a prerequisite for this natural protec-tion mechanism[3]. In cases of a stiffened or a permanently rigid ossicular chain, due to ossicular joint ankylosis, pressure will be directly transferred from the tympanic membrane via the ossicular chain into the internal ear. Therefore, daily situations with ambient pressure changes such as gusts of wind, swallow-ing, flying, or diving, would lead to a three times higher displacement of the stapes footplate into the vestibulum[4]. It is not clear whether these unphysi-ological displacements in daily life are responsible for internal ear disorders such as, *e.g.*, hearing loss, tinnitus or vertigo in cases of ossicular joint ankylo-sis[4,5].

Although the effects of increased atmospheric pressure on middle ear me-chanics have already been described, there are only a few specific descriptions of the effect of ossicular joint fixation[4,6-9]. One possible reason for this could be that diagnosis of ossicular joint ankylosis is difficult in practice. This ex-plains why various authors have only been able to demonstrate suspicious tympanometric findings in patients suffering from rheumatoid arthritis[10-12]. In general, the ossicular joints have a negligible effect on the acoustic transfer function of the middle ear during physiological pressure conditions.

The purpose of our experimental study was to demonstrate acoustic conse-quences arising from ossicular joint ankylosis during altered atmospheric pres-sure changes. It was our goal to evaluate differences between normal and ankylosed ossicular joints, in order to establish this pressure-dependent acoustic method as a diagnostic tool.

Material and methods

Temporal bone measurements

Experiments were carried out on ten fresh temporal bone specimens, all ob-tained within 48 hours after death. The age of the patients at death was, on average, 65 years, ranging from 55 to 75 years. Specimens were kept con-stantly refrigerated at 4°C in Ringer's solution until needed for study. All speci-mens underwent accurate inspection before each experiment, using an operat-ing microscope (Zeiss OPMI 111, Zeiss Co., Oberkochen, Germany) to rule out any middle ear pathology which could interfere with the measurements. Experiments were performed within three days of death in all specimens. All specimens were kept moistened with physiological saline throughout the experimental investigations.

A block diagram of the experimental set-up is shown in Figure 1. After confirmation that the ossicles and tympanic membrane (TM) were normal in appearance, a posterior tympanotomy, including removal of the facial nerve, was performed in order to access the stapes footplate. This was necessary for all measurements concerning stapes vibration amplitude and pressure-induced stapes displacements using LDV (Polytec OFV 3001/ OFV 302; Polytec Co., Waldbronn, Germany). The external auditory meatus was sealed after positioning of a silicone tube with reference to a sound source (Praecitronic Co., Dresden, Germany) and a pressure pump, which was connected to a tympanometer (Phonak Co., Stuttgart, Germany). The sound source was calibrated for sound excitation of 94 dB SPL at 1000 Hz at the TM during normal atmospheric pressure conditions. The voltage necessary to produce this sound pressure of 94 dB SPL was held constant throughout the experiments. The frequency range was between 125 Hz and 5 kHz. A probe microphone (Etymotic Research Inc., Elk Grove Village, IL, USA) was placed through an opening in the external auditory meatus adjacent to the TM to record the first measurement during normal pressure conditions as a control value and was removed afterwards, the opening was then sealed air-tight. This procedure was necessary in order to prevent microphone membrane damage. The influence of altered static pressure on the middle ear input impedance was investigated in separate experiments. Sound pressure in the external auditory meatus produced by earphone was measured while altering atmospheric pressure in the middle ear cavity. After static pressure changes (±10 kPa), the sound pressure in the external auditory meatus increased by as much as 10 dB at 1 kHz with smaller changes at the other frequencies. With equal static pressure values, the sound pressure difference between normal and ankylosed ossicular joints was less than 3 dB. Therefore, equal sound pressure characteristics can be assumed for comparable static pressure conditions. The sound source's case contained an opening which guaranteed equal pressure conditions in front of and beyond the earphone membrane. Due to this pressure compensation, the earphone's frequency characteristics were kept stable during static pressure changes in the external auditory meatus. Altered static pressure in the external auditory meatus was monitored by a connected pressure measuring instrument (Ziegler Co., Germany). Pressure changes were standardized in steps of 2 kPa and ranged from ±10 kPa. Measurements were carried out at each step up to ±10 kPa. All specimens underwent the standardized experiments for LDV measurements of the stapes footplate under pressure changes of ±10 kPa during sound excitation before and after ankylosing the ossicular joints.

The first part (I) included the measurement of the stapes vibration amplitude while the condition of the ossicular joints was normal. This was accomplished by sound excitation of 94 dB SPL using multisinusoidal excitation in the range of 250-5000 Hz, and LDV measurements of the stapes footplate via the poste-

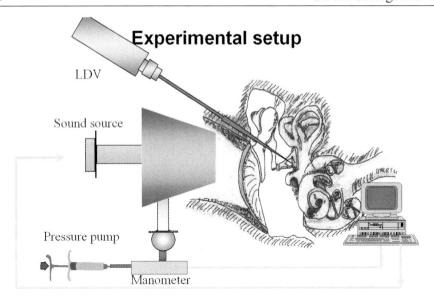

Fig. 1. Schematic view of the experimental set-up used for temporal bone investigations. The external auditory meatus was sealed air-tight after insertion of a sound source and a pressure pump. Measurements were performed by means of laser Doppler vibrometry.

rior tympanotomy approach. Reflection foil was placed onto the middle part of the footplate. Measurements were carried out at each of the steadily increasing positive and negative pressure steps of 2 kPa in the external auditory meatus until the maximum of ±10 kPa was reached.

The second part (II) included measurement of stapes displacement during static pressure changes. LDV measurements of the stapes footplate displacement were performed through the posterior tympanotomy approach, as already described in Part I. Continuous pressure changes of up to ±10 kPa in the external auditory meatus were obtained under steady conditions.

After accomplishing these first two parts, the third part with artificial fixation of the ossicular joints was initialized. The posterior area of the tympanic tegmen was removed in order to prepare the incudo-malleal joint. Using this technique, the suspensory ligament of the malleus, which can be found anteriorly, remains undamaged while obtaining excellent access to the joint. After opening the superior joint capsule, the synovial fluid was removed by suction and a droplet of Cyanoacrylate (Histoacryl®) was administered to the joint cleft. Tiny mechanical movements of the ossicles led to the correct distribution of cyanoacrylate throughout the incudo-malleal joint (intracapsular fixation), with no danger of fixation of ligaments, ossicles, tympanic membrane and/or tympanic cavity from leakage of glue material. Details of this procedure have already been described in the literature[4]. The same procedure was carried out to fix the incudo-stapedial joint via the posterior tympanotomy approach. After completing artificial ankylosis of the ossicles, standardized experimental investigations concerning acoustic transfer characteristics during static pressure variations were repeated in all the prepared specimens, as previously described in Parts I and II using sound excitation, LDV, and defined static pressure changes.

Results

Stapes footplate vibration amplitude

Figures 2 to 5 show examples of temporal bone measurements in one specimen (normal and prepared measurement conditions) with regard to stapes footplate vibration amplitude during defined sound excitation and pressure changes of ±10 kPa in the external auditory meatus. The differently marked curves indicate measurement results for regular ossicular joints during normal pressure conditions, as well as for ossicular joints during positive (Fig. 2) and negative pressure (Fig. 3) application of ±10 kPa. They also demonstrate measurement results with regard to positive (Fig. 4) and negative pressure (Fig. 5) in the external auditory meatus after artificial ankylosis of the ossicular chain.

In normal ossicular joints, a decrease in the stapes footplate vibration amplitude was observed in the low and middle frequency region between 250 Hz and 3 kHz after altering pressure changes. This decrease, mainly seen in the low frequency range, means a maximum threshold shift/drop of 20 dB at ±10 kPa.

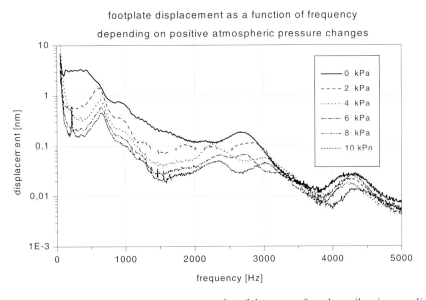

Fig. 2. Diagram demonstrating measurement results of the stapes footplate vibration amplitude in temporal bone specimens following acoustic excitation of 94 dB SPL. The middle ear is normal, positive static pressure was altered up to +10 kPa, consequently leading to a stepwise decrease of transfer function.

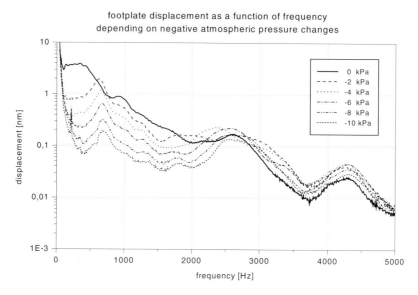

Fig. 3. Diagram demonstrating measurement results of the stapes footplate vibration amplitude in temporal bone specimens following acoustic excitation of 94 dB SPL. The middle ear is normal, negative static pressure was altered down to –10 kPa. The decrease of transfer function follows stepwise in accordance with increasing pressure values.

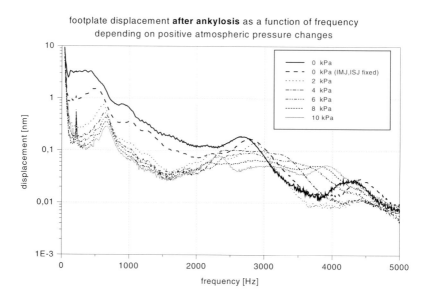

Fig. 4. Diagram demonstrating measurement results of the stapes footplate vibration amplitude in temporal bone specimens following acoustic excitation of 94 dB SPL. The ossicular joints were ankylosed artificially, positive static pressure was altered up to +10 kPa. Maximum values for decrease of transfer function were already reached at pressure levels of 2 kPa.

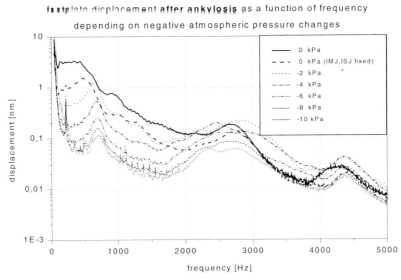

Fig. 5. Diagram demonstrating measurement results of the stapes footplate vibration amplitude in temporal bone specimens following acoustic excitation of 94 dB SPL. The ossicular joints were ankylosed artificially, negative static pressure was altered down to –10 kPa. The transfer function decreases at pressure levels of 6 kPa to the maximum.

An increase of the transfer characteristics towards the normal pressure controls was demonstrable in the high frequency range, starting from 2.5 kHz.

After artificial fixation of the joints, a decrease of about 5 dB was evident in the transfer function compared to normal joint conditions. Even moderate pressure changes (2 kPa) in the external auditory meatus led to a more accentuated and sudden decrease in the vibration amplitude (meaning a drop of middle ear transfer function of up to 20 dB), mainly in the low frequency range with improvement in the high frequency region (Figs. 4 and 5). This is in contrast to normal ossicular chains in which comparable maximum values of decrease were only achieved at a pressure of 10 kPa (Figs. 2 and 3).

Stapes footplate displacement during static pressure changes

Figure 6 demonstrates the static displacement of the stapes footplate under defined pressure changes before and after ankylotic fixation of the ossicular joints. In normal ossicular chains, displacement of the stapes footplate is greater with negative pressure. This is even more accentuated after ankylosing the ossicular joints. Due to ossicular joint fixation, footplate displacement is clearly elevated during application of positive as well as of negative pressure in the external auditory meatus, with footplate displacements of up to 40 μm compared to normal ossicles. Although the increase in footplate displacement is greater in total for negative pressure, positive pressure application also shows a multiple-fold elevation of footplate displacement compared to untreated speci-

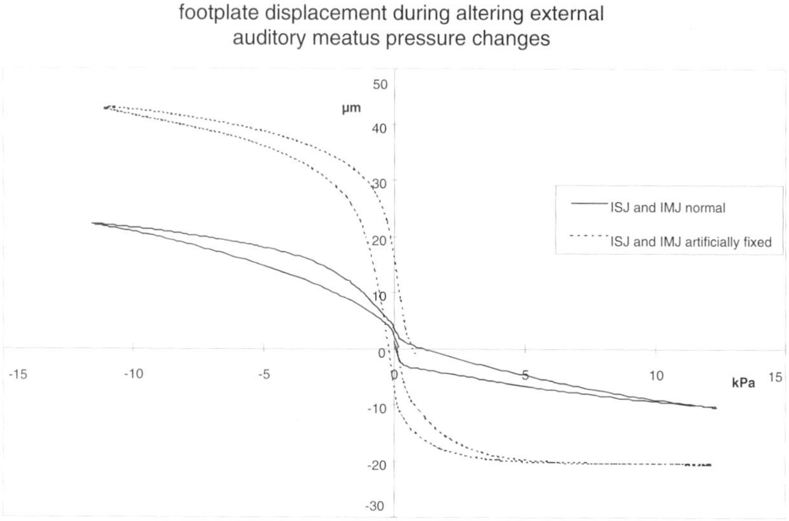

footplate displacement during altering external
auditory meatus pressure changes

Fig. 6. Diagram demonstrating stapes footplate displacement during altering static pressure. The displacement was elevated multiple-fold compared to controls, after artificially ankylosing the ossicular joints.

mens. These experimental results of a two-to-three-fold increase in the magnitude of stapes footplate displacement compared to normals were reproducible in all prepared specimens.

Discussion

A sudden decrease in acoustic middle ear transfer function was found in temporal bone specimens after artificial ankylosis of the ossicular joints and positive atmospheric pressure changes in the external auditory meatus. In contrast to normal middle ears, saturation of the transfer loss was observed at 2 kPa during positive static pressure changes at frequencies of less than 2 kHz (Figs. 2 to 5). The maximal transfer loss in ankylosed ossicular joints was 20 dB at frequencies ≤2 kHz.

The effect of transfer loss in the low frequency range during altering atmospheric pressure changes is well known in clinical practice (*e.g.,* the valsalva maneuver) and has already been described in temporal bone and animal experiments[6,13]. Murakami *et al.*[6] found an acoustic transfer loss of 10 dB after decreasing atmospheric pressure in the tympanic cavity. Wever and Lawrence[14] and Rahm *et al.*[15] confirmed a loss of response of up to 42 dB in the low frequency range and an increase of loudness in the high frequency range, using guinea pigs in their experiments. They concluded that these effects were mainly due to increasing stiffness and damping of the tympanic membrane. This fact coincides with our measurements of non-acoustic footplate displacement during low atmospheric pressure changes. However, at pressure changes beyond 4 kPa, our experimental results suggest that the annular ligament stiffness continues to rise in the normal middle ear. In contrast, a continued increase of the annular ligament stiffness was not observed in cases of ankylosed ossicular joints. These prepared specimens showed maximum footplate displacement even at an atmospheric pressure of 2 kPa. The measured values of 10-30 μm for footplate inward displacement coincide with the results of earlier studies by Hüttenbrink[2,4]. This phenomenon of maximum annular ligament stiffness is considered to be responsible for the sudden acoustic transfer loss of 20 dB at low atmospheric pressure changes in our experimental set-up. Compared to Murakami *et al.*'s study[6], our experimental results demonstrate a higher magnitude of transfer loss. However, it has to be taken into consideration that those authors performed measurements by limiting the atmospheric pressure application to 2 kPa. In comparison to our study, no investigation of acoustic sound transfer after artificial joint fixation was performed.

A surprising but reproducible effect in all our temporal bone specimens was a slight decrease in the stapes vibration magnitudes, as well as a resonance frequency shift to the high frequency range after ankylosis during normal atmospheric pressure conditions. This effect was considered to be a consequence of increased ossicular chain stiffness after gluing of the joints. It demonstrated that the normal ossicular chain is probably not absolutely stiff for acoustic sound transfer. As already described in the literature, the incus, malleus and stapes perform three-dimensional movements during sound excitation that are independent of each other in the high frequency region[9]. It can be assumed that these complex movements require a certain degree of freedom in the ossicular joint cleft. Therefore, fixation of the joints leads to a change in the optimal transfer characteristics. The experimental results of Huber *et al.* support this theory[16]. They found differences in displacement and phase angles between umbo, incus and stapes, and assumed a slippage in the incudo-malleal and incudo-stapedial joint during acoustic transfer function in the high frequency range.

Summarizing our results, we conclude that a combination of altering atmospheric pressure changes in the external auditory meatus and acoustic sound excitation is suitable for detection of ossicular joint ankylosis in temporal bone experiments. However, due to the fact that pressure and ankylosis-induced differences are only 5-10 dB in magnitude, it will be difficult to use these differences in clinical evaluation of the ear. Therefore, it is uncertain whether audiometric investigations with altered pressure changes will be sensitive enough to detect ossicular joint ankylosis. The quest for a clinical tool to investigate and prove the above-mentioned experimental results will be part of our future work to reach the goal of ossicular joint ankylosis detection. These experimental results contain basic experimental data for future investigations of this kind.

References

1. Hüttenbrink KB: The middle ear as a pressure receptor. In: Hüttenbrink KB (ed) Middle Ear Mechanics in Research and Otosurgery, pp 15-20. Dresden: UniMedia 1997

2. Hüttenbrink KB: The mechanics of the middle ear at static air pressure. Acta Otolaryngol (Stockh) Suppl 451:1-36, 1988

3. Cancura W: On the statics of malleus and incus and on the function of the malleus-incus joint. Acta Otolaryngol (Stockh) 89:342-344, 1980

4. Hüttenbrink KB: Ossicle chain mechanics at static air pressures. II: Impaired joint function and reconstructed ossicle chain. Laryngol Rhinol Otol 67:100-105, 1988

5. Mosnier I, Bouccara D, Sterkers O: Sudden hearing loss 1997: etiopathogenic hypothesis, management, prognostic factors and treatment. Ann Otolaryngol Chir Cervicofac 164(7/8):251-266, 1997

6. Murakami S, Gyo K, Goode RL: Effect of middle ear pressure change on middle ear mechanics. Acta Otolaryngol (Stockh) 117:390-395, 1997

7. Marquet J: The incudo-malleal joint. J Laryngol Otol 95:541, 1981

8. Kitahara M, Kodama A, Ozawa H, Iukura H: Mechanism of hearing disturbance due to alteration in atmospheric pressure. Acta Otolaryngol (Stockh) Suppl 510:92-95, 1994

9. Decreamer WF, Khanna SM: Vibration on the malleus measured through the ear canal. In: Hüttenbrink KB (ed) Middle Ear Mechanics in Research and Otosurgery, pp 32-40. Dresden: UniMedia 1997

10. Megighian D, Menegus T, Todesco S, Rossi M: Contribution à l'étude de la fonction de l'oreille moyenne dans l'arthride rhumatoide. Cah Oto-Rhino-Laryngol Chir Cerv Fac 18:685-690, 1983

11. Moffat DA, Ramsden RT, Rosenberg JN, Booth JB, Gibson WPR: Otoadmittance measurements in patients with rheumatoid arthritis. J Laryngol Otol 91:917-927, 1977

12. Reiter D, Konkle DF, Myers AR, Schimmer B, Sugar JO: Middle ear imittance in rheumatoid arthritis. Arch Otolaryngol 106:114-117, 1980

13. Bekesy GV: Zur Theorie des Hörens. Phys Zeits 30:115-125, 1929

14. Wever EG, Lawrence M: Physiological Acoustics. Princeton, NJ: Princeton Univ Press 1954

15. Rahm WE, Strother W, Crump JF: The effects of pressure in the external auditory meatus. Ann Otol Rhinol Laryngol 65:657-664, 1956

16. Huber A, Assai M, Ball G, Goode RL: Analysis of ossicular vibration in three dimensions. In: Hüttenbrink KB (ed) Middle Ear Mechanics in Research and Otosurgery, pp 82-88. Dresden: UniMedia 1997

MIDDLE-EAR RECONSTRUCTION

HISTOPATHOLOGICAL CORRELATES OF RESIDUAL AND RECURRENT CONDUCTIVE HEARING LOSS FOLLOWING TYMPANOPLASTY AND STAPEDECTOMY

Joseph B. Nadol, Jr

Department of Otology and Laryngology, Harvard Medical School; Department of Otolaryngology, Massachusetts Eye and Ear Infirmary, Boston, MA, USA

Abstract

Hearing results following tympanoplasty for chronic otitis media and following stapedectomy for otosclerosis commonly result in either residual or recurrent conductive hearing loss. The purpose of this study was to review the histopathology of human temporal bone specimens from patients who in life had undergone surgery for chronic otitis media or otosclerosis in order to identify probable causes of this hearing loss. In chronic otitis media, these pathological changes include tympanosclerosis, resorptive osteitis of the ossicles, fibrocystic sclerosis and sclerosing osteitis of the temporal bone, fibrous thickening or atrophic changes in the tympanic membrane. In addition, ossicular replacement grafts and prostheses are subject to an inflammatory response and resorption.

Following stapedectomy, the most common causes of residual and recurrent conductive hearing loss include resorptive osteitis of the incus, obliteration of the round window by otosclerosis, unremoved footplate fragments in contact with the prosthesis, contact of the prosthesis with the bony margin of the oval window, adhesions in the middle ear, and new bone formation within the oval window.

Better control of the inflammatory responses in chronic otitis media and following surgical manipulation of the middle ear, either for chronic otitis or for otosclerosis, may decrease the occurrence of residual and recurrent conductive hearing loss and must be considered in modification of procedures and prostheses for these surgeries.

Keywords: residual/recurrent conductive hearing loss, tympanoplasty, stapedectomy

Introduction

Hearing results following tympanoplasty for chronic otitis media, as evaluated by the ability to close the air-bone gap, leave significant room for improve-

Supported by the Lynch Research Endowment Fund

Address for correspondence: Joseph B. Nadol, Jr, MD, Department of Otolaryngology, Massachusetts Eye & Ear Infirmary, 243 Charles Street, Boston, MA 02114, USA

The Function and Mechanics of Normal, Diseased and Reconstructed Middle Ears, pp. 189–203
edited by J.J. Rosowski and S.N. Merchant
© 2000 Kugler Publications, The Hague, The Netherlands

ment. The postoperative air-bone gap is closed to within 20 dB in approximately 50-70% of cases[1-3]. With longer-term follow-up, most authors agree that the results are even poorer[3,4]. Most authors agree that loss of the stapes superstructure is correlated with poorer initial and long-term results[3,5]. Doubtless, improvements in postoperative hearing results can be achieved by improvement of surgical technique and design of implanted devices to improve the motion mechanics of the ossicular chain[6-8]. However, pathological changes induced in the middle ear and mastoid by the chronic suppurative process also limit the hearing results[9-11].

Hearing results following primary stapedectomy are much better than has been reported for tympanoplasty or ossiculoplasty, with initial closure of the air bone gap to 10 dB or less in 90-95% of patients[12]. Over time, however, most authors agree that the air-bone gap increases significantly[12-14], and the ability to the close the air-bone gap to within 10 dB in revision stapedectomy has been reported to be in the range of 18-80% with a mean of approximately 50%[15]. Thus, residual and recurrent conductive hearing loss following stapedectomy remains a significant clinical problem.

It is the purpose of this report to review the histopathology of the middle ear in chronic otitis media and following stapedectomy to provide an overview of the pathological changes that may be correlated with residual and recurrent conductive hearing loss following surgery for these disorders. The pathology of chronic otitis media has been reported previously[16-21]. In this report, pathological alteration of the middle ear which may reasonably be expected to influence the motion mechanics of the tympanic membrane and ossicular chain will be emphasized. Likewise, there have been previous studies of the temporal bones from patients who in life had undergone stapedectomy. Most focused on postoperative complications[22,23], with little attempt to correlate postoperative air-bone gap with the histopathological findings[24-27].

Findings

Histopathology of chronic otitis media

Although some pathological changes, such as mucosal edema, infiltrates of inflammatory cells, and bone resorption, can be expected to be at least partially reversible following control of cholesteatoma and/or the suppurative process, other pathological changes in chronic otitis media cannot be expected to resolve spontaneously and may be very difficult or impossible to reverse surgically. Examples of such pathologies include tympanosclerosis, resorptive osteitis of ossicles, fibrocystic sclerosis and sclerosing osteitis of the temporal bone, and fibrous thickening or atrophic changes in the tympanic membrane.

Tympanosclerosis

Tympanosclerosis results from the deposition of collagen fibrils and subsequent calcification in a submucosal plane of the tympanic membrane, middle ear and mastoid[28]. The pathogenesis of tympanosclerosis is not completely understood. However, most authors agree that it is most commonly seen in temporal bones with other evidence of an inflammatory process[29,30], and that immunological factors[31] may play a role. Certain types of major histocompatibility given complex (HLA) antigens may predispose the patient to formation of tympanosclerosis[32]. By chemical analysis, tympanosclerotic plaques reveal a partially calcified organic matrix with a calcium/phosphate molar ratio similar to hydroxyapatite[33]. Although the most common site of occurrence of tympanosclerosis is the tympanic membrane[30] (Fig. 1), it may be found throughout the middle ear and epitympanum and may cause fixation of the stapes (Fig. 2) and/or malleus and incus (Fig. 3). Tympanosclerosis is not an absolute contraindication to ossiculoplasty. In limited disease, removal of the tympanosclerotic plaque may result in adequate mobilization of the ossicular chain including the stapes[34,35]. In extensive disease, the involved ossicles, including stapes, may require removal[34,36,37]. Closure of the air-bone gap to within 10 dB was achieved in 15% of 311 cases[34] reconstructed for tympanosclerosis.

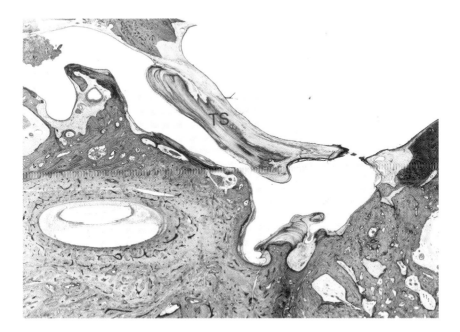

Fig. 1. Tympanosclerosis (TS) of the anterior segment of the right tympanic membrane. The tympanosclerosis extended to the lateral epitympanic wall causing firm fixation of malleus and incus. The patient had a history of chronic inactive otitis media for many years with a conductive hearing loss. (magnification, 11.5x)

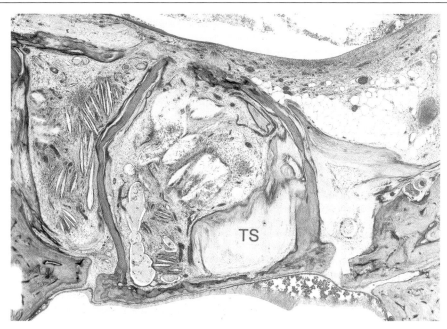

Fig. 2. Tympanosclerosis (TS) causing ankylosis of the stapes in the left ear in a 67-year-old woman. There was a history of chronic otitis media for many years. A canal-down mastoidectomy had been performed eight years before death. Audiometry demonstrated a conductive hearing loss. (magnification, 36x)

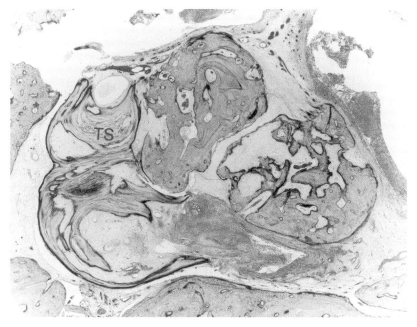

Fig. 3. Tympanosclerosis of the epitympanum. This 35-year-old man had a history of long-standing chronic active otitis media. The ossicles were embedded in fibrous tissue with tympanosclerosis (TS) within the epitympanum in the left ear. (magnification, 26x)

Resorptive osteitis

The term resorptive osteitis seems to have been coined by Schuknecht[20] and refers to an inflammatory process of the ossicles leading to loss of osseous integrity. It is most commonly seen in chronic active otitis media with and without cholesteatoma (Fig. 4). However, it may also occur without evidence of other inflammatory or suppurative process in the tympanomastoid compartment (Fig. 5) where, presumably, it is the result of aseptic necrosis. The cause of this focal bone resorption is probably multi-factorial, including osteolysis caused by inflammatory cells[38,39]. In cases with cholesteatoma, an enzymatic process such as collagenase[40] may also play a role. The degree of resorption of the ossicles cannot always be evaluated clinically at the time of surgery and progression of the osteitis may occur despite control of the inflammatory and suppurative process (personal observation).

Fibrocystic sclerosis

Early inflammatory changes in the middle ear and mastoid caused by chronic otitis media include edema and leukocytic infiltration of the subepithelial plane of middle ear mucosa[21]. Progression of this process leads to extensive submucosal fibrosis and micro-cyst formation in the pneumatized spaces of the middle

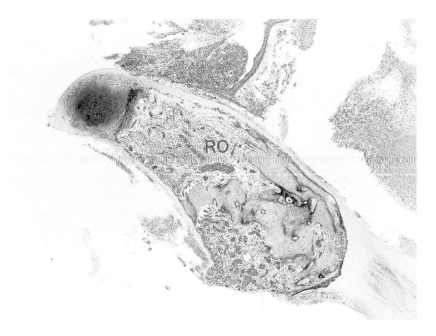

Fig. 4. Resorptive osteitis (RO) of the malleus. This 23-year-old woman had a history of chronic otitis media of the left ear and succumbed to cardiac arrest during mastoid surgery. Advanced resorptive osteitis of both the malleus and incus were found. (magnification, 55x)

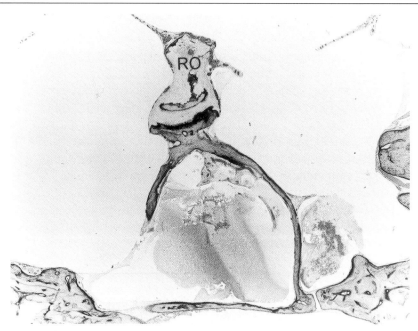

Fig. 5. Resorptive osteitis (RO) of the incus of the right ear. There was no history of chronic otitis media in either ear in this 92-year-old woman. There was no evidence of an active inflammatory process in the middle ear or mastoid. (magnification, 28x)

ear and mastoid[20]. This process may encase ossicles within the epitympanum (Fig. 6) and may extensively involve the middle ear including the oval (Fig. 7) and round windows (Fig. 8). This process is only partially reversible by surgical debridement because of the formation of postoperative cicatrix and difficulty in total removal from the oval and round window areas.

Sclerosing osteitis

New bone formation in response to chronic inflammatory change is common in chronic active otitis media. When extensive, it may be visualized by computerized tomography as sclerosis of the tympanomastoid compartment. Such new bone formation (Fig. 9) may result in sequestration of the tympanomastoid compartment compounding poor pneumatization and may interfere with motion of the ossicular chain.

Fibrosis of the tympanic membrane

Chronic inflammatory change in the tympanomastoid compartment may result in thickening of the fibrous layer of the tympanic membrane. When advanced, it may be expected to interfere with the motion mechanics of the tympanic membrane.

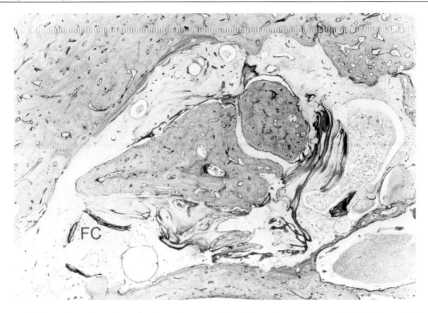

Fig. 6. Fibrocystic sclerosis and sclerosing osteitis of the epitympanum in the left ear. This 89-year-old woman had a history of chronic otitis media of the left ear without cholesteatoma. The pneumatized space of the epitympanum and the aditus were obliterated by fibrocystic change (FC) with areas of tympanosclerosis and new bone formation. (magnification, 16.6x)

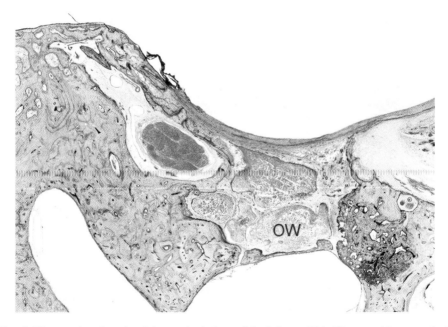

Fig. 7. Fibrocystic sclerosis of the oval window of the left ear. This 76-year-old woman had a history of chronic otitis media of both ears. She underwent a canal-wall tympanomastoidectomy of the left ear 15 years prior to death. The oval window niche (OW) is obliterated by fibrocystic sclerosis (FS). (magnification, 15x)

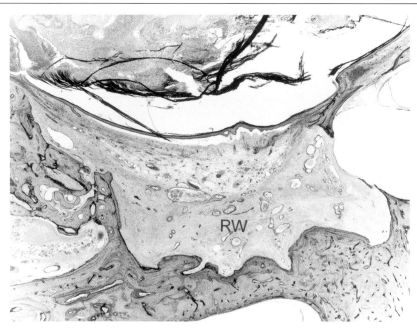

Fig. 8. Fibrocystic obliteration of the left round window (RW) niche. This 71-year-old man had a history of chronic active otitis media of both ears since childhood. He underwent a canal wall down tympanomastoidectomy of the left ear 16 years prior to death. (magnification, 21x)

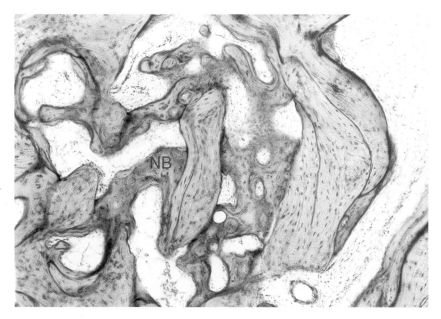

Fig. 9. Sclerosing osteitis of the right temporal bone. This 69-year-old diabetic male had a four-year history of chronic suppuration from the right ear resulting in chronic petrositis. Active bone resorption and osteoneogenesis (NB) were seen. (magnification, 105x)

Atrophic (dimeric) tympanic membrane

Spontaneous healing of a perforation of the tympanic membrane caused by chronic otitis media may result in a secondary membrane which is frequently thin, atrophic, or dimeric. When such atrophic segments of the tympanic membrane are large, interference with transmission of acoustic energy through the tympanic membrane and ossicular chain may be anticipated.

Histopathology of ossicular replacement grafts and prostheses

Bone resorption and surgical necessity to remove components of the ossicular chain in order to remove disease in the medial epitympanum require reconstruction of the ossicular chain. The most commonly used materials are autologous bone grafts or a variety of alloplastic materials, including polyethylene (Plastipore®) and hydroxyapatite. Even in cases in which the suppurative process has been successfully managed, such implanted materials often undergo resorption. Autogenous grafts seem to maintain their osseous integrity for long periods of time, despite death of osteocytes[41] (Fig. 10). Although cartilage grafts may be quite satisfactory in stiffening or reinforcing the tympanic membrane, cartilage is less reliable as an ossicular replacement graft because its propensity for progressive chondromalacia (Fig. 11) results in changes in size and mechanical properties of the graft[41].

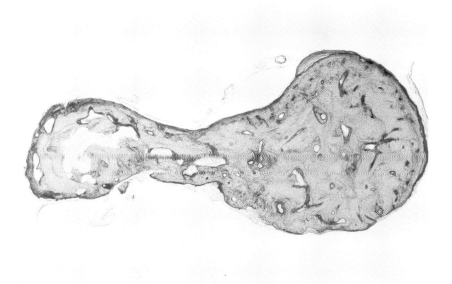

Fig. 10. Malleus autograft. This 52-year-old woman underwent a left mastoidectomy for chronic otitis media and repositioning of a malleus as a sculptured strut. The prosthesis was removed 11 years later for recurrent conductive hearing loss due to fixation of the stapes. Although the bone appears devitalized with loss of osteocytes, there was no evidence of significant bone resorption or inflammatory response. (magnification, 27x)

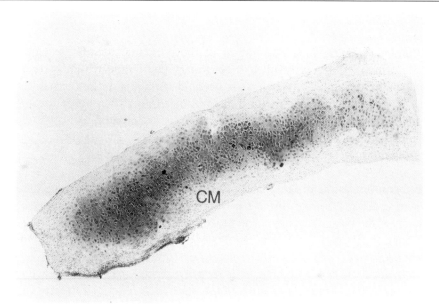

Fig. 11. This patient underwent a revision tympanomastoidectomy with a conchal cartilage graft between a mobile footplate and the tympanic membrane graft. This procedure was revised four years later and the cartilage graft submitted for histopathological study. The cartilage was no longer in contact with the footplate. There was evidence of chondromalacia (CM), particularly at the outer margins of the implant. (magnification, 45x)

Polyethylene (Plastipore®) ossicular replacement prostheses incite a vigorous inflammatory response consisting of plasma cells, lymphocytes and foreign body giant cells (Fig. 12), resulting in frequent resorption and displacement. Although hydroxyapatite prostheses appear to be better tolerated, partial resorption is commonly encountered[42,43].

Histopathology of the middle ear following stapedectomy

Review of the histopathology of the middle ear from patients who in life had undergone stapedectomy provides some insight into the causation of both residual and recurrent conductive hearing loss. In our temporal bone collection, there are 22 cases with a post-stapedectomy air-bone gap greater than or equal to 10 dB (average at 500, 1000, 2000, 3000 and 4000 Hz, using postoperative air and bone conduction thresholds). In 19 cases, there was a residual conductive hearing loss; in two, there was a recurrent conductive loss, and in one case, both residual and recurrent losses. The most common causes of residual and recurrent conductive hearing loss following stapedectomy included resorptive osteitis of the incus (64%) (Fig. 13), obliteration of the round window by otosclerosis (23%) (Fig. 14), the prosthesis lying on an unremoved footplate fragment (23%), the prosthesis abutting a bony margin of the oval window (18%),

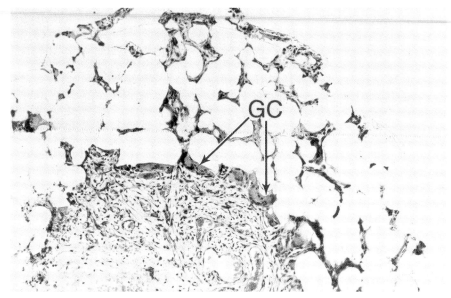

Fig. 12. This 44-year-old woman underwent ossiculoplasty for chronic inactive otitis media using a Plastipore® PORP. Because of residual conductive hearing loss, the procedure was revised within two months. There was a brisk inflammatory response including foreign body giant cells (GC) within the shaft of the prosthesis. (magnification, 83x)

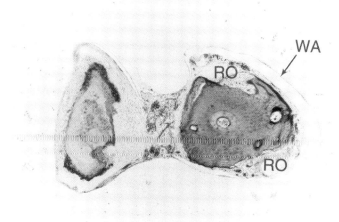

Fig. 13. At the age of 54 years, this patient underwent a total stapedectomy with a drill and the placement of a gel wire incus to oval window prosthesis of the right ear. The first postoperative audiogram at two months showed an average air-bone gap of 0 dB compared to 35 dB preoperatively. However, at 132 months postoperatively, there was a 19 dB recurrent average air-bone gap. He died at 70 years of age. In addition to new bone formation in the oval window, resorptive osteitis (RO) of the incus was seen underlying the wire attachment (WA). (magnification, 60x)

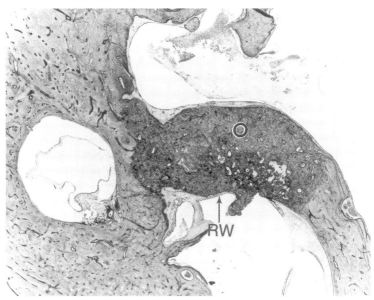

Fig. 14. At the age of 63 years, this patient underwent a stapedectomy using a drill out technique and the placement of a fat-wire incus to oval window prosthesis. There was no apparent improvement of the approximate 30 dB air-bone gap present preoperatively. The patient died at the age of 68 years. Otosclerosis (O) was found to have totally obliterated the round window (RW). (magnification, 19x)

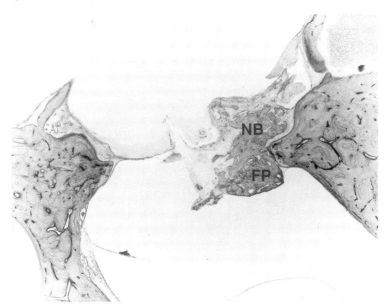

Fig. 15. At the age of 54 years, this man underwent a total stapedectomy using a drill to saucerize the oval window and the placement of an incus to oval window gel wire prosthesis. The postoperative audiogram done at two months, showed an average air-bone gap of 0 dB compared to 35 dB preoperatively. However at 132 months, a 19 dB recurrent average air-bone gap had developed. He died at the age of 70 years. Examination of the temporal bone showed evidence of new bone (NB) in the oval window abutting an otosclerotic footplate fragment (FP). The new bone formation appears to be lamellar bone rather than otosclerosis. (magnification, 22x)

adhesions in the middle ear (14%), or new bone formation within the oval window (14%) (Fig. 15).

Discussion and conclusions

In surgery for chronic otitis media, residual and recurrent conductive hearing loss may be attributed in part to surgical technique and inefficiencies in the motion mechanics of the reconstructed tympanic membrane and ossicular chain. However, the biological response to chronic otitis media, including tympanosclerosis, resorptive osteitis, fibrocystic sclerosis, sclerosing osteitis, and, of course, residual dysfunction of the Eustachian tube, also contribute to residual and recurrent conductive hearing loss.

In primary stapedectomy, residual conductive hearing loss occurs in approximately 10% of cases and, over time, recurrent conductive hearing loss is common. The most common causes of residual and recurrent conductive hearing loss following stapedectomy include resorptive osteitis of the incus and malposition of the prosthesis abutting bony margins of the oval window, due to imperfect original placement or postoperative migration of the device or new bone formation.

Better control of the inflammatory responses in chronic otitis media and following surgical manipulation of the middle ear may decrease the occurrence of residual and recurrent conductive hearing loss.

References

1. Shelton C, Sheehy JL: Tympanoplasty: review of 400 staged cases. Laryngoscope 100(7):69-81, 1990
2. Vartiainen E, Nuutinen J: Long-term hearing results of one-stage tympanoplasty for chronic otitis media. Eur Arch Otorhinolaryngol 249(6):329-331, 1992
3. Farrior JB, Nichols SW: Long-term results using ossicular grafts. Am J Otol 17(3):386-392, 1996
4. Donaldson I, Snow DG: A five year follow up of incus transposition in relation to the first stage tympanoplasty technique. J Laryngol Otol 106(7):607-609, 1992
5. Mills RP: The influence of pathological and technical variables on hearing results in ossiculoplasty. Clin Otolaryngol 18(3):202-205, 1993
6. Merchant SN, Ravicz ME, Puria S, Voss SE, Whitemore KR Jr, Peake WT, Rosowski JJ: Analysis of middle ear mechanics and application to diseased and reconstructed ears. Am J Otol 18(2):139-154, 1997
7. Merchant SN, Ravicz ME, Rosowski JJ: Mechanics of type IV tympanoplasty: experimental findings and surgical implications. Ann Otol Rhinol Laryngol 106(1):49-60, 1997
8. Merchant SN, Ravicz ME, Voss SE, Peake WT, Rosowski JJ: Toynbee Memorial Lecture 1997: Middle ear mechanics in normal, diseased and reconstructed ears. J Laryngol Otol 112(8):715-731, 1998
9. Ojala K, Sorri M: The preoperative state of infection in chronic otitis media correlated with postoperative hearing results. Arch Otorhinolaryngol 234(3):253-262, 1982
10. Ojala K, Sorri M: Late post-operative hearing results correlated with the severity of tissue

changes in ears with chronic otitis media. J Laryngol Otol 97(2):131-139, 1983

11. Merchant SN, McKenna MJ, Rosowski JJ: Current status and future challenges of tympanoplasty. Eur Arch Otorhinolaryngol 255(5):221-228, 1998

12. Shea JJ Jr: Forty years of stapes surgery. Am J Otol 19(1):52-55, 1998

13. Portmann D, Arramon-Tucoo JF: Stapedectomy and micro-stapedotomy in the treatment of otospongiosis: a comparative study. Rev Laryngol Otol Rhinol (Bordeaux) 110(3):317-322, 1989

14. Langman AW, Jackler RK, Sooy FA: Stapedectomy: long-term hearing results. Laryngoscope 101(8):810-814, 1991

15. Han WW, Incesulu A, McKenna MJ, Rauch SD, Nadol JB Jr, Glynn RJ: Revision stapedectomy: intraoperative findings, results and review of the literature. Laryngoscope 107:1185-1192, 1997

16. Friedmann I: The comparative pathology of otitis media-experimental and human. II. The histopathology of experimental cholesteatoma. J Laryngol Otol 69:588-601, 1955

17. Friedmann I: The pathology of otitis media. J Clin Pathol 9:229-236, 1956

18. Friedmann I: The pathology of otitis media III. With particular reference to bone changes. J Laryngol Otol 71:213-220, 1957

19. Meyerhoff WL, Kim CS, Paparella MM: Pathology of chronic otitis media. Ann Otol Rhinol Laryngol 87(6/1):749-760, 1978

20. Schuknecht HF: Pathology of the Ear, 2nd edn. Philadelphia, PA: Lea & Febiger 1993

21. Wright CG, Meyerhoff WL: Pathology of otitis media. Ann Otol Rhinol Laryngol (Suppl) 163:24-26, 1994

22. Wolff D: Untoward sequelae eleven months following stapedectomy. Ann Otol 73:297-304, 1964

23. Schuknecht HF, Jones DD: Stapedectomy: postmortem findings. Ann Otol Rhinol Laryngol 88(Suppl 55):1-43, 1979

24. Lindsay JR: Histologic findings following stapedectomy and polyethylene tube inserts in the human. Ann Otol 70:785-807, 1961

25. Subotic R, Kaufman RS: Human temporal bone findings post stapedectomy: a review of ten cases. Acta Otolaryngol (Stockh) 71(5):385-391, 1971

26. Gibbin KP: The histopathology of the incus after stapedectomy. Clin Otolaryngol 4(5):343-354, 1979

27. Himi T, Igarashi M, Kataura A: Temporal bone histopathology over 15 years post-stapedectomy. Acta Otolaryngol Suppl (Stockh) 447:126-134, 1988

28. Sørenson H, True O: Histology of tympanosclerosis. Acta Otolaryngol (Stockh) 73:18-26, 1971

29. Friedmann I, Galey FR: Initiation and stages of mineralization in tympanosclerosis. J Laryngol Otol 94(11):1215-1229, 1980

30. Bhaya MJ, Schachern PA, Morizono T, Paparella MM: Pathogenesis of tympanosclerosis. Otolaryngol Head Neck Surg 109(3/1):413-420, 1993

31. Schiff M, Poliquin JF, Catanzaro A, Ryan AF: Tympanosclerosis: a theory of pathogenesis. Ann Otol Rhinol Laryngol 89(Suppl 70):1-16, 1980

32. Dursun G, Acar A, Turgay M, Calgüner M: Human leukocyte antigens in tympanosclerosis. Clin Otolaryngol 22(1):62-64, 1997

33. Buyanover D, Tietz A, Luntz M, Sadé J: The biochemical composition of tympanosclerotic deposits. Arch Otorhinolaryngol 243(6):366-369, 1987

34. Kinney SE: Postinflammatory ossicular fixation in tympanoplasty. Laryngoscope 88(5):821-838, 1978

35. Tos M, Lau T, Arndal H, Plate S: Tympaosclerosis of the middle ear: late results of surgical treatment. J Laryngol Otol 104(9):685-689, 1990

36. Morgan WC Jr: Tympanosclerosis. Laryngoscope 87(11):1821-1825, 1977

37. Emmett JR, Shea JJ: Surgical treatment of tympanosclerosis. Laryngoscope 88(10):1642-1648, 1978

38. Endó I, Berco F: Bone destruction in chronic otitis media: a histopathological study. J Laryngol Otol 88(5):413-422, 1974
39. Berger G, Hawke M, Ekem JK: Bone resorption in chronic otitis media: the role of mast cells. Acta Otolaryngol (Stockh) 100(1/2):72-80, 1985
40. Abramson M, Sugita T, Huang CC: The natural history of cholesteatoma. In: Alberti PW, Ruben RJ (eds) Otologic Medicine and Surgery, Vol 1, pp 803-811. New York, NY: Churchill Livingstone 1988
41. Merchant SN, Nadol JB Jr: Histopathology of ossicular implants. Otolaryngol Clin N Am 27(4):813-833, 1994
42. Reck R, Störkel S, Meyer A: Bioactive glass-ceramics in middle ear surgery: an 8-year review. Ann NY Acad Sci 523:100-106, 1988
43. Blayney AW, Williams KR, Erre J-P et al: Problems in alloplastic middle ear reconstruction. Acta Otolaryngol (Stockh) 112:322-327, 1992

SHORT- AND LONG-TERM HEARING RESULTS AFTER MIDDLE EAR SURGERY

John Hamilton and James Robinson

Gloucestershire Royal Hospital, Gloucester, UK

Abstract

The aims of surgical reconstruction of the middle ear conducting apparatus are: to restore an acoustic line between the external meatus and the inner ear; to minimize the acoustic energy absorbed or reflected by such a reconstruction over as wide a range of frequencies as possible; to ensure that the reconstruction is durable; and, by such work, to benefit the patient.

The range of defects presented for reconstruction are many, and the reconstructive techniques and materials diverse. There are few properly conducted scientific comparisons of either techniques or materials to define the optimal approach to any given defect. Even for a given technique, the results of tympanoplasty are unpredictable, and most reconstructions result in a conductive hearing loss. Data relating to long-term outcome are scarce. These issues demand consideration prior to any planned middle ear surgery for hearing loss alone.

This review emphasises the wide distributions of results after tympanoplasty, in order to encourage a more scientific approach to the evaluation of hearing results after middle ear surgery.

Introduction

Wullstein introduced the concept and practise of tympanoplasty nearly half a century ago[1]. Thereafter, reconstructive middle ear surgery progressed rapidly. Within a few years, ossicular surgery[2] and the use of synthetic prostheses[3] were established. Likewise, modern techniques in tympanic membrane reconstruction were introduced[4]. It became apparent that the status of the middle ear prior to surgery should underlie any categorization of middle ear surgery[5]. A natural consequence of such a model is a series of subclassifications describing appropriate reconstructions. This framework could be employed in the meaningful comparison of outcomes in middle ear surgery. In other words, given any basic situation at surgery, it should be possible to establish the relative merits of techniques proposed to reconstruct that situation.

Address for correspondence: John Hamilton, FRCS, Department of Otolaryngology, Gloucestershire Royal Hospital, Great Western Road, Gloucester GL1 3EE, UK. *email:* john.hamilton@dial.pipex.com

The Function and Mechanics of Normal, Diseased and Reconstructed Middle Ears, pp. 205–214
edited by J.J. Rosowski and S.N. Merchant
© *2000 Kugler Publications, The Hague, The Netherlands*

Comparison of surgical interventions in middle ear surgery

The comparison of interventions in medicine is a well-established science[6]. A proposed comparison of two surgical techniques should ensure that the outcome genuinely reflects the difference between the techniques. In other words, there should be no bias in the composition of the two study groups, the personnel providing treatment, or in the measurement of their respective outcomes. If any such bias does exist, the outcome may reflect this rather than the surgery. The gold-standard method for achieving this aim is the prospective, randomized, double-blind controlled trial. A Medline search and review of publications from cholesteatoma and otitis media meetings was performed to identify all prospective randomized controlled trials in tympanoplasty surgery. Only two such trials were found.

Mangham and Lindemann intended to compare the outcomes of ossicular reconstruction using two materials well established for this purpose, ceravital and plastipore[7]. They used a power analysis to define the number of patients needed to test their hypotheses and enrolled patients randomized for treatment over a two-year period. Outcomes were assessed according to postoperative air-bone gap at six months and three years. Results were analyzed at a number of test frequencies and, correcting for multiple outcomes, no difference between the two materials was statistically discernible for either PORPs or TORPs. An unexpected, but extremely important, finding was that a statistically significant difference between the results obtained by the two surgeons was found.

Maassen and Zenner compared the results of different means of reconstructing a deficient long process of incus[8]. They studied incus interposition and two methods of reconnecting the long process to the stapes. They showed that incus interposition was a less effective technique than either means of reconstructing the long process, as measured by air-bone gap. They also showed that only a small test population was required to demonstrate this. Bearing in mind the finding of Mangham and Lindemann, this study is weakened because the surgeons performing the procedures differed between the trial groups.

No other prospectively randomized studies were uncovered. The vast bulk of comparative trials in middle ear reconstructive surgery utilize historical controls. These have been shown in cancer trials to favor the more recent trial wing[9], and this may reflect improvements in nursing and other paramedical care rather than the intended differences in technique. Quite how helpful or misleading such studies are, is therefore not clear. Of course, the other main type of source for information regarding outcomes of middle ear surgery is retrospective tabulation of large personal series.

Information provided by a single large series of operations on the middle ear

A single well-documented large personal series provides considerable useful information regarding the outcomes of reconstructive middle ear surgery. In addition, it illustrates the features which confound this approach.

In the proceedings of the Second International Conference on Cholesteatoma and Mastoid Surgery, Tos published his results with ossiculoplasty in cholesteatomatous ears[10]. This paper was notable by its immense detail of audiometric information. It should be noted that 622 patients were initially included, but that details of 98 were excluded from presentation by virtue of reoperation. It is therefore likely that the results of the presented 524 patients represent a slightly favorable sample from the whole.

Figure 1 shows the results of tympanoplasty as measured by air-bone gap in the range 500-2000 Hz in all 524 ears. It is immediately apparent that there is a wide distribution of outcomes, and that it is uncommon for the conductive hearing loss to be completely eliminated even though the air-bone gap is small for most of these results. In Figure 2, the results are re-analyzed according to preoperative status and reconstructive technique. The air-bone gap is generally least for the intact chain, greatest after round window protection tympanoplasty, and intermediate for intermediate ossicular chain residue prior to surgery. This confirms assertions regarding the importance of preoperative status[5]. Of equal importance is the fact that the distribution of results remains wide for all subgroups. In other words, there is considerable uncertainty regarding audiometric outcome, regardless of preoperative status or operative technique. This uncertainty has a number of significant corollaries. It is difficult to provide a patient with accurate information concerning postoperative hearing status. It is especially difficult to provide a patient with such accurate information if the ossicular chain is badly damaged prior to surgery. Under such circumstances, consideration could be given to the more predictable outcome offered by a hearing aid if there is no indication for surgery other than hearing loss. Further, it may be unwise to be dogmatic about many aspects of reconstructive middle ear surgery when the uncertainty regarding outcome is so large.

Because the distributions above are so wide, the prognostic information they offer is limited, even though statistical tests may show the subgroups to differ significantly. This simply means that these tests can identify differences in the shape of the distributions. In order to have a positive predictive value, the demands on the distributions are more stringent in that they should have very little common data.

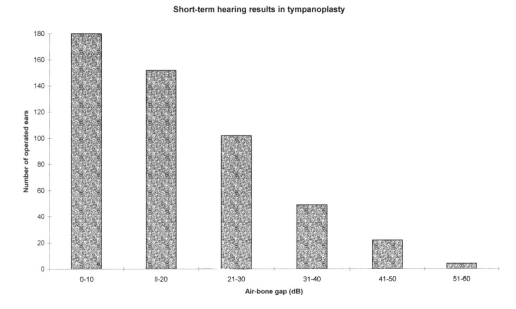

Fig. 1. Initial air-bone gap after middle ear reconstruction. Data from Tos[10].

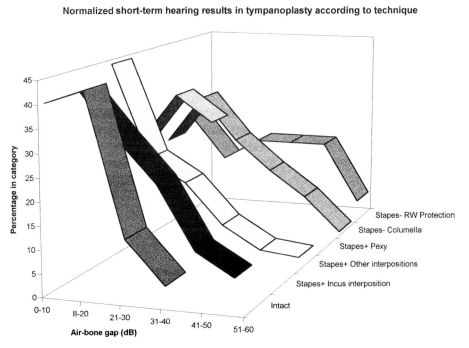

Fig. 2. Initial air-bone gap after middle ear reconstruction. Results stratified according to pre-operative status and nature of reconstruction. Data from Tos[10].

Prognosis in middle ear surgery

Whilst the arguments above indicate the difficulty of identifying prognostic variables based on the retrospective analysis of surgical results, attempts have nonetheless been made to offer prognostic information regarding hearing outcome in middle ear surgery since the early days of tympanoplasty[11]. Sophisticated prognostic indexes have been constructed on the basis of statistical inference from retrospective data[12]. Such data cannot confirm causality and, without some modelling, cannot indicate causal structures within the data. Multivariate analysis of data has been little used after middle ear surgery, and only one paper has specifically investigated this aspect of retrospectively collected information[13]. Babighian and coworkers analyzed their results collected from 540 tympanoplasties, and used multiple logistic regression to identify the principle prognostic factors. They subdivided their procedures according to pathological process prior to analysis, and therefore obtained results separately for simple chronic otitis media, granulating otitis media and cholesteatoma (*see* Table 1). Whilst such data is useful, it only reflects the nature of the data collected. At present, the fundamental variables affecting surgical outcome remain unknown, uncertain or unmeasurable, and so prognostic information based on retrospective data can only have limited application.

Long-term results in tympanoplasty

A very considerable problem complicates the formation of firm conclusions regarding long-term results in tympanoplasty. This is the loss of patients from follow-up (*see* Fig. 3). Because of the incompleteness of the data, the confidence that can be gained from long-term data is limited. Some have even concluded that this lack of information places in question the long-term value of tympanoplasty altogether.

One way of limiting this uncertainty, which maximizes the information provided by the incomplete data, is to reorganize the information as a series of conditional

Table 1. Prognostic factors for tympanoplasty by disease process, according to multivariate analysis of 544 patients. Data according to Albu *et al.*[13]

Simple COM	Granulating COM	Cholesteatoma
mastoidectomy -	manubrium +	intact canal wall
manubrium +	mastoidectomy -	manubrium +
perforation <0.5	revision = 0	stapes arch +
revision = 0	perforation <0.5	revision = 0
stapes arch +	stapes arch +	perforation <0.5

COM: chronic otitis media

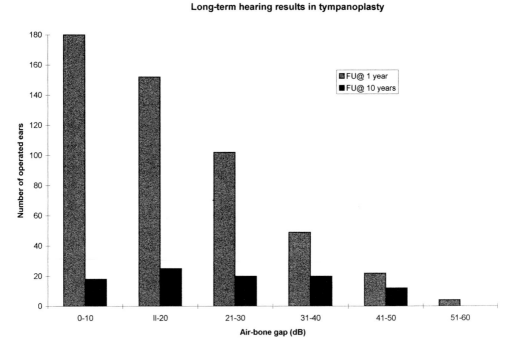

Fig. 3. Comparison of early and late results of tympanoplasty. Note the markedly different numbers in the two distributions. The two distributions also differ significantly (χ^2=26.29; df=5; p<0.001). Data from Tos[10].

probabilities[14]. For instance, the overall probability of good results at year three depends on the overall status at year two. As this procedure is repeated year by year, the information available to furnish early results continues to contribute to late results. This technique is known as life table analysis and has rarely been used to study results in tympanoplasty[15]. So far as we are aware, it has not been used to study ossiculoplasty at all.

We retrospectively analyzed the hearing results of middle ear reconstructions in 332 cholesteatoma operations performed over a 23-year period. Thirty ears had intact ossicular chains. The long process of the incus was eroded in 73 ears, and the interval between the long process and the stapes head was reconstructed with bone pate in all of these. More extensive defects in which the stapes superstructure was retained numbered 103. There were 126 ears in which the stapes superstructure was absent. These four groups were considered separately, even though there were multiple different techniques employed to reconstruct the middle ear within the last two.

A variety of outcome measures was considered. The air-bone gap is considered simple to measure and an index of technical success. However, bone conduction is, in reality, frequently very difficult to measure. The air-bone gap is also an incomplete measure of surgical competence, as it will not identify even a significant deterioration in bone conduction due to technically poor surgery. In the present era,

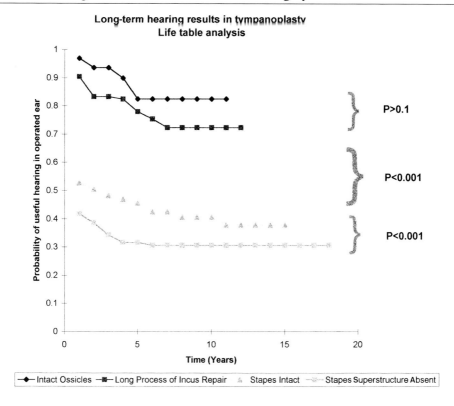

Fig. 4. Life table analysis of long-term audiometric follow-up data of middle ear reconstruction after cholesteatoma. The endpoint denoting failure was defined as air-conduction threshold of 30 dBHL or less. *P* values obtained from log rank tests performed on adjacent survival curves. The apparent difference obtained for long process of incus reconstruction compared with the intact chain is not in fact discernible on formal testing.

patient satisfaction plays an important role in the measurement of surgical success, and so we used a parameter (postoperative air conduction threshold >30 dBHL) shown to be related to patient satisfaction to measure the success of surgery[16]. Hearing <30 dBHL was regarded as a failure, and this endpoint was used to construct the life table analysis. The conditional probability curves are shown in Figure 4.

Strikingly, in the groups with substantial ossicular damage at the time of surgery, reconstruction often did not provide useful hearing in even the short term. In addition, all the curves show some deterioration with time. However, this appears to be small in all groups and is principally limited to the early years of follow-up. It is possible to compare entire probability curves using the log-rank test, and this identifies no difference between the results of the intact chain and reconstructed long process of incus groups. All the other groups are significantly different from one another.

When confidence intervals are added to the curves, a clearer image of the uncer-

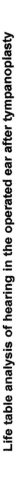
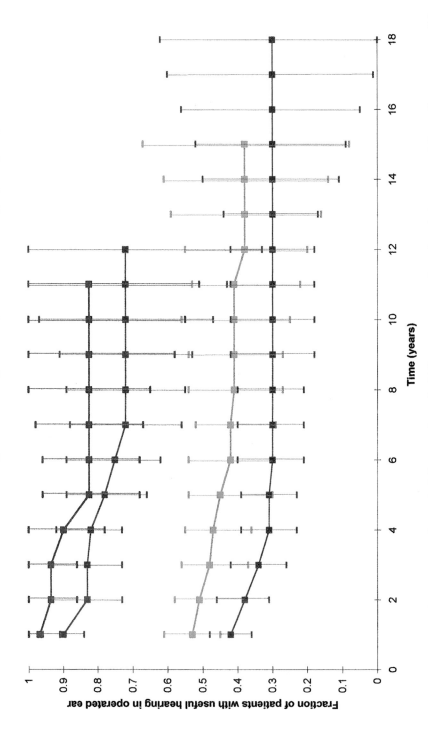

Fig. 5. Life table analysis of long-term audiometric follow-up data of middle ear reconstruction after cholesteatoma. Ninety-five percent confidence intervals included.

tainty associated with the data is obtained (*see* Fig. 5). It is doubtful whether any firm conclusions can be drawn from the last third of the conditional probability curves.

Conclusions

The distribution of hearing results in middle ear surgery is wide, regardless of preoperative status or operative technique.

There is a tendency to better and less variable hearing results, the less the ossicular chain is diseased.

Whilst observational studies on large series provide basic data on the outcomes of surgery, they do not provide unequivocal answers, and provide only the most rudimentary prognostic information. Consequently, further observational studies on large series are unlikely to answer any fundamental questions in tympanoplasty.

Answers to fundamental questions in tympanoplasty are more likely to result from advances in basic science and a more scientific approach to testing hypotheses in clinical practice.

The collection of long-term results requires an immense amount of effort. Firm conclusions regarding results beyond eight to ten years cannot yet be drawn, even from observational studies.

Humility and caution are required when considering middle ear hearing reconstruction in severely damaged ears. The value of the reconstruction to the patient may be modest, particularly if there is even minor sensorineural hearing loss prior to surgery.

References

1. Wullstein HL: Theory and practice of tympanoplasty. Laryngoscope 66:1076, 1956
2. Hall A, Rytzner C: Stapedectomy and auto-transplantation of ossicles. Acta Otolaryngol (Stockh) 47:318-324, 1957
3. Shea JJ: Fenestration of the oval window. Ann Otol Rhinol Laryngol 67:932, 1958
4. Ortegren U: Trumhinneplastik. Forhandlinger i Svensk Otolaryngol Forening 1958/1959
5. Farrior JB: Classification of tympanoplasty. Arch Otolaryngol 93:548-550, 1971
6. Bradford Hill A: A Short Textbook of Medical Statistics, 11th edn. London: Hodder and Stoughton 1984
7. Mangham CA, Lindemann RC: Ceravital versus Plastipore in tympanoplasty: a randomized prospective trial. Ann Otol Rhinol Laryngol 99:112-116, 1990
8. Maassen MM, Zenner HP: Tympanoplasty type II with ionomeric cement and titanium-gold-angle prostheses. Am J Otol 19:693-699, 1998
9. Sacks HS, Chalmers TC, Smith H: Sensitivity and specificity of clinical trials: randomized versus historical controls. Arch Int Med 143:753-755, 1983
10. Tos M: Short- and long-term results with ossiculoplasty in cholesteatomatous ears. In: Sadé J (ed) Cholesteatoma and Mastoid Surgery, pp 547-558. Amsterdam: Kugler Publ 1982

11. Bellucci RJ: Basic considerations for success in tympanoplasty. Arch Otolaryngol 90:732-741, 1969

12. Black B: Ossiculoplasty prognosis: the SPITE method of assessment. Am J Otol 13:544-551, 1992

13. Albu S, Babighian G, Trabalzini F: Prognostic factors in tympanoplasty. Am J Otol 19:136-140, 1998

14. Peto R, Pike MC, Armitage P: Design and analysis of randomised clinical trials requiring prolonged observation of each patient. I. Introduction and design. Br J Cancer 34:585-612, 1976

15. Smyth GDL: Results of middle ear reconstruction: do patients and surgeons agree? Am J Otol 6:276-279, 1985

16. Halik JJ, Smyth GDL: Long-term results of tympanic membrane repair. Otolaryngol Head Neck Surg 98:162-169, 1988

SURGERY FOR CONGENITAL CONDUCTIVE DEAFNESS

A retrospective study of 37 cases

Tsun-Sheng Huang

Department of Otolaryngology – Head & Neck Surgery, Chang Gung Memorial Hospital, Chang Gung University, Taipei, Taiwan

Abstract

A retrospective study was conducted of 37 cases of surgery for congenital conductive deafness where anomalies were confined to the middle ear, in order to assess the efficacy and applicability of corrective surgical procedures. Reconstructive surgery was performed in 25 cases (68%) with the expectation of good hearing results and without complications, and in five additional cases (14%) in which good hearing results were not expected, but in which no complications were anticipated. Corrective procedures were abandoned in the remaining seven cases (19%) because of conditions observed during exploratory surgery which were judged to pose a risk of complications. For the above-mentioned 25 cases, a mean postoperative hearing level of 23.2 dB (average gain of 30.3 dB pure-tone average) was achieved, as well as complete or near closure of the air-bone gap in almost all cases. As expected, little or no hearing gain was achieved in the five additional cases, although there were no complications. Notable in this series is the relatively high incidence of misdiagnosis of fenestral otosclerosis (ten cases or 27%), which may be attributed mainly to a lack of audiological testing in childhood. Also of interest was cholesteatoma-like material in place of the incus or of both the incus and stapes (five cases) and fibrous material in place of the incus or incus long process (two cases). On the basis of these results, it can be concluded that reconstructive surgery, in cases in which conditions are favorable, offers consistently excellent hearing results, and late detection of conductive deafness increases the possibility of the misdiagnosis of otosclerosis.

Keywords: congenital conductive deafness, ossicular reconstruction

Introduction

As reported in the literature[1], congenital abnormalities of the ear are rare, with a reported estimated incidence of only one case in 15,000 people, while con-

Address for correspondence: Tsun-Sheng Huang, MD, Department of Otolaryngology – Head & Neck Surgery, Chang Gung Memorial Hospital, 199 Tung Hwa North Road, Taipei, Taiwan, Republic of China

The Function and Mechanics of Normal, Diseased and Reconstructed Middle Ears, pp. 215–224
edited by J.J. Rosowski and S.N. Merchant
© 2000 Kugler Publications, The Hague, The Netherlands

genital anomalies of the middle ear are even rarer. In our experience, however, it would seem that such anomalies are not so infrequently observed in daily practice.

Symptomatically, congenital conductive deafness is typically characterized by a nonfluctuating conductive hearing loss in the range 40-60 dB pure-tone average (PTA), an air-bone gap over 40 dB PTA, a type D or A tympanogram, and onset in early childhood, assuming the absence of a history of trauma or serious middle ear infection or effusion, which may produce similar symptoms. External auditory canal atresia, microtia, and other abnormalities of the external ear are strong indicators of probable middle ear anomalies inasmuch as the external and middle ears are closely linked developmentally[1]. However, congenital middle ear abnormalities can occur without any concomitant malformation of the external ear. Although developmentally linked, the inner ear is not intimately linked with the middle ear, and the associated frequency of inner ear and middle ear anomalies has been estimated to be 10-30%[2,3], for which reason congenital inner ear abnormalities must nevertheless be taken as signs of possible congenital middle ear abnormalities.

The most obvious radiographic indication of congenital conductive deafness is a gap in the ossicular chain, sometimes in conjunction with a small tympanic cavity. Radiological examination is also useful for eliminating the possibility that conductive deafness is caused by congenital cholesteatoma of the middle ear, as well as for checking for congenital inner ear abnormalities. However, radiological testing does not definitely reveal various types and degrees of anomalous conditions of the middle ear ossicles, oval window, or facial nerve, even when advanced high-resolution computed tomography (HRCT) techniques are employed.

When aural anomalies are confined to the middle ear, the most common surgical procedure used for the treatment of congenital conductive deafness is ossiculoplasty. In uncommon cases of footplate fixation, stapedectomy or stapedotomy is used, replacing the earlier practice of fenestration of the horizontal semicircular canal. However, the latter procedure is still used by some physicians in extremely rare cases of an anomalous facial nerve occluding the oval window, which precludes ossicular chain reconstruction.

Reports of the results of hearing after the surgical correction of anomalous middle ear conditions are sparse, as are the reported rates of corrective surgical procedures being abandoned intraoperatively, and discussions of the reasons for this abandonment.

The purpose of this paper is to analyze and discuss our experience in a series of 37 cases of surgery for congenital conductive deafness associated with isolated middle ear anomalies, paying particular attention to: the efficacy of reconstructive surgery in cases in which it is applicable; intraoperative decision-making with regard to such applicability; and, the incidence of various types of anomalies. Attention is also given to the possibility of misdiagnosis of otosclerosis among adults who did not receive audiological evaluation during their childhood.

Material and methods

Patient profile and diagnostic indications

Between December 1989 and August 1999, surgery was performed by us on a total of 37 ears (25 right, 12 left) of 36 patients with congenital conductive deafness caused by isolated middle ear anomalies (excluding cases of microtia and/or meatal atresia, but including three ears with minor external ear abnormalities: one instance of a circumferentially contracted tympanic sulcus relative to the external auditory canal, and two of a small, slightly deformed auricle and slightly contracted external auditory canal). The 36 patients included 22 females and 14 males, averaging 28.1 years of age (range, 10-52 years) at the time of operation. Surgery was performed on both ears of only one patient, with an interval of nine years between operations.

Preoperatively, 27 of the 37 ears (26 patients) were diagnosed as having congenital conductive deafness and as being candidates for reconstructive surgery based on: *a.* a history of fixed hearing loss with onset at birth; *b.* normal or near-normal bone conduction thresholds (with the exception of one case of 57 dB loss); *c.* a flat air-conduction loss greater than 40 dB PTA; *d.* a wide air-bone gap; and/or *e.* a type D or A tympanogram; in addition to *f.* a normal mastoid, as indicated either by conventional radiology or, in some cases, by HRCT. Surgery was performed on the remaining ten ears (ten patients) for treatment of clinically diagnosed fenestral otosclerosis. The misdiagnoses mentioned were based on combinations of diagnostic indications contrary to the above-mentioned criteria, the most frequent and misleading of them being adult patients' claims of onset of hearing impairment after childhood and/or progressive hearing loss.

In accordance with the 1995 Guidelines of the American Academy of Otolaryngology – Head and Neck Surgery (AAO-HNS)[4], the PTA was calculated using 0.5, 1, 2 and 3 kHz frequencies (using 4 kHz values in rare cases in which 3 kHz values were not available), and air-bone gaps were calculated with a pure-tone bone-conduction average at 1, 2 and 4 kHz. Preoperatively, the mean air-conduction hearing threshold for the 37 ears was 56.9 dB PTA (range, 24-98 dB) with a mean air-bone gap of 36.3 dB (range, 21-67 dB). Apparently, few if any of the patients had undergone audiological evaluation in childhood.

Intraoperative findings and surgical management

The intraoperatively-observed conditions that determined the decision of whether to perform reconstructive surgery and the expectation of success, are summarized in Table 1. Reconstruction was performed on 25 ears (group 1) with the expectation of hearing improvement, including 24 cases in which there was no fixation of the footplate and one case with a fixed footplate in which it was

Table 1. Conditions accompanying ossicular deformity in 37 cases, determining the decision to perform reconstructive surgery

Condition	Cases (n)	Condition	Cases (n)
Group 1: reconstruction performed with expectation of hearing improvement (n=25)			
Discontinuity; no fixation of footplate	20	Cholesteatoma-like or fibrous material in place of incus or incus/stapes; no fixation of footplate	4
Discontinuity; fixation of footplate; facial nerve under oval window (small fenestra stapedotomy)	1		
Group 2: reconstruction performed with little expectation of hearing improvement (n=5)			
Discontinuity; limited mobility of footplate	4	Discontinuity; footplate mobility uncertain due to partial occlusion of oval window by facial nerve	1
Group 3: reconstruction not performed due to severity of anomalies (n=7)			
Discontinuity; total occlusion of oval window by facial nerve	3	Discontinuity; fixation of footplate	2
Discontinuity; absence of round window	1	Discontinuity; very small oval window	1

judged that stapedotomy could be performed with little risk of complications. Reconstruction was also performed on five additional ears (group 2) in which little or no hearing gain could realistically be expected, due to limited mobility or suspected immobility of the footplate. Reconstruction was not attempted in seven of the 37 cases (group 3) because of various congenital anomalous conditions observed during exploratory surgery which, in our judgment, posed considerable danger of complications and/or offered little chance of hearing improvement. These included an anomalous facial nerve occluding the oval window, a fixed footplate, absent round window, or a very small oval window.

The frequency of ossicular involvement observed intraoperatively in this series is shown in Table 2. In addition to deformities or the absence of ossicles, grainy, whitish cholesteatoma-like material was found in place of the incus in three cases, and in place of both the incus and stapes in two cases. Fibrous material was found in place of the incus in one case and in place of the incus long process in another case. Nonossicular aural irregularities included an anomalously coursing facial nerve (five cases, occluding the oval window in four cases, inferior to the oval window in one case), a small oval window (two cases), and absence of the round window (one case).

The main procedure used in the 30 cases of reconstruction surgery was ossiculoplasty, with either homograft incus interposition (21 cases) or autograft incus interposition (five cases). Ossiculoplasty with total ossicular replacement prostheses (TORP) was used in three cases, all prior to March 1995. In the

Table 2. Incidence of ossicular involvement (deformity or absence)

Ossicle	Single ossicle			Multiple-ossicle combination			Overall incidence per ossicle		
	I	S	M	IS	ISM	SM	I	S	M
No. of cases	8	3	0	20	5	1	33	29	6
Percentage of cases*	21.6	8.1	0	54.1	13.5	2.7	89.2	78.4	16.2

I: incus; S: stapes; M: malleus; *percentage of 37 cases

Table 3. Hearing thresholds (dB PTA) and air-bone gaps* pre- and postoperatively in group 1 (25 cases in which reconstruction was performed with the expectation of hearing improvement)

	Air conduction average (range)		Bone conduction average (range)		Air-bone gap average (range)		Hearing gain average (range)	
Preoperative	53.5	(24-98)	11.9	(3-57)	41.6	(21-62)	—	
Postoperative**	23.2	(3-62)	12.3	(3-52)	10.9	(0-44)	30.3	(6-45)

*In accordance with AAO-HNS (1995) guidelines; **at latest follow-up (average, 5.4 months)

remaining case, a small fenestra stapedotomy using a Teflon® piston was carried out. The postauricular approach was used in all cases.

Results

Follow-up audiological testing was typically performed at one-, three-, six- and 12-monthly intervals, and irregularly at later times (average follow-up period, 5.5 months).

At the latest follow-up, the five ears for which there seemed to be little chance of success had indeed shown no hearing gain, but also little or no worsening.

In the 25 ears upon which ossicular reconstruction was performed with a good chance of success (Table 3), postoperative audiometry showed, a. a mean 23.2 dB hearing threshold (range, 3-62 dB), representing a mean gain of 30.3 dB, and b. a mean air-bone gap of 10.9 dB (range, 0-44 dB), representing a mean air-bone gap closure of 30.7 dB. Five of these 25 operations resulted in a hearing threshold greater than 30 dB (average, 45.3 dB; range, 33-62 dB), but nevertheless achieved a mean gain of 26.6 dB. Only four of the 25 operations resulted in a hearing gain of less than 20 dB (average, 11.8 dB), and only four operations resulted in an air-bone gap exceeding 15 dB (average, 26.1 dB), representing a mean air-bone gap reduction of 20.0 dB.

No complications occurred intra- or postoperatively in any of the operations.

Discussion

Efficacy and applicability of surgical procedures

Reconstructive surgery in the 25 cases (64.1%) in which it was deemed to have a good chance of success, without the risk of complications (group 1), resulted in a mean hearing threshold of 23.2 dB, representing an average hearing gain of 30.3 dB, and complete or near closure of the air-bone gap in almost all cases, without complications. This mean hearing level falls within the range of hearing levels (20–25 dB) which others have stated to be normally attainable after reconstructive surgery[5]. A 'comfortable' hearing level better than 30 dB was achieved in 20 (80%) of these 25 cases, while in the remaining five cases (20%), a significant average gain of 26.6 dB was obtained. Overall, including the 12 cases in which reconstructive procedures were either abandoned or performed with little expectation of hearing improvement, the end result in 21 of the total 37 cases (56.8%) was a hearing threshold better than 30 dB.

Based on this series, therefore, it can be concluded that ossicular reconstructive surgery for congenital conductive deafness, in cases of isolated middle ear anomalies where conditions are judged favorable, provides consistently excellent results. Moreover, in our experience, hearing gains confirmed within the first few months of follow-up are almost always maintained over the long term.

It is our guiding principle to attempt reconstructive or other corrective procedures only when intraoperatively observed conditions do not pose a serious risk of complications, especially in view of the fact that, in our experience, and as emphasized by others[5,6], hearing aids can provide excellent rehabilitation of conductive hearing loss (which patients must be made to understand before making the decision to undergo an operation). Also, for this reason, we use relatively riskier procedures such as stapedectomy sparingly, and never use fenestration of the horizontal semicircular canal. With regard to the latter procedure, some physicians choose to perform it rather than to abandon corrective surgery when an anomalously coursing facial nerve occludes the oval window. However, this operation is tricky, and should only be undertaken by physicians who have become highly skilled in its performance through extensive laboratory experience[5].

In connection with surgical procedures, it is also worth noting that the external auditory canals and eardrums of Oriental people tend to be smaller than those of Caucasians. For this reason, we prefer to use the postauricular approach when possible in surgery for congenital conductive deafness as well as for other surgically treatable ear maladies, although other authors report that an external endaural incision is the preferred approach in reconstructive ear surgery[6,7].

Incidence of anomalies

In contrast with other reports stating that the stapes is the most commonly involved ossicle in congenital conductive deafness[8-10], the ossicle most commonly involved in this series (limited to cases of isolated middle ear anomalies) was the incus, in 33 of the 37 cases (89.2%), whereas stapes-related irregularities occurred in 29 cases (78.4%). The malleus was only involved in six cases (16.2%), and *no* isolated malleus anomalies were found, which was only to be expected, given the fact that all eardrums in this series were intact and that development of a normal tympanic membrane implies development of a normal or near-normal malleus connected to the eardrum. The most common combination of ossicular anomalies was incus-stapes, occurring in 20 cases (54.1%). Overall, incus-stapes anomalies were also the most common congenital ossicular problem in this series, as was also the case in an earlier series (18 of 68 cases)[9].

A rather interesting and relatively common finding in this series with respect to ossicles, apparently not yet reported in the literature, was whitish, grainy cholesteatoma-like material in place of the incus (three cases) or in place of both the incus and stapes (two cases), which was so fragile that it was easily removed by suction. Regrettably, the nature of this material is uncertain as no histological studies were conducted. Findings of fibrous material in place of the incus or incus long process (two cases) parallel earlier findings of a fibrous incudostapedial joint[11,12].

Also of interest, with respect to the incidence of associated, nonossicular anomalies of the middle ear, is the fact that in five of the 37 cases (13.5%) an anomalously coursing facial nerve was involved (three of which have been reported previously[13]). This associated frequency seems surprisingly high, in view of the extreme rarity of reports of this phenomenon (in our estimation, and including the present five cases, no more than 50 cases have been reported in the literature by us[13] and by others since it was first described by Henner in 1960[14] and observed by others at earlier dates, *e.g.*, as cited by Durcan *et al.*[15]). In consideration of this finding, it is worth emphasizing that in all cases where congenital conductive deafness is a possibility, it is imperative *a.* to maintain a high index of suspicion of a dangerously dislocated facial nerve in order to obviate damage to it, and *b.* routinely to use HRCT to check for the presence of this and/or other anomalies.

Reasons for and implications of delayed diagnosis

While in other countries, corrective surgery for congenital conductive deafness is less often conducted in adulthood than in childhood or adolescence[16], in the present series only 11 patients were under 20 years of age, and only four of these were under 12 years old. Furthermore, as previously mentioned, it appeared that few, if any, of the patients had undergone audiological evaluation in childhood.

Although there are no published statistical analyses to prove this, it is our impression that the delayed detection and surgical treatment of various ear diseases is more common in Taiwan than in other countries. For example, as earlier reported by us[17], while in the past two or more decades, there has been a trend in other countries toward the detection and surgical treatment of congenital cholesteatoma in early childhood, of the 12 patients presenting with this disease at Chang Gung Memorial Hospital between 1984 and 1992 (out of a total of 1611 cases of surgery for cholesteatoma during that period), eight were adults, ranging in age from 20 to 35 years, one was a teenager of 15 years, and only three were children, aged ten, seven and five years.

It may reasonably be conjectured that the major reason for this pattern of delayed diagnosis and surgical treatment is the fact that Taiwan has only in recent years become an affluent country with relatively well-developed health services, including widespread health insurance coverage, widely available medical facilities, and referring physicians experienced in the diagnosis of various ear diseases. One indication of the likely validity of this sociological interpretation is the fact (Table 4) that 20 of the 37 operations in this series (54.1%) were performed during the seven-year period from December 1989 to December 1996, representing a rate of 2.8 operations per year; whereas, in contrast, the remaining 17 operations (45.9%) were performed during the much shorter 2.75-year period from January 1997 to August 1999, at a rate of 6.2 operations per year. This represents a 100%-plus increase in the average yearly number of cases of isolated middle ear abnormalities in the more recent period compared to the earlier period, far out-pacing the growth in Taiwan's population.

It might reasonably be expected that, as the result of improved health care standards, the average age of patients in the more recent period mentioned above would be lower than that of those in the earlier period. In fact, however, the average age in the more recent period was higher, 28.1 years, compared to 27.1 years in the earlier period (Table 4). This probably reflects the fact that routine audiological testing of young children, common in other countries, has yet to be instituted in Taiwan, despite improvements in health care.

Table 4. Time period versus number of operations for congenital conductive deafness involving isolated middle ear anomalies and average age of patients at time of surgery

Time period	December 1989- December 1996 (7.08 years)	January 1997- August 1999 (2.75 years)	December 1989- August 1999 (total, 9.83 years)
Operations (*n*)	20	17	37
Average operations/year	2.8	6.2	3.8
Average age (years)	27.1	29.3	28.1

Besides making earlier improvement in hearing possible, routine audiological evaluation in childhood, including tympanometric testing, may have the added advantage of helping to avoid misdiagnosis of otosclerosis, so common in the present series (ten of 37 cases, or 27%). Because the audiometric indications for congenital conductive deafness and those for fenestral otosclerosis are often similar, and because ears with either of these maladies commonly manifest a normal mastoid, misdiagnosis of otosclerosis is possible when HRCT does not clearly indicate middle ear anomalies, and especially when patients are adults who, for whatever reason, have reported onset of deafness after early childhood and/or progressive hearing loss. Among children, conductive hearing impairment is a much stronger indication of congenital conductive deafness than of fenestral otosclerosis, whereas among adults the reverse is true. Therefore, delayed detection of conductive deafness increases the likelihood of a misunderstanding arising from a patient's faulty reporting of their history, as appears to have occurred in most of the ten misdiagnoses in this series, where the patients ranged in age from 16 to 49 years (average age, 32.2 years).

Conclusions

In cases of congenital conductive deafness associated with isolated middle ear anomalies, where intraoperatively observed conditions are judged favorable, ossicular chain reconstructive surgery offers a consistently effective, safe alternative to hearing amplification.

In all cases where congenital conductive deafness is a possibility, a high index of suspicion of an anomalously coursing facial nerve must be maintained, requiring extreme caution in the exploratory phase of surgery, and HRCT should routinely be used in order to check for this and for other aural congenital anomalies.

Routine audiological evaluation and detection of conductive deafness in childhood, in addition to enabling earlier hearing improvement, can significantly reduce the possibility of misdiagnosis of otosclerosis in cases of congenital conductive deafness arising from a patient's inaccurate reporting of his or her history.

References

1. Nager GT, Levin LS: Congenital aural atresia: embryology, pathology, classification, genetics and surgical management. In: Paparella M, Shumrick D (eds) Otolaryngology, Vol 2, pp 1303-1344. Philadelphia, PA: WB Saunders Co 1980
2. Jafek BW, Nager GT, Strafe J, Gayler RW: Congenital aural atresia: an analysis of 311 cases. Ann Otol Rhinol Laryngol 80:588-595, 1975
3. Patterson ME, Linthicum FH: Congenital hearing impairment. Otol Clin N Am 3:201-219, 1970
4. Committee on Hearing and Equilibrium: Committee on Hearing and Equilibrium guide-

lines for the evaluation of results of treatment of conductive hearing loss. Otolaryngol Head Neck Surg 113(3):186-187, 1995

5. Farrior JB: Fenestration of the horizontal semicircular canal in congenital conductive deafness. Laryngoscope 95:1029-1036, 1985

6. De La Cruz A, Doyle KJ: Ossiculoplasty in congenital hearing loss. Otolaryngol Clin N Am 27:799-811, 1994

7. Jahrsdoerfer RA: Congenital atresia of the ear. Laryngoscope 88(Suppl 13):1-48, 1978

8. Cavo JW, Pratt LL, Alonso WA: First branchial cleft syndromes and associated congenital hearing loss. Laryngoscope 86:739, 1976

9. Jahnke K, Schrader M: Surgery for congenital aural atresia. Adv Otorhinolaryngol 40:1, 1988

10. Swartz JD, Faerber EN: Congenital malformation of the external and middle ear: high-resolution CT findings of surgical import. AJR 144:501-506, 1985

11. Maran AGD: The Treacher-Collins syndrome. Arch Otolaryngol 78:135, 1964

12. Brackmann DE, Sheehy JL, Luxford WM: TORPs and PORPs in tympanoplasty: a review of 1042 operations. Otolaryngol Head Neck Surg 92:32, 1984

13. Huang TS: Anomalously coursing facial nerves above and below the oval window: three case reports. Otolaryngol Head and Neck Surg 116:438-441, 1997

14. Henner F: Congenital middle ear malformations. Arch Otolaryngol 71:454-461, 1960

15. Durcan DJ, Shea JJ, Sleeckx JP: Bifurcation of the facial nerve. Arch Otolaryngol 86:619-631, 1976

16. Sperling NM, Patel N: A patient-benefit evaluation of unilateral congenital conductive hearing loss presenting in adulthood: should it be repaired. Laryngoscope 109:1386-1391, 1999

17. Huang TS, Lee FP: Congenital cholesteatoma: review of twelve cases. Am J Otol 15:276-281, 1994

INACTIVATED HOMOGRAFTS IN RECONSTRUCTIVE MIDDLE EAR SURGERY

Michel A. Hotz[1], Tracy Orr[2], Andrew D. Speirs[2] and Rudolf Häusler[1]

[1]Department of Ear, Nose and Throat Surgery; [2]M.E. Müller Institute for Biomechanics, Inselspital, Bern, Switzerland

Abstract

This study examined the effects of NaOH inactivation techniques on mechanical homograft properties. The clinical data of ten implanted patients are presented. Thirty-three normal ossicles received either treatment with *1.* NaOH, *2.* NaOH followed by autoclaving, *3.* NaOH followed by freeze-drying, or *4.* no treatment. All ossicles underwent destructive axial compression in a mechanical testing machine measuring force and displacement. Compared to controls, NaOH-treated ossicles showed a significant decrease in material properties' ultimate strength and elastic modulus. The additional treatments of freeze-drying and autoclaving caused no significant deterioration of mechanical properties. The anatomical and audiological results of implanted patients were comparable to those of patients implanted with untreated or formalin-cialit treated homografts. No adverse effects or extrusions were observed. The combined NaOH-autoclave inactivation procedure produces similar material homograft changes and clinical and audiological results that are similar to NaOH treatment alone and also to effects of older formaldehyde/cialit treatments.

Keywords: ossicle, homograft, structure, inactivation, middle ear surgery

Introduction

When pathological conditions exist in the middle ear, autograft (where the donor is also the recipient), homo- or allograft (human ossicles from an organ donor program) ossicles are used to replace diseased ossicles in middle ear reconstruction[1]. Allografts offer good functional results at a low cost[2-6]. Even though they are graded class 4 (non-detectable) in the World Health Organization (WHO) classification for spongioform encephalopathies[7], allograft ossicles may involve a minimal risk of viral, bacterial, and/or prion disease transmission from donor to recipient. The recommended screening procedures to use only intact tissues cannot guarantee safety; some diseases may be undetectable

Address for correspondence: M.A. Hotz, MD, Clinic of ENT, Head and Neck Surgery, Inselspital, 3010 Bern, Switzerland. *email:* michael.hotz @insel.ch

The Function and Mechanics of Normal, Diseased and Reconstructed Middle Ears, pp. 225–230
edited by J.J. Rosowski and S.N. Merchant
© 2000 Kugler Publications, The Hague, The Netherlands

during the incubation period. Therefore, homograft ossicles have to undergo a safe and effective treatment in order to inactivate infection agents and yet maintain proper preservation. Until recently, formaldehyde was most frequently used as a disinfectant, and cialit (2-ethylmercuriothio-5-benzoxolcarboxylic acid) as a preservative for ossicle homografts[8]. Unfortunately, this combination is not only ineffective in preventing human immunodeficiency virus (HIV), but also may even propagate Creutzfeldt-Jakob (CJD) infections[9]. The recommended sterilizing or inactivating procedures in the literature that also inactivate the more resilient germs, such as the nucleotide-free putative infectious prions causing CJD[10,11], include autoclaving and NaOH treatment.

In a former study, we tested the mechanical and radiological ossicle structures and material changes induced by different inactivation procedures, and identified alkaline NaOH treatment as a suitable method for ossicle homograft inactivation[12]. This procedure has the disadvantage of potentially dangerous and time-consuming handling conditions during the operation procedure. Combined ossicle treatment with NaOH and autoclaving or freeze-drying may solve this practical problem.

The purpose of this study was to test the effects of these combination treatments on the mechanical properties of ossicle homografts. Moreover, the first clinical results of implanted NaOH treated ossicles will be reported.

Material and methods

Mechanical testing

Thirty-four normal human incuses and malleuses were obtained from autopsies and from the organ donor program at the Inselspital. Transcanalicular tympanotomy was performed under microscope control to remove the ossicles from the middle ear. The ossicles were kept frozen at -20°C for several weeks. After thawing, ten ossicles were exposed to 1N NaOH for 60 minutes at room temperature. Additionally, six ossicles were treated for NaOH and then autoclaved for eight minutes at 134°C (NaOH-Au), and six ossicles were treated for NaOH and then underwent freeze-drying (NaOH-FD). The control group ($n=12$) received no further treatment after thawing.

All ossicles were drilled manually under the microscope into a similar cylindrical shape (average size: 3.5×2 mm) with a diamond burr, and then underwent mechanical testing. This consisted of destructive axial compression in a mechanical testing machine (Mini Bionix, MTS, Minneapolis, MN) at a rate of 0.05 mm/sec, while measuring the force and displacement[13]. The ultimate strength, highest stress on the stress-strain curve and elastic modulus, and ratio of stress to strain below the elastic limit, were the material properties of interest. The elastic modulus was obtained by performing a linear regression on the linear part of the stress-strain curve. This method had been validated in a previous study by synthetic bone and normal untreated ossicles[13].

Statistical analysis involved a one-way ANOVA across treatment groups for each parameter. A Student Newman-Keuls (SNK) *post-hoc* test was performed to determine treatment differences. The protocol was reviewed and approved by the ethics committee of the Inselspital Bern, Switzerland.

Clinical study

Indications for an ossicle implant in patients included an intact stapes suprastructure and destroyed incus, usually due to extensive cholesteatoma. All implanted ossicles were provided by the organ donor program at the Inselspital. All patients underwent a pure-tone audiogram, including air and bone conduction hearing levels, one day before the operation. The operation consisted of a canal wall-down mastoidectomy and tympano-ossiculoplasty. All patients underwent follow-up, which included a pure-tone audiogram six to eight weeks after the operation. The pre- and postoperative air-bone gaps at the frequencies of 0.5, 1, 2 and 4 kHz were compared in each patient.

Results

Mechanical testing

Analysis of variance of mechanical testing revealed a significant difference for the material property of ultimate strength between control and NaOH treated ossicles. No further decrease in material properties was observed after additional autoclaving or freeze-drying. Elastic modulus and the other material properties showed no significant difference compared to controls. One specimen of NaOH-freeze-drying failed during testing the set up. Figures 1 and 2 show the ultimate strength and elastic modulus exhibited by the samples.

The SNK *post-hoc* test was performed to detect any differences between individual groups. The results for ultimate strength and elastic modulus are shown in Tables 1 and 2, respectively.

Clinical study

Since 1998, six male and four female patients (mean age, 44 year; range, 12-69 years) have received an NaOH-treated ossicle implant. The mean follow-up time was ten months (range, 5-24 months). The average air-bone gap gains by frequency for the ten patients with NaOH-treated ossicle implants are shown in Figure 3. No adverse effects or homograft extrusion were observed during the operation or the follow-up. No notable postoperative sensorineural hearing loss was observed.

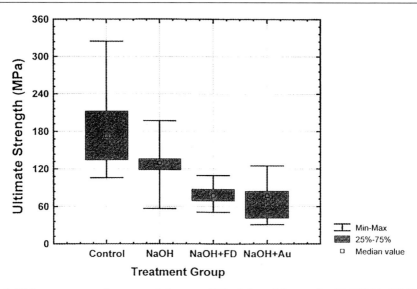

Fig. 1. Ultimate compressive strength (mean ± SD) of shaped incus after NaOH, NaOH/freeze-drying (NaOH+FD) and NaOH/autoclave (NaOH+Au) inactivation treatments.

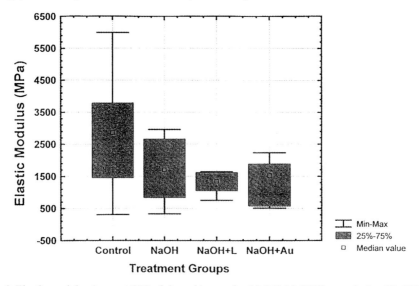

Fig. 2. Elastic modulus (mean ± SD) of shaped incus after NaOH, NaOH/freeze-drying (NaOH+FD) and NaOH/autoclave (NaOH+Au) inactivation treatments.

Table 1. p values of between-treatment ultimate strength differences (SNK)

	Control	NaOH	NaOH+FD
NaOH	0.039*		
NaOH+FD	0.001*	0.062	
NaOH+Au	0.001*	0.092	0.815

*significant

Table 2. p values of between-treatment elastic modulus differences (SNK)

	Control	NaOH	NaOH+FD
NaOH	0.073		
NaOH+FD	0.077	0.788	
NaOH+Au	0.061	0.611	0.884

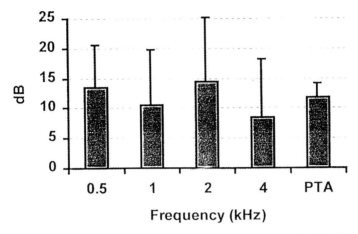

Fig. 3. Postoperative air-bone gap reduction (average values + standard deviations) for frequencies 0.5/1/2/4 kHz and for the pure-tone average (PTA) combination, respectively.

Discussion

In a former study, we found significant NaOH-induced changes in the properties of mechanical ossicles[12]. The extent of these changes were similar to those treated by the formalin-cialit procedure. Based on the successful clinical experience with cialit, NaOH-treated ossicles emerged as a suitable method for future ossicle inactivation. In practical terms, 1N NaOH has considerable drawbacks concerning handling and safety. Additional short-term autoclaving or freeze-drying after NaOH treatment could resolve this problem, because ossicles could then be stored for a longer time period in the freezer or at room temperature. The mechanical testing showed no significant changes in mechanical properties between the exclusive NaOH and the combined NaOH-autoclaving and NaOH-freeze-drying procedure. In addition, the physiological mechanical load of the implanted homograft ossicle at normal hearing levels is more than ten orders of magnitude smaller than the maximum load applied in this study to assess differences in material properties. Based on the infectious guidelines[10,11], and from the point of view of structural properties, 60 minutes of 1N NaOH treatment followed by eight minutes of autoclaving allows the adequate preservation of mechanical properties and inactivation of pathogens. The method is simple, practical for routine use, and non-ototoxic[14]. For the surgeon and nurse, such inactivated ossicles do not imply any changes in operative technique or ossicle handling. The senior surgeon (RH) even subjectively describes a better malleability of NaOH-treated homografts.

The limited number of patients implanted with homografts treated in this way, showed clinical and audiological results comparable to those described in earlier studies still using the formalin-cialit-technique[2-6]. Moreover, in the future, the inactivation procedure will remain the critical step in homograft preparation, because infectious profiles may undergo rapid and considerable changes.

In conclusion, the NaOH-autoclaving inactivation procedure causes mechanical changes in thawed ossicle homografts. The extent of the changes in material properties is comparable to those found during the formaldehyde/cialit procedure, which has been used successfully for over 30 years in otosurgery. Even though the first clinical results of NaOH-autoclaving ossicle inactivation encourage further application of this inactivation method, further investigations are necessary to re-evaluate the clinical long-term use of ossicle homografts in middle ear reconstructive surgery.

References

1. Hough JVD: Incudostapedial joint separation: etiology, treatment and significance. Laryngoscope 69:644-654, 1959
2. Marquet JFE: Twelve years experience with homograft tympanoplasty. Otolaryngol Clin N Am 10:581-593, 1977
3. Chiossone E: Homograft ossiculopasty: Long term results. Am J Otol 8:54, 1987
4. Roulleau P, Lacher G: 20 years of tympano-ossicular homografts: results. Acta Otorhinolaryngol Belg 45:87-94, 1991
5. Messerli A, Altermatt HJ, Vischer MW, Häusler R: Incus Homograft Ossiculoplastik. Aktuelle Probleme Otorhinolaryngol 18:77-85, 1994
6. Farrior JB, Nichols SW: Long-term results using ossicular grafts. Am J Otol 17(3):386-392, 1996
7. Bagot d'Arc M: L'oto-rhino-laryngologiste et la maladie de Creutzfeldt Jakob. Rev Laryngol Otol Rhinol 119:1-12, 1998
8. Perkins R: Grafting materials and methods in reconstructive ear surgery. Ann Otol 84:518-526, 1975
9. Bujia J, Wilmes E, Kastenbauer E, Gürtler L: Influence of chemical homograft preservation procedures on the human immunodeficiency virus. Laryngoscope 106:645-647, 1996
10. Steelman V: Creutzfeldt-Jakob disease: recommendations for infection control. Am J Infect Control 22:312-318, 1994
11. Ernst DR, Race RE: Comparative analysis of scrapie agent inactivation methods. J Vir Methods 41:193-202, 1993
12. Hotz MA, Speirs AD, Oxland T, Müller M, Hämmerle C, Häusler R: Radiologic and mechanical properties of inactivated ossicle homografts. Laryngoscope 109:65-69, 1999
13. Speirs AD, Hotz MA, Oxland TR, Häusler R, Nolte LP: Biomechanical properties of human ossicles. J Biomechanics 32:485-491, 1999
14. Sataloff RT, Roberts B: Preservation of otologic homografts. Am J Otol 7:214-217, 1986

CARTILAGE INTERPOSITION IN OSSICULOPLASTY WITH HYDROXYLAPATITE PROSTHESES

A histopathological study in the guinea pig

Astrid G.W. Meijer, Jolanda Verheul, Frans W.J. Albers and Hans M. Segenhout

Department of Otorhinolaryngology, University Hospital Groningen, Groningen, The Netherlands

Abstract

In this experimental animal study, a cartilage disc was interposed between a synthetic middle ear prosthesis and the tympanic membrane of guinea pigs to investigate its effect on the extrusion process of the implant. Two groups of guinea pigs were studied. One group consisted of animals in which the prosthesis was directly in contact with the tympanic membrane, the other consisted of animals in which a cartilage disc had been inserted between the head of the prosthesis and the tympanic membrane. Before histological processing, *in situ* inspection was performed using an operation microscope. After fixation and embedding, light microscopical and transmission electron microscopical examination were performed. The authors studied the histopathological aspects of the tympanic membrane with regard to the protrusion and extrusion processes of the middle ear implant. In this experimental model, protrusion and extrusion of a hydroxylapatite middle ear prosthesis was greatly reduced by interposition of a cartilage disc. Further clinical evaluation of these experimental results is needed in the human middle ear.

Keywords: ossiculoplasty, hydroxylapatite, cartilage interposition

Introduction

In tympanoplasty, otological surgeons have successfully used biocompatible synthetic materials to reconstruct the middle ear air conduction system. Synthetic implants are greatly preferred to autografts and allografts[1]. At this time, hydroxylapatite is the most used synthetic material for reconstruction of the ossicular middle ear chain in tympanoplasty. Hydroxylapatite is a calcium phosphate ceramic, which resembles the mineral matrix of living bone tissue. It is rapidly covered by epithelial cells and permits differentiation into goblet and

Address for correspondence: A.G.W. Meyer, MD, Department of Otorhinolaryngology, University Hospital Groningen, P.O. Box 30001, 9700 RB Groningen, The Netherlands

The Function and Mechanics of Normal, Diseased and Reconstructed Middle Ears, pp. 231–241
edited by J.J. Rosowski and S.N. Merchant
© 2000 Kugler Publications, The Hague, The Netherlands

ciliated cells without any foreign body reaction. Hydroxylapatite is completely bioactive, biocompatible and osteoconductive[2-6].

In the past, there were intrinsic problems of rejection and extrusion for all synthetic implants. However, these days, with the introduction of highly biocompatible materials, rejection is seldom observed. Extrusion of a biocompatible ceramic middle ear implant in direct contact with the tympanic membrane is probably not caused by a foreign body reaction, but by decubital necrosis of the membrane[7-11]. Extrusion rates can be lowered by interposing a small cartilage disc between a synthetic implant and the tympanic membrane[1,7-16]. Cartilage has the advantage of being well tolerated by the tympanic membrane. It can be placed under some tension, with a very low risk of extrusion. The literature refers to average extrusion rates of biocompatible implants varying from 15-22%; interposing a cartilage disc reduces extrusion rates to 3-6%, making them comparable to those of transplants[1,7-13].

In this study, we implanted hydroxylapatite middle ear prostheses in the bullae of guinea pigs. The guinea pig temporal bone and its contents are similar to those of humans, but there are some minor differences. In relation to the dimensions of the temporal bone, those of the eardrum and tympanic ring are greater in the guinea pig than in humans, and the tympanic membrane is devoid of a pars flaccida[17].

Two groups of guinea pigs were investigated: the first consisted of cases in which a hydroxylapatite prosthesis was directly in contact with the tympanic membrane, the second of cases in which a cartilage slice had been inserted between the head of the hydroxylapatite prosthesis and the tympanic membrane. The purpose of this study was to evaluate the histopathological aspects of the tympanic membrane, and the differences in extrusion and protrusion between the groups of guinea pigs operated on.

Material and methods

In this study, middle ear surgery was carried out on 21 female pigmented guinea pigs, weighing about 450 g. Animal care and use were approved by the Experimental Animal Committee of the University of Groningen, protocol No. 1174, in accordance with the principles of the Declaration of Helsinki.

Operation technique

The animals were anesthetized by an intramuscular injection of Ketalar-Rompun (0.7:0.3). All operations were performed by the same surgeon, using a Zeiss stereo microscope. Body temperature was maintained by using an electric heating pad. Tympanotomy was performed by the inferior approach[18,19]. After stripping off the perichondrium covering, the bulla was opened by creating a square shutter (0.4×0.4 mm). The hydroxylapatite prosthesis (diameter, 2.0 mm) with a spiral spring shaft was implanted between the tympanic membrane and the bulla wall, under minimal tension. The shaft had no contact with middle ear structures other than the bulla wall at its end. In half the cases, a slice of cartilage, 0.3-0.5 mm thick, was interposed between the prosthesis head and the tympanic membrane, with the perichondrium covering opposed to the tympanic membrane. The cartilage disc with the overlying perichondrium was obtained from the auricle. After adequate positioning of the prosthesis, the square shutter was replaced on the bulla defect and fixed with histoacryl tissuecol, and wound closure was performed. After six months, the guinea pigs were sacrificed by decapitation.

Histological processing

After sacrifice by decapitation, the bullae were opened and fixed in 2.5% glutaraldehyde in 0.1 M sodium cacodylate buffer, pH 7.4. The specimens were then decalcified for five days in 10% EDTA, pH 7.4, postfixed in 1% OsO_4 with 1% $K_4Ru(CN)_6$ for two to three hours, carefully rinsed in distilled water, dehydrated in a graded ethanol series followed by propylene oxide, and infiltrated using a mixture of 1:1 propylene oxide and Spurr's low viscosity resin for two hours, followed by pure resin infiltration overnight. One specimen was embedded in HPMA (hydroxypropyl methacrylate) and stained for elastin. Polymerization took place at 70°C after desiccation in a vacuum. The specimens were cut in semi-thin slices (2 µm) and stained with toluidine blue for evaluation by light microscopy (LM). Six selected pieces were further examined by transmission electron microscopy (TEM). Ultra-thin 100-nm sections were contrast-stained with 7% uranyl acetate in 70% methanol and lead citrate. Evaluation was performed using a Philips 201 transmission electron microscope operating at 40 kV.

Examination

Before histological processing, *in situ* inspection of the position, protrusion and extrusion of the prosthesis was performed using a Zeiss stereo operation microscope. After fixation and embedding, light microscopy (LM) was performed. We studied the histopathological aspects of the tympanic membrane, including signs of protrusion or extrusion of the middle ear prosthesis. Protrusion was defined as prominence of the prosthesis in the tympanic membrane, with the tympanic membrane still intact. Extrusion was defined as prominence of the prosthesis in the tympanic membrane, resulting in discontinuity of the tympanic membrane. In addition to the light microscopical evaluation, we also performed transmission electron microscopy (TEM) evaluations in selected cases. Six cases (five with cartilage interposition, one without) of apparently normal tympanic membranes, as observed with LM, were further investigated with TEM, as were three left control ears which had not had any intervention.

Results

We initially implanted hydroxylapatite middle ear prostheses in the right bullae of 21 guinea pigs (11 without cartilage interposition, ten with). During the six months' follow-up period, three guinea pigs died, two in which cartilage was interpositioned, and one in which it was not. There was no clear cause of death. Moreover, two guinea pigs (with cartilage interposition) were excluded after being prepared for evaluation, for technical reasons: in one, the prosthesis was situated against the bulla wall and therefore had no contact with the tympanic membrane; in the other, the fixation and embedding procedure had failed. Consequently, we studied 16 guinea pigs: group A consisted of ten animals in which the prosthesis was directly in contact with the tympanic membrane, group B consisted of six animals in which a cartilage disc had been inserted between the head of the prosthesis and the tympanic membrane. Apart from the two implantation groups, we studied the histological aspects of a group of six left control ears which had not had any intervention.

In situ *inspection*

In the 16 right bullae, we observed 15 healthy middle ear cavities with no sign of infection or inflammation. Only one bulla, in which cartilage was positioned between the prosthesis head and the tympanic membrane, showed a purulent otitis media. In all 16 bullae, the prostheses were in an adequate position and directly or indirectly in contact with the tympanic membrane.

We estimated the extrusion and protrusion rates of the prostheses (Table 1): eight cases of extrusion/protrusion (varying between mild and severe) were observed (seven without cartilage interposition, one with). One protrusion/extrusion was questionable (no cartilage interposition) and the resulting seven showed no clear signs of protrusion/extrusion (two without cartilage interposition, five with). It was impossible to differentiate between extrusion and protrusion.

Table 1. In situ inspection and LM examination of the tympanic membrane after implantation of hydroxylapatite middle ear prostheses with or without cartilage interposition

	In situ *inspection*	LM
No cartilage *n*=10	7 protrusion/extrusion 1 questionable pro-/extrusion 2 normal	3 extrusion 7 protrusion
Cartilage *n*=6	1 protrusion/extrusion 5 normal	1 extrusion 1 protrusion 4 normal

Light microscopy

Control group (n=6)
We studied the tympanic membranes of six left control ears which had not had any intervention. The tympanic membrane is built up of three layers: the outer epidermal layer, the middle lamina propria (fibrous layer), and the inner mucous layer, as reported in the literature[20-22]. All the tympanic membranes studied had an entirely normal appearance with no sign of atrophy. The HPMA-embedded tympanic membrane showed elastin in the epidermal and mucosa layer, but not in the fibrous layer.

Group A (no cartilage interposition, n=10)
All ears except one showed severe histopathological changes in the tympanic membrane (Fig. 1). The most prominent changes took place in the middle fibrous layer. The outer epidermal layer was less affected. Of the ten prostheses, three were actually extruded, while the remainder were seen to protrude (Table 1). The changes in the middle fibrous layer consisted of mild to severe reduction in thickness (atrophy) and discontinuity of the middle fibrous tissue layer to total absence of this layer. The middle fibrous layer of the tympanic membrane was questionably atrophic in one case, atrophic in five, and absent in four (Table 2).

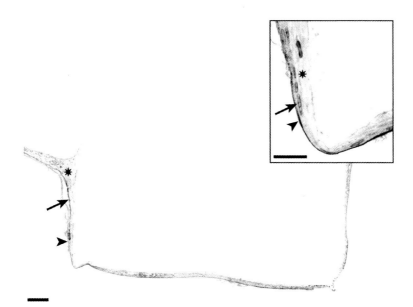

Fig. 1. Light microscopy photograph of a tympanic membrane after implantation of a hydroxylapatite middle ear prosthesis without cartilage interposition. The prosthesis protrudes into the tympanic membrane. The middle fibrous layer (arrow) is atrophic with discontinuity at the edge (inset), the outer epidermal layer (arrow head) and the inner mucosal layer (asterisk) are less affected. Bar: 100 µm; bar inset: 20 µm.

Table 2. LM and TEM examinations of the tympanic membrane after implantation of hydroxy-lapatite middle ear prostheses with or without cartilage interposition, with emphasis on the middle fibrous layer of the tympanic membrane

	LM	*TEM*
No cartilage	4 absent	
n=10	5 atrophic	
	1 questionable atrophy	1 with continuous fibers
Cartilage	1 absent	
n=6	1 questionable atrophy	1 with continuous fibers
	4 normal	3 with fiber intermissions
		1 with continuous fibers

Group B (cartilage interposition, n=6)

Histopathological examination of these six guinea pigs showed one case of extrusion, *i.e.*, the one with purulent otitis media. In only one animal did we observe protrusion of the prosthesis and a tympanic membrane with questionable atrophy of the middle fibrous layer (Tables 1 and 2). The remaining tympanic membranes were all normal with no signs of atrophy, protrusion or extrusion (Fig. 2). The interposed cartilage discs showed some signs of degradation, but all had an intact extracellular matrix.

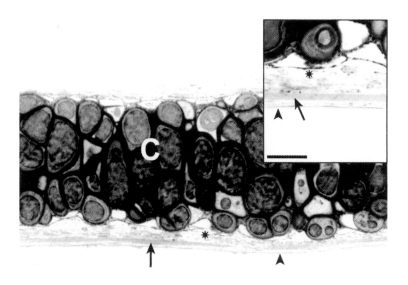

Fig. 2. Light microscopy photograph of a tympanic membrane after implantation of a hydroxy-lapatite middle ear prosthesis with cartilage interposition (C). There are no signs of protrusion or extrusion of the prosthesis. No sign of atrophy of the middle fibrous layer (arrow) can be observed. Neither the outer epidermal layer (arrow head) nor the inner mucosal layer (asterisk) are affected. Bar: 20 μm; bar inset: 20 μm.

Transmission electron microscopy

Control group
The tympanic membranes of the three left control ears showed an outer epidermal layer, an inner mucosal layer, and a middle fibrous layer (Fig. 3). The fibrous layer consisted of two types of fibers: outer radial and inner circular. The outer radial layer, which was by far the largest, was arranged in radially orientated fibers and was about 2-3 µm thick. The inner circular layer was much thinner. The fibers of both layers consisted of very thin, approximately 20 nm thick, fibrils which did not seem to display the typical collagenous crossbanding patterns; this is in accordance with data from the literature[20,21]. Few interruptions of the (radial)fibers were observed. Some cells were present in the middle layer between the fibers. In one case, which was close to the malleus, the lamina propria of the epidermal layer showed cell-cell contacts, and many small vesicles were present below. The radial fibers were loose at that location, and many cells could be seen in between.

Research group
The group investigated consisted of five cases with cartilage interposition and one case without. In all cases, LM examination revealed an apparently normal histological aspect of the tympanic membrane, including the two cases with a

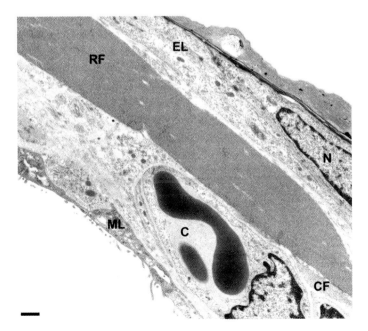

Fig. 3. Transmission electron microscopy photograph of the tympanic membrane of a control ear without intervention. The tympanic membrane is built up of the outer epidermal layer (EL), the middle fibrous layer consisting of radial fibers (RF) and smaller circular fibers (CF), and the inner mucosal layer (ML). N: nucleus; C: capillary; Bar: 1 µm.

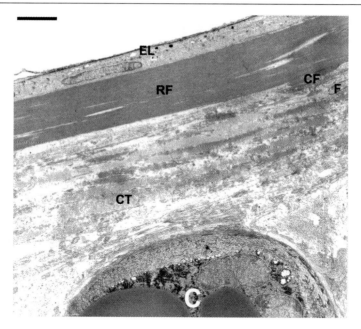

Fig. 4. Transmission electron microscopy photograph of the tympanic membrane after implantation of a hydroxylapatite middle ear prosthesis with cartilage interposition (C). The aspect of the outer epidermal layer (EL) is normal. The middle fibrous layer has a normal appearance with the radial fibers (RF) and the smaller circular fibers (CF) still intact. The inner mucosal layer has been replaced by connective tissue (CT) containing fibrocytes (F: fibrocyte nucleus) surrounded by collagen. Bar: 5 μm.

questionable atrophic fibrous layer. All tympanic membranes showed a normal appearance of the epidermal layer on TEM (Fig. 4). The mucosal layer was absent in all cases, and was replaced by a connective tissue layer that connected the tympanic membrane to the underlying cartilage or prosthesis. The connective tissue layer contained fibrocytes, and collagen fibers with the characteristic crossbanding pattern. The fibrocytes were the end result of an active process of remodelling of the tympanic membrane (fibroblasts) which had been stabilized by this point. The basal lamina on the mucosal side was no longer recognizable in half the cases, while in the other half, it was still partly intact. The middle fibrous layer was present in all cases (Table 2). In half the cases, including the two with questionable atrophy of the fibrous layer on LM, the fibers were continuous. The other half showed some interruptions. Apart from this finding, the histological appearance of this layer was normal.

Discussion

In this experimental study, a cartilage disc was interposed between a synthetic middle ear prosthesis and the tympanic membrane of guinea pigs to investigate its effect on the extrusion process of the implant. Two groups of guinea pigs were studied: one with and the other without cartilage interposition between the implant and the tympanic membrane. A control group was also included.

A synthetic middle ear implant that is shielded by cartilage can easily extrude or become liable to extrusion when the cartilage is displaced or resorbed. Clinical and experimental evidence suggests that, when alone, cartilage softens and is either absorbed or replaced by fibrous tissue[7,15]. Preservation with perichondrium on one side improves the viability of the cartilage graft[7,15,23,24]. All our cartilage discs were covered with perichondrium on the side opposed to the tympanic membrane. Histological examination of the interposed cartilage discs with a perichondrium covering showed no evidence of resorption. All the interposed cartilage discs had an intact extracellular matrix. It is clear that neither the extrusion of a ceramic implant, nor liability to extrusion can be prevented with any certainty by interposition of a cartilage disc. The role of the interface is particularly important in cases of relative eustachian tube insufficiency, because the negative pressure inside the middle ear can cause the head of the prosthesis to exert increased pressure against the tympanic membrane[8-10]. This may interfere with the nutrition of the overlying tympanic membrane.

The mechanism of extrusion can be infection or inflammation, a foreign body reaction to the prosthesis material, or decubital necrosis of the tympanic membrane[7-9]. In our present series, there was one case of extrusion as a result of inflammation. The other protrusions/extrusions were not related to an inflammatory process. No lymphocytic infiltration or foreign body giant cells were observed in any cases, suggesting that no foreign body reaction to the hydroxylapatite material was involved. However, the histopathological observations strongly indicated a process of decubital necrosis of the tympanic membrane. The most prominent changes indicating this necrosis consisted of atrophy of the middle fibrous layer or total absence of this layer. Abnormal pressure of the prosthesis on the tympanic membrane may have interfered with the nutrition of the overlying tympanic membrane. Cartilage interposition may have caused less decubital necrosis of the tympanic membrane than a synthetic prosthesis would have done when in direct contact with the tympanic membrane.

Conclusions

In this experimental model, protrusion and extrusion of a hydroxylapatite middle ear prosthesis could frequently be prevented by interposition of a cartilage disc. Higher extrusion/protrusion rates and severe histopathological changes of the middle fibrous layer of the tympanic membrane were observed in the group without cartilage interposition compared to the one with. This means that autologous cartilage does indeed provide a good interface material between two systems with different elastic modules. On the basis of our observations, we strongly recommend the interposition of an autologous cartilage disc between a hydroxylapatite middle ear prosthesis and the eardrum. Further clinical evaluation of these experimental results is needed in the human middle ear, including a study of the sound conduction mechanism in tympanoplasty after cartilage interposition between the prosthesis and the tympanic membrane.

Acknowledgments

This study was supported by the Heinsius Houbolt Foundation and is part of our Department's research program, Communication through Hearing and Speech. This program is incorporated into the Sensory Systems Group of the Groningen Graduate School for Behavioral and Cognitive Neurosciences (BCN).

References

1. Meijer AGW, Westerlaken BO, Albers FWJ: The Groningen cartilage cutting device: a new instrument for tympanoplasty. Laryngoscope 109:2025-2027, 1999
2. Blitterswijk CA van, Kuijpers W, Daems Th, Grote JJ: Epithelial reactions to hydroxyapatite. Acta Otolaryngol (Stockh) 101:2331-2341, 1986
3. Blitterswijk CA van, Kuijpers W, Daems Th, Grote JJ: Epithelial reactions to hydroxyapatite: an in vivo and in vitro study. Acta Otolaryngol (Stockh) 101:231-241, 1986
4. Goldenberg RA: Hydroxylapatite ossicular replacement prostheses: results in 157 consecutive cases. Laryngoscope 102:1091-1096, 1992
5. Simon JP, Fabry G: An overview of implant materials. Acta Orthop Belg 57:1-5, 1991
6. Bonfield W: Composites for bone replacement. J Biomed Eng 10:522-526, 1988
7. Zöllner C: Interposed cartilage as a precaution against extrusions of ceramic ossicular replacement implants. Ann Otol Rhinol Laryngol 96:207-209, 1987
8. Sanna M, Gamoletti R, Magnani M, Baccinu S, Zini C: Enhanced biofuntionality of plastipore ossicular prostheses with the use of homologous cartilage. Am J Otol 4:138-141, 1982
9. Jahnke K: Extrusion of middle ear implants. Clin Otolaryngol 12:227-232, 1987
10. Zöllner C, Strutz J: Mittelohrimplantate aus Al2O3-keramik. Laryngorhinootologie 66:517-521, 1987
11. Zöllner C: Aluminiumoxid-keramik implantate (typ Tübingen) in der mittelohrchirurgie. Laryngol Rhinol Otol 64:233-237, 1985
12. Niparko JK, Kemink JL, Graham MD, Kartush JM: Bioactive glass ceramic in ossicular reconstruction: a preliminary report. Laryngoscope 98:822-825, 1988
13. Brackmann DE, Sheeny JL, Luxford WM: TORPs and PORPs in tympanoplasty: A review of 1042 operations. Otolaryngol Head Neck Surg 92:32-37, 1984
14. Nikolaou A, Bourikas Z, Maltas V, Aidonis A: Ossiculoplasty with use of autografts and synthetic prosthetic materials: a comparison of results in 165 cases. J Laryngol Otol 106:692-694, 1992
15. East CA, Mangham CA: Composite tragal perichondrial/cartilage autografts vs cartilage or bone paste grafts in tympanoplasty. Clin Otolaryngol 16:540-542, 1991
16. Yamamoto E: Long term observations on ceramic ossicular replacement prostheses (CORP). Laryngoscope 98:402-404, 1988
17. Goksu N, Haziroglu R, Kemaloglu Y, Karademir N, Bayramoglu I, Akyildiz N: Anatomy of the guinea pig temporal bone. Ann Otol Rhinol Laryngol 101:699-704, 1992
18. Asarch R, Abramson M, Litton WB: Surgical anatomy of the guinea pig ear. Ann Otol Rhinol Laryngol 64:250-255, 1971

19. Wells JR, Gernon WH, Ward G, Davis K, Hays LL: Otosurgical model in the guinea pig (Cavia porcellus). Otolaryngol Head Neck Surg 4.450-457, 1986
20. Lim DJ: Tympanic membrane. Electron microscopic observations. Part I: pars tensa. Acta Otolaryngol (Stockh) 66:181-198, 1968
21. McMinn RH: Electron microscopic observations on the repair of perforated tympanic membranes in the guinea pig. J Anat 120:207-217, 1975
22. Reijnen CJH, Kuijpers W: The healing pattern of the drum membrane. Acta Otolaryngol (Stockh) Suppl 287:1-74, 1971
23. Schuknecht HF, Shi SR: Surgical pathology of middle ear implants. Laryngoscope 95:249-258, 1985
24. Steinbach E, Pusalkar A: Long-term histological fate of cartilage in ossicular reconstruction. J Laryngol Otol 95:1031-1039, 1981

TITANIUM IN OSSICULAR CHAIN RECONSTRUCTION

Morphological results in animal experiments and after implantation in the human middle ear

Konrad Schwager

Department of Otolaryngology, Head and Neck Surgery, University of Würzburg, Würzburg, Germany

Abstract

Titanium ossicular replacement prostheses were studied using light and scanning electron microscopy. An animal study was performed in the middle ear of the rabbit: titanium pins were used as middle ear prostheses, and morphological studies were performed up to 504 days after implantation. In a subsequent clinical study, a total of 536 ears were implanted and 23 prostheses removed at revision surgery were studied morphologically. Tissue reactions in animal and in human middle ears looked similar. An inflammatory reaction was seen in the early postoperative stage in the animal study and in chronic ear disease. The material's surface was covered with regular mucosa and submucosal connective tissue. In cases of chronic ear disease, high cylindrical epithelium with ciliated and goblet cells was detected. From the experimental standpoint and clinical experience so far, titanium seems to be a favorable biomaterial for ossicular replacement.

Keywords: titanium, middle ear, ossicular replacement

Introduction

Appropriate reconstruction of the ossicular chain in chronic ear disease is a major challenge in middle ear surgery. Often, the patient's own ossicles cannot be used, due to underlying disease. Homografts carry the risk of potentially transmitting infectious diseases. Thus, alloplastic materials have been introduced for reconstruction.

Address for correspondence: Priv.-Doz. Dr. med. Konrad Schwager, Klinik und Poliklinik für Hals-, Nasen- und Ohrenkranke, Bayer. Julius-Maximilians-Universität Würzburg, Josef-Schneider-Strasse 11, D-97080 Würzburg, Germany. *email:* K.Schwager@mail.uni-wuerzburg.de

The Function and Mechanics of Normal, Diseased and Reconstructed Middle Ears, pp. 243–254
edited by J.J. Rosowski and S.N. Merchant
© *2000 Kugler Publications, The Hague, The Netherlands*

A variety of biomaterials have been used in ossicular reconstruction, including different types of ceramics (aluminumoxid, bioglasses, hydroxyapatite), carbon materials, glass ionomer cement, and synthetic materials such as Plastipore® (high-density-polyethylene-sponge, HDPS) and Proplast® (polytetrafluorethylene-vitrous carbon). Metals also have been implanted, mostly as composite prostheses using platinum, stainless steel, tantalum, or gold.

Titanium has been an accepted prosthetic material for decades in craniofacial and orthopedic surgery. The special environment in the middle ear makes it necessary to assess biocompatability in this potentially infected implantation site, even if the material is well tolerated elsewhere in the body. A preclinical study was performed first to demonstrate the biocompatibility of titanium in the mammalian middle ear. Since starting implantation in humans, several prostheses from revision surgery are available for morphological investigation.

Material and methods

Animal experiments

The biomaterial for the animal experiments consisted of commercially pure titanium (purity 99.427%, Leibinger, Freiburg, Germany). The titanium implant was pin-shaped, measuring 4 mm in length and 0.4 mm in diameter.

A total of 36 female rabbits (New Zealander, Charles River Germany, Sulzfeld, Germany) were housed one per cage and given food and water *ad libitum* until they were six months old (weight, 2-3 kg). At this time, the animals were anesthetized with Rompun® (Xylacin-HCL + parahydroxy-benzoeacidmethylester; Bayer, Leverkusen, Germany) and Ketanest® (ketamine-hydrochloride, Parke-Davis, Berlin, Germany). Middle ear exposure was performed, raising a tympanomeatal flap from the left ear, partially removing the lateral attic wall, and dissecting away the incus and head of the malleus.

The titanium pins were then interposed as a total ossicular replacement prosthesis (TORP) between the stapes footplate and the handle of the malleus. The tympanic membrane was then closed by underlaying perichondrium and cartilage. A sham-operated animal was prepared as a control for each animal group. In this case, after opening the middle ear, the incus was removed, and the head of the malleus and the crura of the stapes were dissected away. In addition, the non-operated ear of each animal served as a negative control.

The animals were sacrificed on days 28 (*n*=8), 84 (*n*=7), 168 (*n*=7), 336 (*n*=8) or 504 (*n*=6) post-surgery, and the temporal bones were removed and fixed in formalin. The specimens were embedded in epoxy resin, and histological slides were cut with a sawing microtome (Leica, Wetzlar, Germany) to a thickness of 30-80 μm (average, 50 μm). Staining was performed using the Giemsa technique for light microscopy[1]. One animal from each time period was prepared for scanning electron microscopy.

Implantation in humans

Since June 1997, titanium PORPs (partial ossicular replacement prostheses, 'Bell', Heinz Kurz, Dusslingen, Germany) and TORPs (total ossicular replacement prostheses, 'Aerial', Heinz Kurz, Dusslingen, Germany) have been implanted in human middle ears at our institution. Of 536 operated ears, 34 (6.3%) ears had to undergo revision surgery for several reasons. Twenty-three of these explanted prostheses were studied morphologically. The reasons for revision surgery and the clinical diagnosis are listed in Tables 1-3. Seventeen of the removed middle ear prostheses were prepared for scanning electron microscopy (SEM). After SEM, six of these prostheses together with six others were prepared for light microscopy using a sawing microtome, and stained according to the Giemsa technique.

Results

Animal experiments

Light microscopy
All prostheses were covered by epithelium. Epithelialization was completed as early as day 28. Granulation tissue and free inflammatory cells and macrophages could be seen in the tympanum four weeks postoperatively. The macrophages were fused to giant cells in a few cases.

From day 84 on, no postoperative inflammation was noted. There was no difference between the mucosa covering the prostheses and the mucosa in the tympanum in any of the specimens examined, and vascularization of the tympanum was unremarkable (Fig. 1). Unusual findings seen were bone growth in one specimen on day 168 and another with new bone formation by day 336 (Fig. 2).

Medialization of the tympanic membrane was noted in several specimens (12/36), most commonly at day 336 (4/6). Huge amounts of cellular debris in the outer ear canal forced the tympanic membrane medially. Thus, non-aerated spaces developed in the tympanon, such as those in atelectatic ears, and became chronically inflamed.

Scanning electron microscopy
From the start (day 28), scanning electron microscopy revealed a normal tympanum, with the prosthesis covered by fibrous tissue and mucosa. Squamous epithelium cells were the only cells found on the biomaterial at any time point. Neither ciliated cells nor mucus producing cells were seen. The epithelium showed regular squamous cells covered by microvilli (Fig. 3). No inflammatory cells were seen.

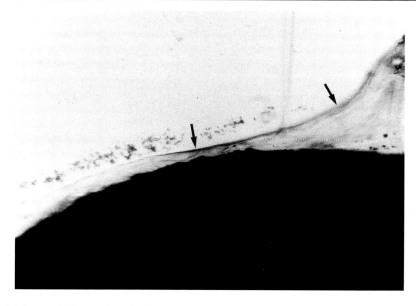

Fig. 1. Mucosa (←) covering titanium pin. 84 days, rabbit, Giemsa, ×54.

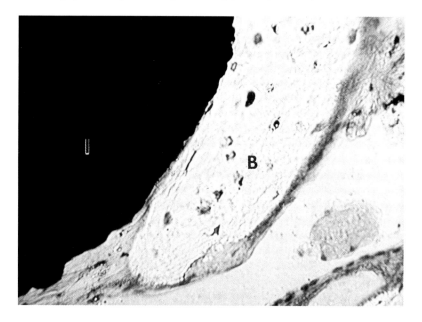

Fig. 2. Growth of bone (B) around the implant (I). 168 days, rabbit, Giemsa, ×80.

Controls

The non-operated ear of each animal showed no visible disorders. All the ears of the sham-operated controls showed remarkable amounts of cerumen, and one animal had a cholesteatoma in the outer ear canal, which was not morphologically different from the other cholesteatomas noted.

Table 1. Clinical diagnosis and morphological findings: explanted prostheses from the human middle ear (SEM)

Specimen no.	Clinical diagnosis	Implantation time (months)	PORP	TORP	Connective tissue	Hornifying squamous epithelium	Squamous epithelium	Cuboidal epithelium	Ciliated cells	Goblet cells	Inflammatory cells
1	fibrosis	7	+		+						
2	perforation	4		+	++						
3	cholesteatoma	8	+		+						+
4	vestibular disorder	2		+	+	+					
5	cholesteatoma	6	+		++	+	+				+
6	atelectasis, fibrosis	13	+		+	+	+				
7	cholesteatoma	13	+		++		+				
8	cholesteatoma	12	+		+	+	+				++
9	protrusion	4	+		++		+				++
10	fibrosis	9			++		+				
11	protrusion	9		+	++				+	+	
12	protrusion	8	+		+	+		+			
13	cholesteatoma	10	+			++	+				+
14	cholesteatoma	15	+		+						
15	cholesteatoma	5		+	+		+				
16	protrusion, atelectasis	10		+	++	+	+	+	+		+
17	fibrosis	10		+	+		+		+		+

Table 2. Clinical diagnosis and morphological findings: explanted prostheses from the human middle ear (light microscopy)

Specimen no.	Clinical diagnosis	Implantation time (months)	PORP	TORP	Connective tissue	Hornifying squamous epithelium	Squamous epithelium	Cuboidal epithelium	Ciliated cells	Goblet cells	Inflammatory cells
18	atelectasis, radical cavity	2	+		++						
19	protrusion	8		+	+						+
20	cholesteatoma	2	+		++	+	+				+
21	cholesteatoma	5	+		++	+	+				
22	atelectasis	8	+		++						
23	protrusion	10	+		+						

Table 3. Clinical diagnosis and morphological findings: explanted prostheses from the human middle ear (light microscopy after SEM)

Specimen no.	Clinical diagnosis	Implantation time (months)	PORP	TORP	Connective tissue	Hornifying squamous epithelium	Squamous epithelium	Cuboidal epithelium	Ciliated cells	Goblet cells	Inflammatory cells
5*	cholesteatoma		+		+	+	+				+
9*	protrusion		+		+						++
10*	fibrosis		+		+						+
12*	protrusion		+		+			+	+	+	
13*	cholesteatoma				+	+	+				+
16*	protrusion, atelectasis			+	+	+					

Implantation in humans (Tables 1-3)

Twenty-three implants were examined. The average implantation time was eight months.

Light microscopy

Six explanted prostheses (five PORPs, one TORP) were studied primarily by light microscopy (Table 2). A further six were studied after SEM (Table 3). Most of the prostheses from infected middle ears showed amounts of connective or granulation tissue. Some specimens showed lymphocyte infiltration. No inflammatory cells were seen close to the material's surface. Some connective tissue appeared to be rather thickened, but the cell layer on the surface revealed regular fibrocytes (Fig. 4). Even in cases of inflammatory infiltration, no foreign body giant cells were seen on any of the specimens. Most implants showed squamous epithelium. In one specimen, respiratory epithelium with ciliated cells and mucus-producing goblet cells was seen, in agreement with the SEM findings regarding this prosthesis (specimen #12). No formation of new bone was noted in any of the human specimens.

Scanning electron microscopy

Most explanted prostheses showed regular connective tissue on the surface, but the amount differed between the specimens (Fig. 5, Table 1). Regular squamous epithelium was detected on several implants (Fig. 6). Respiratory

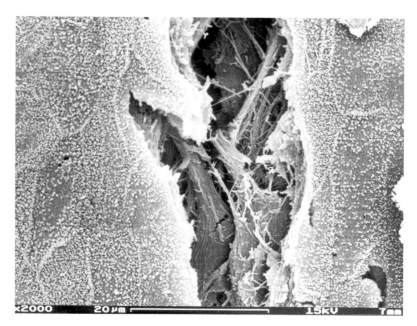

Fig. 3. Squamous epithelium covering titanium pin. Artificial crack opens submucosal tissue layer. 168 days, rabbit, SEM, ×2000.

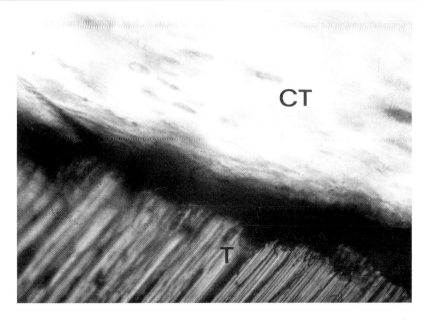

Fig. 4. Connective tissue (CT) covering TORP (T). Human specimen #2. Giemsa ×320.

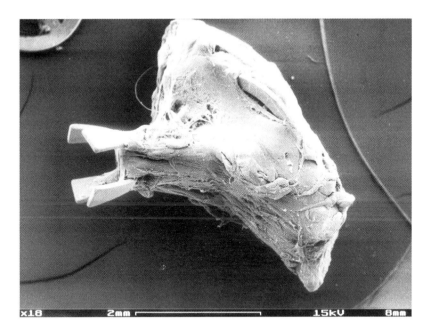

Fig. 5. PORP embedded in connective tissue. Human specimen #9. SEM ×18.

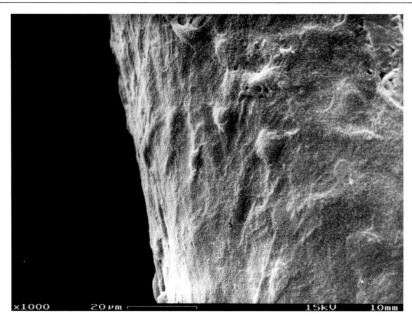

Fig. 6. Squamous epithelium covering shaft of TORP. Human specimen #11. SEM ×1000.

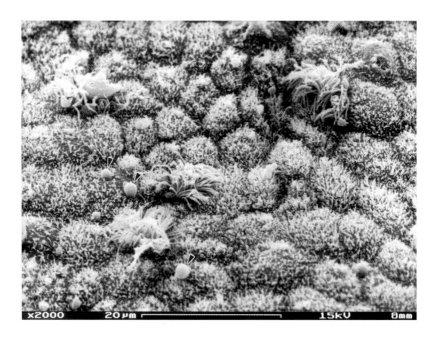

Fig. 7. Respiratory epithelium with ciliated cells. Mucus produced from goblet cells ◄. Human specimen #12. SEM ×2000.

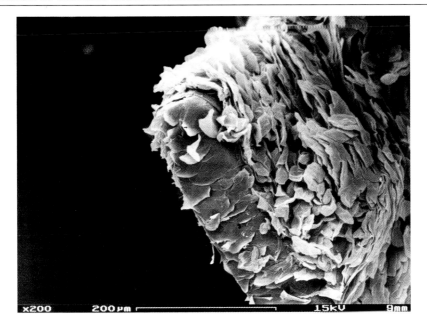

Fig. 8. Cholesteatoma. Rosette-like configured hornifying squamous epithelium. Base of PORP. Human specimen #5. SEM ×1000.

epithelium with ciliated cells and mucus-producing goblet cells were seen in two specimens (Fig. 7).

In cases of cholesteatoma, the explanted prostheses showed a typical rosette-like conformation of hornifying squamous epithelium (Fig. 8).

Discussion

Before an alloplastic material can be used in the middle ear space, its reactions to the surrounding tissue and special environment of the middle ear must be examined. One important consideration is the epithelialization of an implant material. In the animal experiment, all implants were covered by mucosa by day 28. Some of the prostheses explanted from human middle ears did not show adequate epithelial cover, but presented with normal subcutaneous fibrous tissue. This may represent a problem of completely removing implants with their covering mucosa from middle ears.

Histological criteria for judging the biocompatibility of alloplastic materials are the amount of fibrous tissue, the number and distribution of inflammatory and giant cells, and the vascular state of tissues adjacent to and surrounding the implant[2]. In our animal study, round cell infiltration was noticeable at day 28. This was considered to be a normal condition of the wound healing process, during which macrophages and consecutive giant cells remove cellular debris[1]. Inflammatory cells also were noted in trapped areas of medialized eardrums by ceruminal masses. But there was no hint of the material's surface being a reason for an inflammatory reaction. No macrophages or giant cells were detected at the submucosa biomaterial interface. The amount of fibrous tissue and inflammatory cells noted on specimens from human middle ears was probably due to the underlying disease. Large amounts of cellular debris was a recognized phenomenon in several rabbits operated on. This was probably due to a self-cleaning disorder in the rabbit's outer ear canal after surgery.

Animal studies of polymers tested for middle ear implants, Plastipore® and Proplast®, showed huge amounts of giant cells on their surfaces, and these resulted in prostheses being extruded[3-6], and large amounts of fibrous tissue[7-9] being seen after human middle ear surgery. Aluminumoxid, a bioinert ceramic, has been used with success in middle ear surgery[10]. However, in animal studies, macrophages and giant cells have been reported on the surface of this biomaterial during the primary postoperative period[11,12]. The bioglass, Ceravital® (Smith & Nephew, Bartlett, TN, USA) a bioactive calcium-silicon ceramic, is known to biodegrade, particularly in infected middle ears showing giant cells in the fibrous tissue surrounding the biomaterial[13].

Because of its similarity to human bone, hydroxyapatite has been recognized as an excellent ossicular replacement material[14,15]. However, biodegradation has been observed in experimental studies, with macrophages and giant cells displayed in the rat middle ear after implantation[16,17]. More recently, ionomeric cement was introduced in middle ear surgery[18-21]. In animal studies, biodegradation could not be assessed after two years of implantation[22].

Gold has been used as a biomaterial for stapes prostheses, as well as for TORPs and PORPs[23,24]; however, the bioinertness of gold has not been proven histologically. Giant cells have been seen close to the surface of gold implants that had been removed from human middle ears[25].

It is important to recognize the special conditions of the middle ear as an implantation site[26]. Polymers, or the bioactive ceramic Ceravital®, are well tolerated in normal middle ears, but show degradation in infected surroundings. Any material for reconstruction of the ossicular chain has to be tested under chronic ear disease conditions. Therefore, after animal studies that demonstrate biocampatibility in mammalians, implants from human middle ears should be consequently examined morphologically.

Titanium has been used as prosthesis in combination with gold[27], and a clinical study has reported favorable results in human middle ear surgery[28]. The affinity of titanium towards bone, known as osseointegration in bone-anchored devices[29], seems to occur in a similar way in the middle ear. Bone growth towards the prosthesis was recognized in our own animal experiments, and was also observed in clinical studies[28]. We did not find any bony fixation of the prostheses in revision cases. From this we can conclude that osseous fixation is possible, but is not an often-to-be-expected phenomenon.

Two types of epithelium were found on implants from human middle ears: flat polygonal squamous and high cylindrical respiratory epithelium with ciliated cells and mucus producing goblet cells. In the human middle ear, goblet cells are normally found in the hypotympanum and towards the eustachian tube. Chronic otitis media leads to the transformation of regular squamous cell epithelium to high cylindric respiratory epithelium with secretory and ciliated cells[30]. The finding of this respiratory epithelium on the specimens is probably a transformation due to chronic ear disease. The regular epithelium that would be expected on the material's surface is flat polygonal epithelium, as shown in the non-infected middle ears of rabbits.

Conclusions

1. The excellent coverage by normal middle ear mucosa and the lack of macrophages and giant cells on the material's surface are histological signs of the good acceptance of titanium in the middle ears of rabbits.
2. The histological study of prostheses removed during revision surgery in humans did not show signs of the non-acceptance of this material, even in cases of chronic ear disease.
3. The animal study, as well as the investigation of explanted prostheses from human middle ears, demonstrates that titanium can successfully be used as a biomaterial in middle ear surgery.

Acknowledgments

Special thanks to Ms P. Joa for carrying out the light microscopy procedures, and to Ms C. Gehrig for preparing the prostheses for scanning electron microscopy.

References

1. Homsy CA: On alloplasts for otology. In: Grote JJ (ed) Biomaterials in Otology, pp 9-17. Boston, MA: Martinus Nijhoff Publ 1984
2. Geyer G: Glasionomerzement als Knochenersatz in der Ohrchirurgie. Tierexperimentelle und klinische Untersuchungen. Habilitationsschrift (Thesis), Würzburg 1990
3. Cousins VC, Jahnke K: Light and electronmicroscopic studies on Polycel™ ossicular replacement prostheses. Clin Otolaryngol 12:183-189, 1987
4. Gjuric M, Mladina R, Koscak J: Die Plastipore-Prothese im Tierexperiment. Laryngol Rhinol Otol 66:522-525, 1987
5. Kerr AG: Six years experience of Plastipore®. Clin Otolaryngol 9:361-367, 1984
6. Kuijpers W: Behavior of bioimplants in the middle ear: an experimental study. In: Grote JJ (ed) Biomaterials in Otology, pp 18-28. Boston, MA: Martinus Nijhoff Publ 1984
7. Coletti V, Fiorino GF, Sittoni V: Rilievi istopatologici su protesi in Proplast e in Plastipore. Acta Otorhinol Ital 4:689-696, 1984
8. Spector M, Teichgraeber JF, Per-Lee JH et al: Tissue response to porous materials used for

ossicular replacement prostheses. In: Grote JJ (ed) Biomaterials in Otology, pp 29-40. Boston, MA: Martinus Nijhoff Publ 1984

9. Teichgraeber JF, Spector M, Per-Lee JH et al: Tissue response to Plastipore and Proplast otologic implants in the middle ears of cats. Am J Otol 5:127-136, 1983

10. Plester D, Jahnke K: Ceramic implants in otologic surgery. Am J Otol 3:104-108, 1981

11. Jahnke K, Galic M: Zur Verträglichkeit bioinerter Aluminiumoxidkeramik im Mittelohr. Arch Oto-Rhino-Laryngol 227:624-627, 1980

12. Jahnke K, Plester D, Heimke G: Aluminiumoxid-Keramik, ein bioinertes Material für die Mittelohrchirurgie. Arch Oto-Rhino-Laryngol 223:373-376, 1979

13. Reck R: Tissue reactions to glass ceramics in the middle ear. Clin Otolaryngol 6:63-65, 1981

14. Grote JJ: Tympanoplasty with calcium phosphate. Am J Otol 6:269-271, 1985

15. Wehrs RE: Incus replacement prostheses of hydroxylapatite in middle ear reconstruction. Am J Otol 10:181-182, 1989

16. Grote JJ, Van Blitterswijk CA, Kuijpers W: Hydroxyapatite ceramic as middle ear implant material: animal experimental results. Ann Otol Rhinol Laryngol (Suppl) 123:1-5, 1986

17. Grote JJ, Kuijpers W, De Groot K: Use of sintered hydroxylapatite in middle ear surgery. ORL 43:248-254, 1981

18. Bagot d'Arc M: Alloplastische Materialien in der Ohrchirurgie. In: Hagen R, Geyer G, Helms J (eds) Knochenersatz in der Mittelohr- und Schädelbasischirurgie. Band 1: Chirurgie, pp 47-54. München: Sympomed 1996

19. Geyer G, Helms J: Ionomer-based bone substitute in otologic surgery. Eur Arch Otorhinolaryngol 250:253-256, 1993

20. McElveen JT: Ossiculoplasty with polymaleinate ionomeric prostheses. Otolaryngol Clin N Am 27:777-784, 1994

21. McElveen JT Jr, Feghali JG, Barrs DM et al: Ossiculoplasty with polymaleinate ionomeric prosthesis. Otolaryngol Head Neck Surg 113:420-426, 1995

22. Geyer G: Ionomerzement als Knochenersatzmaterial im Mittelohr des Kaninchens. HNO 4:222-226, 1997

23. Jaehne M, Hartwein J: Erfahrungen mit Gold-Prothesen bei der Stapesplastik. In: Hagen R, Geyer G, Helms J (eds) Knochenersatz in der Mittelohr- und Schädelchirurgie. Band 1: Chirurgie, pp 63-65. München: Sympomed 1996

24. Steinbach E, Pusalkar A: Goldossikel zur Mittelohrrekonstruktion: histologische Befunde aus dem Mittelohr nach Implantation. In: Hagen R, Geyer G, Helms J (eds) Knochenersatz in der Mittelohr- und Schädelbasischirurgie. Band 1: Chirurgie, pp 58-62. München: Sympomed 1996

25. Hoppe F, Pahnke J: Rasterelektronenmikroskopische und histologische Befunde an alloplastischem Gehörknöchelchen-Ersatz. In: Hagen R, Geyer G, Helms J (eds) Knochenersatz in der Mittelohr- und Schädelbasischirurgie. Band 1: Chirurgie, pp 104-109. München: Sympomed 1996

26. Schwager K: Mittelohrprothesen und das biologische Umfeld. Biomaterialen (in press)

27. Pusalkar A, Steinbach E: Titan-Gold-Implantate in der Kettenrekonstruktion. In: Hagen R, Geyer G, Helms J (eds) Knochenersatz in der Mittelohr- und Schädelbasischirurgie. Band 1: Chirurgie, pp 55-57. München: Sympomed 1996

28. Stupp CH, Stupp HF, Grün D: Gehörknöchelchenersatz mit Titan-Prothesen. Laryngol Rhinol Otol 75:335-337, 1996

29. Albrektsson T, Brånemark P-I, Hansson H-A, Ivarsson B, Jönsson U: Ultrastructural analysis of the interface zone of titanium and gold implants. In: Lee AJC, Albrektsson T, Brånemark P-I (eds) Advances in Biomaterials, Vol. 4, Clinical Applications of Biomaterials, pp 167-177. New York: John Wiley & Sons, 1982

30. Arnold W: Reaktionsformen der Mittelohrschleimhaut. Arch Otorhinolaryngol 216:537-553, 1977

GOLD AND TEFLON IN THE OVAL WINDOW

A comparison of stapes prostheses

Rinze A. Tange[1], Arthur J.G. de Bruijn[1] and Wouter A. Dreschler[2]

Departments of [1]Otolaryngology – Head and Neck Surgery, Division of Otology, and [2]Audiology, Academic Medical Center, University of Amsterdam, Amsterdam, The Netherlands

Abstract

This paper present the results of a study in which retrospective analyses were carried out on the pre- and postoperative hearing results obtained after primary stapedotomy. One hundred and three gold pistons and 97 Teflon piston implantations were evaluated. The results were compared according to mean audiometrical parameters. Furthermore, the individual audiological results were demonstrated with the 'Amsterdam Hearing Evaluations Plot' (AHEP). This method is a visual presentation of the hearing result for each operated ear. These AHEPs clearly show the results of this comparative study and the authors conclude that there is a trend towards the heavier gold piston (shaft diameter, 0.4 mm; weight, 10.2 mg) giving more overclosure (35.9%) gain than the lightweight (shaft diameter, 0.4 mm; weight, 3.2 mg) Teflon piston (27.8% cases of overclosure). Because of the different properties of the two pistons (gold is very malleable; Teflon rather stiff), a choice can be made for different anatomical or pathological situations in the operated middle ear.

Keywords: otosclerosis, stapedectomy, audiometry, Teflon, gold

Introduction

During the evolution of otosclerosis surgery, various materials have been used to compose the stapes prostheses. Current prostheses are most commonly composed of three materials: fluoroplastic (Teflon type polymer), stainless steel, or platinum. Of these, Teflon remains the most frequently used material. Recently, a new prosthesis composed of gold became available on the market. Gold has the same advantage of not being reactive with tissue. One of the most important differences between Teflon and gold is the specific gravity of the material.

Address for correspondence: Prof. R.A. Tange, UHD MD, Department of Otolaryngology – Head and Neck Surgery, Academic Medical Center, University of Amsterdam, Meibergdreef 9, 1105 AZ Amsterdam, The Netherlands. *email:* R.A.Tange@amc.uva.nl

The Function and Mechanics of Normal, Diseased and Reconstructed Middle Ears, pp. 255–260
edited by J.J. Rosowski and S.N. Merchant
© 2000 Kugler Publications, The Hague, The Netherlands

In our clinic, the Teflon piston was the most frequently used. However, since the golden piston became available in 1995, we have started to use this prosthesis for implantation, and the first results were promising[1]. The purpose of this study was to analyze retrospectively the audiological results of the heavier gold piston compared to the lighter Teflon piston. For data analysis, *mean* values of several audiological parameters are most often taken into account, and we also analyzed our results in this way. However, it is also illustrative to evaluate the hearing results of each *individual* ear in separate analyses for the ears that received a gold or a Teflon piston. Therefore, we used the 'Amsterdam Hearing Evaluation Plot' (AHEP)[2] as a method of simple visual presentation of the audiometric results of each individually operated ear. Presenting results with AHEPs opens up the possibility of interpreting and analyzing audiometric data in whatever way desired.

Material and methods

In the two-year period from January 1994 to December 1995, a Teflon stapes replacement prosthesis was the first choice in primary stapes surgery, and in the following two-year period from January 1996 to December 1997, a gold stapes replacement prosthesis was the first choice. All operations were performed by one experienced surgeon who had performed more than 500 stapes operations before the period of this study, and therefore the selection bias caused by a learning curve, due to the fact that the surgeon would be more experienced during the second set of surgeries, only played a minor role. Ninety-seven Teflon pistons (shaft diameter, 0.4 mm; weight, 3.2 mg) and 103 gold pistons (shaft diameter, 0.4 mm; weight, 10.2 mg) were implanted. The patients receiving a Teflon piston consisted of 31 males and 66 females, with a median age of 39.7 years at the time of surgery. The patients receiving a gold piston consisted of 34 males and 69 females, with a median age of 41.9 years at the time of operation. The transcanal surgical approach to the middle ear was used in all cases. In all cases, the micro-pick technique described by Marquet[3] was used to create a small area fenestra in the stapes footplate. The pistons were inserted directly into the opening of the stapes footplate. No soft tissue grafts were used to cover or fill the oval window for sealing purposes. Oral antibiotic prophylaxis was given during surgery in all cases. Each patient had audiometric testing of both air-conduction (AC) thresholds and bone-conduction (BC) thresholds before and after the operation. All audiograms were performed by classified personnel according to the ISO-389 (1975) standard. The mean follow-up time after surgery was 18.2 months in the gold piston group and 24.5 months in the Teflon group. For evaluation of the effects on the air-bone gap (ABG), we used the AC and BC from the same test session (*i.e.*, postoperative audiogram) to compute the postoperative ABG, as recommended by the AAO-HNS. All data were entered into a computer database and analyzed with a spreadsheet program. Inferential statistics (paired t tests) were used to study the hearing changes per group. Our criterion for statistical significance was set at a p value ≤ 0.05.

Results

The results are presented with regard to mean postoperative changes in BC, ABG and AC. Furthermore, the hearing results of each individual ear were analyzed separately for the gold piston and Teflon piston groups. Preoperatively, there were no clear differences in BC thresholds between the groups. Postoperatively, there was an average improvement in mean BC levels at all frequencies for both prostheses, with exception of 0.25 kHz in the Teflon piston. The most obvious improvements in mean BC thresholds were at 2 kHz, being 8.4 dB for the gold piston and 7.4 dB for the Teflon piston group. In the gold piston group, the mean improvements in BC hearing were statistically significant (paired t test) for the individual frequencies in the range from 0.5-2 kHz, whereas the mean improvement in the Teflon piston group was statistically significant (paired t test) for the frequency 2 kHz. However, none of the inter-group differences according to the repeated measures analysis of variance were statistically significant for any of the frequencies.

Before surgery, the mean ABG for the three frequency pure tone audiograms (PTAs) was 30.9 dB in the gold piston group and 29.4 dB in the Teflon piston group. Postoperatively, these values were 6.9 and 7.7 dB, respectively. After a repeated measures analysis of variance, there was no evidence of a significantly better ABG reduction between the groups. Taking ABG closure within 10 dB as a measure of success, the gold piston had a small advantage. Before surgery, there were no clear differences in the mean AC thresholds between the groups. Postoperatively, there were statistically significant (paired t test) improvements in the AC thresholds at all frequencies for both prostheses, except at 8 kHz. The mean preoperative AC levels for the four frequency PTAs were 52.3 dB in the gold piston group and 49.3 dB in the Teflon piston group. Postoperatively, this improved to 25.7 and 25.6 dB, respectively. We used AHEPs[2] as a method of visual presentation when reporting the hearing results in each individually operated ear that had received a gold and a Teflon piston. To visualize the effect of surgery on each operated case, the AHEP was designed by De Bruijn et al.[2]. The gain in AC after surgery is largely dependent on the preoperative gap between AC and BC levels: the greater the ABG, the more gain there may be expected in AC after a technically successful operation.

To show the relationship between these two parameters, the AC for the PTA combination 0.5, 1, 2, and 4 kHz is plotted against the preoperative ABG of each individually operated ear in Figures 1 and 2 for the gold and Teflon pistons, respectively. In these graphs, the solid diagonal line indicates total closure of the gap between preoperative AC and BC. Consequently, each point below the solid diagonal line indicates a gain in AC larger than what may be expected from the preoperative ABG, and such a result can be regarded as overclosure. The number of overclosures can easily be seen from the plots, being 37 (35.9%) in the golden piston group (Fig. 1) and 27 (27.8%) in the Teflon piston group (Fig. 2). All ears that were considered a technically 'successful' operation (i.e., all points below the thinner diagonal line) had ABG closure to 20 dB or less between postoperative AC and

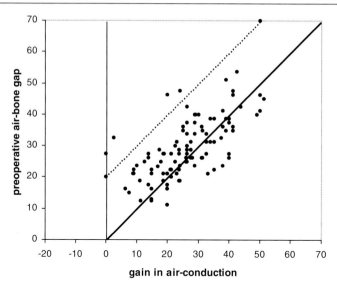

Fig. 1. Audiometric results after implantation of 103 gold pistons visualized with the Amsterdam Hearing Evaluation Plot (AHEP). Postoperative gain in air conduction plotted against preoperative air-bone gap for individual ears. PTA was calculated for the frequency combination at 0.5, 1, 2, and 4 kHz. The thicker diagonal line indicates total closure of the gap between preoperative air conduction and bone conduction. Each point below this line is defined as overclosure. An unsuccessful operation result with regard to air conduction is defined as a negative change in air conduction (indicated by the dotted vertical line at 0 dB gain in air conduction), or a change in air conduction that was not enough to close the gap between postoperative air conduction and postoperative bone conduction to 20 dB or less (indicated by the thin dotted diagonal line).

preoperative BC levels, but also between postoperative AC and postoperative BC thresholds. We defined an 'unsuccessful' result as a negative change in AC threshold, or a change in AC that was not enough to close the gap between postoperative AC and preoperative BC to 20 dB or less. Each point above the thinner diagonal line in Figures 1 and 2 indicates such an 'unsuccessful' result.

Discussion

Since Shea introduced the stapedectomy and interposition of the stapes prosthesis in 1958[4], many different prostheses have become available on the market, and the Teflon piston is now the most widely employed prosthesis for reconstruction of the ossicular chain in cases of otosclerosis. Recently, Pusalkar and Steinbach[5] introduced a new type of stapes prosthesis made of 99.9% pure gold. This new gold piston inhibits bacterial growth due to its ologodynamic properties, and is easy to handle around the long process of the incus. Gold is soft and malleable so that the stapes piston can easily be shaped to the individual condition of the incus and stapes footplate in cases of otosclerosis.

Comparison of stapes replacement prostheses in the literature is difficult

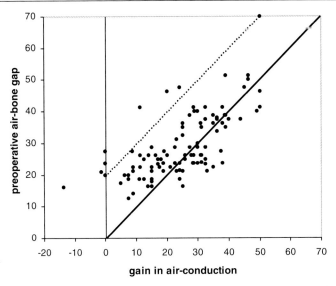

Fig. 2. Audiometric results after implantation of 97 Teflon pistons visualized with the Amsterdam Hearing Evaluation Plot (AHEP). Postoperative gain in air conduction plotted against preoperative air-bone gap for individual ears. PTA was calculated for the frequency combination at 0.5, 1, 2, and 4 kHz.

because different audiological criteria are used to establish success. Some studies report pre- and postoperative AC results with three or four frequency pure-tone averages[6,7]. Other studies used postoperative ABG to evaluate success[8,9]. Using preoperative BC thresholds rather than postoperative BC thresholds to compute the ABG artificially improves hearing results after stapes surgery because ABG overclosure due to the Carhart effect is included. In our results, this improvement was 4.5% for the gold piston and 3.3% for the Teflon piston for a closure rate within 10 dB, averaged at 0.5, 1, 2, and 4 kHz.

We used AHEPs to evaluate the hearing results in each operated ear. The plots show the individual results and visualize the amount of overclosures (Figs. 1 and 2), which is especially interesting when reporting the results of stapes surgery. In addition, the unfavorable hearing results can easily be recognized with regard to cochlear damage and residual conductive hearing loss.

When comparing audiometric results after implanting different prostheses, it is important only to take those prostheses into account that are functioning normally with regard to sound transmission function. By not excluding 'unsuccessfully' performed operations (*i.e.*, all points above the thinner diagonal line in Figures 1 and 2), this could easily lead to misleading results. The exact reason why a substantial ABG still exists postoperatively can only be detected by performing revision surgery. Although definitions of good, moderate, or unsuccessful results are arbitrary issues, we chose to define an 'unsuccessful' result as a negative change in AC threshold or a remaining gap of more than 20 dB between postoperative AC and preoperative BC levels.

In our opinion, analyzing audiometric data with AHEPs is a valuable complementary method for determining technical success after surgery and for comparing the spread in individual results for different populations. The results of a previous comparable study of the two different stapes prostheses have shown that the lighter Teflon piston gives slightly more hearing gain in the higher frequencies, and that the heavier gold piston gives more gain in the lower frequencies. The results of this study with a larger number of patients showed the same outcome. Furthermore, we also found a higher overclosure rate with the heavier gold piston (35.9%) compared to the lighter Teflon piston (27.8%).

In the present study, we were also interested in the postoperative hearing results in the two pistons studied, as well as in the different clinical possibilities of the two pistons. The advantage of the Teflon piston is its stiffness, which is important in cases of adhesion formation. Furthermore, the length of the Teflon piston can easily be altered. Disadvantages of the full Teflon piston are that it cannot be shaped to the individual condition of the middle ear, and that sometimes the positioning of the 'self-thinking' ring can be traumatic to the incus. The advantage of the solid gold piston is that it is malleable, and therefore can easily be shaped to the individual condition of the middle ear. On the other hand, the handle of the gold piston is sometimes too malleable, and therefore difficult to place. Another disadvantage of the piston is the fact that its length cannot be altered.

As a result of this study, we use the Teflon piston in particular in situations of dense fibrous adhesion formations. Because of the stiffness of the Teflon piston, its bending by fibrous tissue is prevented. In cases of anatomical variations in the middle ear, a malleable gold piston can be very useful. Although the overall hearing results were in favor of the gold piston, both types gave good hearing results.

References

1. Tange RA, De Bruijn AJG, Grolman W: Experience with a new pure gold piston in stapedotomy for cases of otosclerosis. Auris Nasus Larynx 25:249-253, 1998
2. De Bruijn AJG, Tange RA, Dreschler WA: Comparison of stapes protheses: a retrospective analysis of individual audioetric results obtained after stapedotomy. Am J Otol 20(5):573-580, 1991
3. Marquet JFE: Technique of stapedotomy. In: Filipo R (ed) Otosclerosis, pp 83-87. Amsterdam/ Milano: Kugler & Ghedini 1990
4. Shea JJ Jr: Fenestration of the oval window. Ann Otol Rhinol Laryngol 67:932-951, 1958
5. Pusalkar AG, Steinbach E: Gold implants in middle ear reconstructive surgery. In: Yanagihara N, Suzuki J (eds) Transplants and Implants Otology, II, pp 111-113. 1992
6. Ginsberg IA, Hoffman SR, White TP, Stinziano GD: Hearing changes following stapedectomy: a six year follow up. Laryngoscope 91:87-92, 1981
7. Schöndorf J, Pilorget J, Gräber S: Der einfluss des Prothesentyps auf das Langzeitergebnis der Stapedektomie; ein Vergleich der Drahtprothese mit der Stahlpistonprothese nach Robinson. HNO 28:153-157, 1980
8. Perkins R, Curto FS: Laser stapedotomy: a comparative study of prostheses and seals. Laryngoscope 102:1321-1327, 1992
9. Elonka DR, Derlacki EL, Harrison WH: Stapes prosthesis comparison. Otolaryngol Head Neck Surg 90:263-265, 1982

MALLEUS-GRIP STAPEDECTOMY
Surgical technique and results

R. Häusler and E. Oestreicher

University Clinic of ENT, Head and Neck Surgery, Inselspital, University of Bern, Bern, Switzerland

Abstract

This is a retrospective evaluation of a series of 44 malleus-grip stapedectomies on 40 patients. Primary malleus-strip stapedectomy was performed because of congenital or inflammatory fixation of the incus and/or malleus head in addition to stapes fixation, or because of a luxated or absent incus. In 31 ears, malleus-grip stapedectomy was a revision procedure because of ankylosis of the incus or malleus head, necrosis of the long process of the incus, luxation of the incus, previous fenestration, or other ear operations. Thirty-nine of the 40 operated patients received follow-up. Thirty-six had a postoperative hearing gain of 14-50 dB. In three patients, a definitive hearing gain was only obtained following revision of their malleus-grip stapedectomy. The residual air-bone gap between 0.5 and 3 kHz was ≤10 dB in 40% and ≤20 dB in 85%. One patient developed a sensory-neural hearing loss of 40 dB with vertigo several weeks following the operation. The results of malleus-grip stapedectomy are less successful compared to primary incus stapedotomy, but the procedure is quite safe and allows a hearing gain to an acceptably good range in most cases.

Keywords: malleus-grip stapedectomy, vestibulo-malleopexy, stapedectomy revision, middle ear malformation, argon laser in otology

Introduction

Conductive hearing loss due to stapes footplate ankylosis may be treated by stapedectomy with fixation of the prosthesis at the long process of the incus. If this is not possible because of an absent incus or luxation or necrosis of the long incus process, it is possible to establish a direct connection between the eardrum and the inner ear by means of an extra-long malleus-grip prosthesis. This so-called 'malleus-grip' stapedectomy, also known as incus replacement stapedectomy or vestibulo-malleopexy, has been used by a small number of otological surgeons since the 1960s[1-4,6-12]. In the present study, we analyzed

Address for correspondence: R. Häusler, MD, Department of Otorhinolaryngology, Head and Neck and Cranio-Maxillo-Facial Surgery, University of Berne, Inselspital, 3010 Bern, Switzerland

The Function and Mechanics of Normal, Diseased and Reconstructed Middle Ears, pp. 261–270
edited by J.J. Rosowski and S.N. Merchant
© *2000 Kugler Publications, The Hague, The Netherlands*

results of 44 consecutive malleus-grip stapedectomies. Our surgical technique is described with presentation of a modified extra-long malleus handle platinum wire-ribbon piston. The results obtained in the present series are compared with those in other published studies.

Patients and methods

Patients

Between 1992 and 1998, 548 stapedectomies were performed by the senior author (RH). Among these, 44 (8%) were malleus-grip stapedectomies, which were carried out on 40 patients (21 females and 19 males, ranging in age from 19-75 years). Of the 44 malleus-grip stapedectomies, 13 (29%) were primary interventions and 31 (71%) revisions. In 13 patients, malleus-grip stapedectomy was their first operation, in 23 patients it was their second, in seven their third, and in one patient it was in fact their fourth, eventually successful, intervention on the same ear.

Indications

Indications for malleus-grip stapedectomy are listed in Tables 1 and 2. The 13 patients who underwent primary malleus-grip stapedectomy were shown to have a fixed stapes and, in addition, a problem with the incus. Nine of these patients had an infectious or congenital ankylosis of the incus and/or malleus head. In the remaining four patients, the intervention was performed because of incus luxation (three cases) due to previous ear trauma or incus malformation, or because of an absent incus (one case). In addition, in three cases there was partial atresia of the external auditory meatus, confirming the presence of an ear malformation. In 31 patients, malleus-grip stapedectomy was a revision procedure. Seventeen of these were cases with a history of a prior stapedotomy with persistent or recurrent conductive hearing loss. In eight cases, there was also ankylosis of the incus or malleus, in six cases necrosis of the long incus process, and in three cases incus luxation which, in most cases, had occurred in conjunction with a previous ear surgery. Four elderly patients underwent malleus-grip stapedectomy after a fenestration operation of the lateral semicircular canal, which had been carried out many years earlier. These patients had a previous radical mastoidectomy cavity with fenestration of the lateral semicircular canal, including removal of the incus and malleus head. Only the malleus handle remained for piston fixation. In six other patients, the malleus-grip stapedectomy was performed after various other middle ear operations for persistent conductive hearing loss. This was often necessary following a previous incus interposition on an undiagnosed simultaneously ankylozed stapes. Malleus-grip stapedectomy was performed twice (once in a primary and once in a revision case) despite a mobile footplate due to fractured stapes crurae, even though a TORP (Total Ossicular Replacement Proteins) reconstruction is usually preferred in this situation in order to avoid an opening into the inner ear. Finally, because only a minimal hearing gain had been obtained or hearing had again decreased, malleus-grip stapedectomy revision was performed in three patients until a persistent hearing gain was achieved. All patients in whom malleus-grip stapedectomy was carried out had a preoperative high grade conductive hearing loss with a negative Rinne and a mean air-conduction threshold between 0.5, 1, 2 and 3 (or 4) kHz of ≥30 dB.

Table 1. Indications for malleus-grip stapedectomy as a primary intervention. In addition, in three ears, there was congenital partial atresia of the ear canal

Stapes fixation with		
fixation of the incus and/or malleus head	9	
luxation of the incus (including one case with a mobile		
footplate and additionally fractured stapes crura)	3	
absent incus	1	
Total	13	(29%)

Table 2. Indications for malleus-grip stapedectomy as revision surgery

After a previous stapedectomy		
ankylosis of the incus and/or malleus head	8	
necrosis of the incus process	6	
incus luxation	3	
After a previous fenestration procedure	4	
Following other ear surgery		
previous incus interposition on a fixed stapes	5	
mobile footplate with broken stapes crura and absent incus	1	
Revision of a previous malleus-grip stapedectomy	4	
Total	31	(71%)

Surgical technique

Malleus-grip stapedectomy was always performed using a transcanal approach without an external skin incision through the fixed ear speculum, which was held in place by an articulated metallic arm. Local anesthesia was used (pre-medication: morphine i.m. in mg corresponding to body weight in kg with 0.2-0.5 mg Scopolamin) with injections of 2-8 ml xylocaine-adrenalin 2% in the four quadrants of the cartilagenous canal, basically according to the Schuknecht technique[4,12,13]. A posterior tympano-meatal flap was elevated. When the indication for malleus-grip stapedectomy became evident, the upper part of the malleus handle, all the way to the neck, was carefully separated from the eardrum with a microtip, and the upper border of the tympano-meatal flap was extended anteriorly over the malleus neck. The connection of the tympanic membrane at the umbo was retained whenever feasible. If there was an additional fixation of the malleus head, the head was detached at the neck superior to the tendon of the *tensor tympani* muscle in order to maintain its stabilizing function on the malleus. Next, total footplate removal or a large opening was created within the posterior part of the stapes footplate. This was usually carried out with the aid of the Skeeter microdrill and a 0.3-mm micro-hook. In revision surgery with fibrous tissue present in the oval window, the argon laser and in one case the erbium laser equipped with a fiberoptic micro-handpiece, were used to carry out the footplate perforation[3-5]. After estimation of distance, an extra-long malleus-grip wire-fluoroplast prosthesis (diameter: 0.6 mm) was selected. Prostheses with lengths of 5.0-6.50 mm were used. This extra-long prosthesis was bent according to the anatomical proportions. With as far as possible a single motion, it was placed in such a way that the loop encircled the uppermost part of the malleus handle and the piston came to rest either at the edge of the oval window or directly within the oval window. The loop was clamped onto the malleus grip as close as possible to the short process, by means of a crimper. Total encirclement of the piston loop around the malleus grip was achieved with a 0.3-mm hook held in the right hand, at the same time securing the piston with

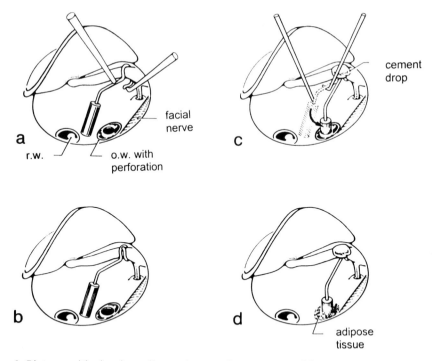

Fig. 1. Piston positioning in malleus-grip stapedectomy. *a and b.* Surrounding the denuded proximal malleus grip with a wire loop with the aid of a 0.3-mm hook held in the right hand, while securing the prosthesis with the aspirator held in the left. *c.* After consolidation of the wire loop around the malleus grip with a drop of dental cement, the piston is advanced into the oval window with two micro-hooks. *d.* Inserted piston of the malleus handle prosthesis. The opening in the footplate is sealed with adipose tissue from the earlobe.

micro-forceps held in the left. The piston was then placed quite deeply into the posterior part of the oval window by progressively bending the wire. Care was taken that the movements did not provoke dizziness.

In the more recent cases, the loop around the malleus grip was additionally secured by a drop of hydroxylapatite and later by Biocem glass polymer bone cement (Corinthian Medical Ltd., Nottingham, UK)[4]. This greatly eased the delicate manipulations necessary to lead the piston into its optimal final positioning.

The oval window was then sealed with adipose tissue harvested from the earlobe. The metal loop and the cement drop at the malleus grip were likewise covered with a small amount of adipose tissue in order to avoid direct contact between cement and eardrum. The tympano-meatal flap was put back in place. Occasionally, if present, fissures in the tympanic membrane, resulting from eardrum detachment from the malleus grip, would also be padded with earlobe adipose tissue. The external ear canal was packed with silk strips and plugged with gauze soaked in Otosporin. Figure 1 is a schematic illustration of the main steps of the malleus-grip stapedectomy technique, as described above.

Description of a specially-designed malleus-handle platinum wire-ribbon fluoroplast piston

For the first 34 malleus-grip stapedectomies, the classical Schuknecht malleus-handle steel wire fluoroplast piston (Fig. 2, left) was used. This has a long wire loop that can be wrapped completely around the malleus grip, as shown in Figure 1. However, the steel wire is somewhat rigid and, because of its memory effect, is quite difficult to place in an optimal position. For this reason, we designed a modified malleus-handle piston in which the steel wire is replaced by a platinum wire that is flattened to a ribbon at the loop, as shown on the right of Figure 2. We have been using this modified malleus-handle stapedectomy piston since 1997, and the fixation of the platinum band around the malleus neck, as well as the following positioning of the piston by bending the platinum wire, has clearly become easier. The modified platinum wire-ribbon Teflon piston is produced by Smith and Nephew®, and is in preparation by Xomed® (Häusler modification of the Schuknecht malleus-handle piston).

Audiological evaluation

A preoperative pure-tone audiogram was performed on the day prior to surgery. All patients were checked again postoperatively after two months. The last audiometric examination considered in this study took place one to six years after the last surgical intervention. The evaluation of the postoperative hearing gain was carried out according to the recommendations of the AAOO[15]. In the examinations that took place before 1994, 4 kHz replaced the 3 kHz frequency in our study.

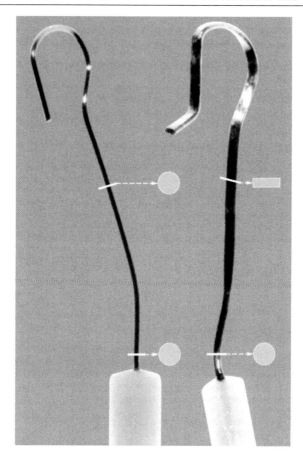

Fig. 2. Magnified view of the wire loop of the classical Schuknecht malleus-handle steel wire fluoroplast piston (left) and of the newly designed modified malleus-handle platinum wire ribbon fluoroplast piston (right) (Smith and Nephew®).

Results

Of the 40 patients operated on, 39 could be followed up. No audiograms were obtained from a patient living abroad, who reported a non-problematic course after malleus-grip stapedectomy. Thirty-six (92%) of the 39 patients had improved hearing (hearing gain: 15-50 dB) postoperatively with a positive Rinne tuning-fork test (512 Hz). Permanent hearing gain was only obtained in three patients after revision surgery because, in the first weeks after malleus-grip stapedectomy, the piston had suddenly extruded from the oval window. Repositioning of the piston somewhat deeper in the vestibulum by additional bending of the wire was non-problematic in these cases, and was performed on an outpatient basis under local anesthesia. One patient, who opted against revision surgery, also has recurring hearing loss, presumably because of a displaced piston. For reasons unknown, another patient only had negligible postoperative hearing improvement. The final patient developed

Table 3. Postoperative hearing threshold with malleus-grip stapedectomy with a follow-up of one to five years

Air-bone gap (0.5,1,2,3 (4) kHz)	n=38*	%
≤10	15	40
11-20	17	45
21-30	4	10
≥30	2	5
Total	38	100

*The patient with postoperatively sensory-neural hearing loss has been excluded

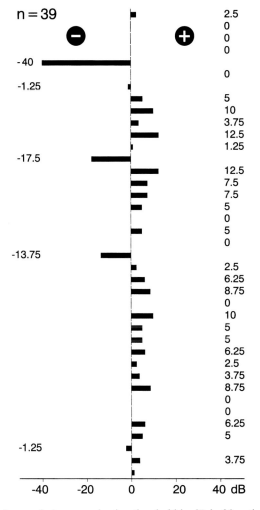

Fig. 3. Postoperative changes in bone conduction threshold in dB in 39 patients after malleus-grip stapedectomy. The values of the bone conduction threshold correspond to the mean value calculated from the frequencies at 0.5, 1, 2, 3 (or 4) kHz.

sudden conductive hearing loss followed by vertigo and additional sensory-neural hearing loss of 40 dB one month following favorable malleus-grip stapedectomy.

Following malleus-handle stapedectomy, patients generally denied having any vertiginous symptoms, even during large pressure changes. Only three patients recounted that they had experienced occasional short translation vertigo during car-door slamming, forceful sneezing, or on driving into a tunnel. However, this did not affect their daily activities. There were no other complications. In particular, there were no wire extrusions through the tympanic membrane.

The postoperative hearing results are summarized in Table 3. Eighty-five percent of the patients had a mean residual air-bone gap of ≤20 dB. An optimal residual air-bone gap of ≤10 dB was reached by only 40% of the patients. The changes in postoperative compared to preoperative bone conduction thresholds are shown in Figure 3 for all 39 patients who underwent follow-up. As well as the patient who developed a sensory-neural hearing loss of 40 dB postoperatively, two others also experienced lesser degrees of high-frequency sensory-neural losses of 10 and 12 dB, respectively.

Discussion

Malleus-grip stapedectomy is technically more difficult than primary, uncomplicated incus stapedotomy. Furthermore, the direct connection between malleus grip and the inner ear is a less optimal acoustic transmission than through an intact malleus and incus. For this reason, it is understandable that the results of malleus-grip stapedectomy are less optimal than those of primary stapedotomy, where an air-bone gap closure of ≤20 dB is reached in over 95% of cases[4]. Nonetheless, 92% of patients enjoyed a considerable postoperative hearing gain after malleus-grip stapedectomy in our series and, in 85%, the mean residual air-bone gap was ≤20 dB. With malleus-grip stapedectomy, there is also a real risk of a significant postoperative sensory-neural hearing loss, which in our series amounted to 2.4% (one case). No total deafness occurred in our small series of 44 operations.

The most prevalent postoperative complication was the extrusion of the piston from the oval window, which occurred in 8% in our series, predominantly in the earlier cases. Rapid repositioning of the piston by a transcanalicular approach under local anesthesia in a previously known middle ear situation led to a nonproblematic outcome with permanent hearing improvement in these cases. Piston extrusion always occurred in the first few weeks following malleus-grip stapedectomy. We did not encounter any late extrusions. We have now learned how better to prevent this complication by placing the piston relatively deeply in the posterior part of the oval window, since no significant inner ear structures are normally found at this location. The problem of optimal piston positioning makes it advisable that malleus-grip stapedectomy should be performed under local anesthesia, so that subjective sensations of the patient with regard to vertigo and hearing may be monitored throughout the procedure. In this respect, it is interesting to note that lasting

Table 1. Comparison of the results of five reports from the literature after malleus-grip stapedectomy

Author	Sheehy	Shea	Schuknecht	Eberle (Fisch's results)	Tange	Present study
Year	1982	1983	1986	1992	1996	1998
No. of patients	146	35	187	123	41	40
Residual air-bone gap						
≤10 dB	51%		36%		70%	40%
≤20 dB	81%	84%	69.1%		88%	85%
Postoperative hearing						
improvement	84%			90%	92.7%	92.2%
				>20 dB hearing		(hearing
				gain in 56% of		gain of
				the patients		15-50 dB)
Sensory-neural						
hearing loss ≥30 dB	4%		8%		0	2.5%
	(≥30 dB)		(≥15 dB)			(*n*=1)
Profound deafness	2%		2%	1.1%	0	0

vertiginous symptoms after piston fixation on the malleus were highly uncommon, even during more important static pressure changes at the eardrum. Apparently, a piston placed deep in the posterior part of the oval window is much less of a problem than the possibility of piston extrusion of a piston placed more superficially. The problem of piston extrusion also prevented us from covering the oval window with an underlying vein graft below the piston. The oval window was sealed with adipose tissue placed around the inserted piston.

In the stapedectomy literature, many otological surgeons indicate that they occasionally carry out malleus-grip stapedectomy, mainly during stapes revision surgery, but without analyzing their results with respect to this special surgical technique[2-6,10]. We have only found five studies that address the topic of malleus-grip stapedectomy specifically[1,8-10,12]. The results of these studies are summarized in Table 4, although direct comparison of the results is difficult because different evaluation criteria were often used. Three papers deal with groups of over 100 patients who were operated on over a period of more than 20 years by well-known otological surgeons. The results of the various studies are relatively similar. The more recent studies possibly show a trend towards better hearing gains and fewer complications. This might be due to improved technical means, such as use of the Skeeter microdrill and the laser. Our introduction of cement to fix the wire loop in malleus-grip stapedectomy proved beneficial and made the final positioning of the piston easier. The specially-designed malleus-handle platinum wire-ribbon fluoroplast piston we have been using since 1997 also turned out to be a significant improvement. This not only has made the procedure of piston fixation and positioning technically less difficult, it also paved the way for the absence of any further piston extrusions in the series performed since 1997. The careful piston fixation procedure on the malleus also explains why wire extrusions through the tympanic membrane, mentioned in other malleus-grip stapedectomy reports[8,12], did not occur in a single instance in our series.

Conclusions

Our analysis confirms that malleus-grip stapedectomy is an adequate surgical alternative when incus attachment stapedectomy is not possible. Postoperative vertigo symptoms were rare in our series of malleus-grip stapedectomy, and the risk of sensory-neural hearing loss appears to be no more frequent than in primary stapedotomy.

References

1. Eberle L: Indikationen and Resultate der Incusersatzstapedotomie bei fixierter and mobiler Fussplatte. ORL Akt Probl Otorhinol 17:91-98, 1994
2. Farrior J: Revision stapes surgery. Laryngoscope 101:1155-1161, 1991
3. Han WW, Incesulu A, McKenna MJ, Rauch SD, Nadol JB, Glynn RJ: Revision stapedectomy: intraoperative findings, results, and review of the literature. Laryngoscope 107:1185-1192, 1997
4. Häusler R: Fortschritte in der Stapeschirurgie. Laryngo Rhino Otol 97(Suppl 2):95-139, 2000
5. Häusler R, Schär PJ, Pratisto H, Weber HP, Frenz M: Advantages and dangers of Erbium laser application in stapedotomy. Acta Otolaryngol (Stockh) 119:207-213, 1999
6. Langmann AW, Lindeman RC: 1993 Revision stapedectomy. Laryngoscope 103:954-958, 1993
7. Lippy WH, Schuring AG, Moshe Z: Stapedectomy revision. Am J Otol 2:15-21, 1980
8. Schuknecht HF, Bartley M: Malleus grip prothesis. Ann Otol Rhinol Laryngol 95:531-534, 1986
9. Shea JJ: Malleus Teflon piston prothesis. Laryngoscope 93:989-991, 1983
10. Sheehy JL: Stapedectomy: incus bypass procedures. A report of 203 operations. Laryngoscope 92:258-262, 1982
11. Silverstein H, Beendet E, Rosenberg S, Nichols M: Revision stapes surgery with and without laser: a comparison. Laryngoscope 104:1431-1438, 1994
12. Tange RA: Ossicular reconstruction in cases of absent or inadequate incus, congenital malformation of the middle ear and epitympanic fixation of the incus and malleus. ORL 58:143-146, 1996
13. Häusler R, Messerli A, Romano V, Burkhaller R, Weber HP, Altermatt HJ: Experimental and clinical results of fiberoptic argon laser stapedotomy. Eur Arch Otorhinolaryngol 253:193-200, 1996
14. Schuknecht HF: Current method of stapes surgery. Adv Otorhinolaryngol 37:101-103, 1987
15. Committee on Hearing and Equilibrium: Committee on hearing and equilibrium guidelines for the evaluation of results of treatment of conductive hearing loss. Otolaryngol Head Neck Surg 113:186-187, 1995

SHORT- AND LONG-TERM RESULTS AFTER STAPES SURGERY FOR OTOSCLEROSIS WITH A TEFLON-WIRE PISTON PROSTHESIS

Izabel Kos, Jean-Philippe Guyot and Pierre B. Montandon

Department of Otolaryngology – Head and Neck Surgery, University Hospital, Geneva, Switzerland

Abstract

The authors analyzed the results of 604 cases of primary stapes surgery performed between 1974 and 1997 with replacement of the stapes by a 0.6 or 0.8 mm Schuknecht Teflon-wire piston. At long term (one to 21 years; mean, seven years), the residual air-bone gap was less than or equal to 10 dB in 78.9% of cases. Hearing results and postoperative complications were comparable to those reported by authors who used the same evaluation criteria. Although the aim of the surgery was to perform a small stapedotomy with a narrow footplate perforation (0.8 mm), a large stapedotomy or a stapedectomy was performed in some cases due to surgical or anatomical conditions. These results show that the larger footplate perforations allowed better correction of the air-bone gap in the lower frequencies. The larger sizes of perforations did not show a higher incidence of complications.

Keywords: stapedotomy, stapedectomy, teaching

Introduction

The surgical technique for the correction of hearing loss caused by otosclerosis has quickly evolved from total extraction of the footplate, so-called stapedectomy[1], to a small perforation in the center of the footplate, stapedotomy[2]. Today, some surgeons use small diameter pistons inserted into the inner ear through a fenestra that is not larger than 0.4 mm[3]. Unless a laser is used, the footplate perforation and placement of the prosthesis demand a high level of technical skill. Several series by prestigious surgeons have been published, demonstrating the accuracy and advantages of stapedotomy compared to other techniques[4]. However, series including operations performed by residents and fellows in-training are rarer[5,6].

The objective of this study was to evaluate the short- and long-term results

Address for correspondence: Izabel Kos, MD, Department of Otolaryngology – Head and Neck Surgery, University Hospital, 24 Rue Micheli-du-Crest, 1211 Geneva 14, Switzerland

The Function and Mechanics of Normal, Diseased and Reconstructed Middle Ears, pp. 271–279
edited by J.J. Rosowski and S.N. Merchant
© *2000 Kugler Publications, The Hague, The Netherlands*

of all cases of stapes surgery performed in our department between 1974 and 1997, and to address the question of whether stapes surgery can be taught safely. In each case, the aim of surgery was to perform a small stapedotomy but, due to surgical or anatomical conditions, a larger stapedotomy or a stapedectomy was necessary in about one of five cases. These cases were initially considered to be surgical accidents but, to our surprise, analysis showed that the functional results and the rate of complications were similar to those of small stapedotomies.

Material and methods

We analyzed the results of 604 cases of otosclerosis operated on between 1974 and 1997 by 19 different surgeons, including residents in-training. The series included 253 (42%) males and 351 (58%) females. The age of the population at the time of surgery ranged from 17 to 72 years, with an average of 43.0 years (±10.7). The diagnosis of otosclerosis was based on the clinical history of progressive hearing loss, normal otoscopy, a negative Rinne test, an audiogram showing a conductive hearing loss >20 dB in the range 0.5-2 kHz, and the absence of a stapedial reflex.

Surgical techniques

All operations were performed as described by Schuknecht[7,8]. A transcanal approach through the ear speculum was standard. A posterior tympanomeatal flap was elevated, the stapedius tendon cut, and the crural arch fractured and removed. The footplate was perforated with a hand drill or a motor-driven sharp-cutting burr. The aim was always to perform a narrow perforation (0.8 mm). Because of surgical or anatomical conditions, a larger perforation was performed in some cases. *A priori*, cases were divided in three groups, according to the size of the footplate perforation: *a.* small stapedotomies with a 0.8 mm perforation; *b.* large stapedotomies with a perforation larger than 0.8 mm; *c.* stapedectomies with total footplate removal. All cases were reconstructed with a Schuknecht Teflon-wire piston. From 1974 to 1983, the wire was made of stainless steel, then of platinum. A 0.6-mm diameter piston was used in most cases, a 0.8-mm piston being used in some cases of stapedectomy. In cases of large stapedotomy or stapedectomy, the oval window was sealed with a piece of ear lobe fatty tissue. The tympanomeatal flap was replaced, and the external ear packed with silk strips and cotton soaked in neomycin, polymyxin and hydrocortisone (Corticosporin®). The packing was removed five to seven days after surgery. In nearly all cases, surgery was performed under local anesthesia and, in a few cases, upon request of the patient, under general anesthesia. Hospital stay was reduced from five days in 1974 to a mostly outpatient procedure from 1994 onwards.

Evaluation of results

Preoperative audiograms (MAICO audiometer) were performed in a soundproof room the day before surgery. A short-term evaluation, including a postoperative audiogram, was performed six weeks after surgery. As a rule, our patients undergo subsequent yearly audiograms. The long-term results are based on the latest available audiogram, one to 21 years (mean, seven years) after surgery. Two values were considered: *a.* a three-frequency average air-bone gap (0.5, 1 and 2 kHz), based on the postoperative air and bone conduction thresholds; and *b.* the postoperative bone conduction threshold at 4 kHz.

Analysis

The Newman and Keuls test was used to determine significant differences between variables involving frequency data, and an analysis of variance (ANOVA) for quantitative data. The assumption of equal variances was tested with an F test[9]. A probability value of $p<0.05$ was the level of significance used for all hypothesis testings.

Results

It was possible to perform a small stapedotomy in 470 cases (77.8%). Surgical and anatomical conditions required a large stapedotomy in 83 cases (13.8%) and a stapedectomy in 51 (8.4%).

Short-term evaluation

The 604 cases were seen six weeks after surgery. The results are shown in Table 1. The number of cases with a residual air-bone gap (rABG) ≤10 dB did not show a statistically significant difference between the small stapedotomies (76.8%), large stapedotomies (87.9%) and the stapedectomies (84.0%), but the mean residual air-bone gap expressed in dB was statistically larger for small stapedotomies (6.2+6.3 dB) than for large stapedotomies (3.5±4.4 dB) or stapedectomies (3.3±4.6 dB) ($p<0.01$). In the high frequency range, the gain was significantly larger in the group of small stapedotomy (20.1±12.3 dB) than in the other two groups (large stapedectomies 15.2±12.1 dB; stapedectomies 15.6±12.3 dB; $p<0.01$).

Postoperatively, Carhart's notch was up to 25 dB lower than preoperatively (mean 3.0±9.1 dB).

A high frequency SNHL >20 dB occurred in 25 cases (4.1%), a low and high frequency SNHL >60 dB in eight (1.1%). The occurrence of SNHL was slightly more frequent and the loss (mean 15.7±12.8 dB) was greater in the group of stapedectomies and large stapedectomies than in the group of small stapedotomies, but the differences did not reach the level of significance.

Revision surgery was scheduled in 32 cases, including 19 of the 23 cases with an

Table 1. Overall results and results according to the size of the footplate perforation. The number of cases with an rABG ≤10 dB is not statistically different between groups, neither is the number of cases with a high frequency loss >20 dB

Primary surgery	Overall		Small stapedotomies		Large stapedotomies		Stapedectomies	
	n	%	n	%	n	%	n	%
Short term	604		470		83		51	
rABG ≤10 dB	477	78.9	361	76.8	73	87.9	43	84.0
rABG >10 ≤20 dB	96	15.8	86	18.2	6	7.2	4	7.8
rABG >20 dB	23	3.8	19	4.0	3	3.6	1	1.9
SNHL >60 dB	8	1.4	4	0.8	1	1.2	3	5.8
SNHL 4 kHz >20 dB	25	4.1	11	2.0	6	7.2	8	15.6
Cases requiring								
revision	32	5.2	27	5.7	3	3.6	2	3.8
rABG >20 dB	19		16		2		1	
vertigo	13		11		1		1	
Long term	441		342		58		41	
rABG ≤10 dB	350	79.3	271	79.2	48	82.0	29	70.7
rABG >10 ≤20 dB	55	9.1	43	12.5	5	8.6	9	21.9
rABG >20 dB	36	5.9	28	8.1	5	8.6	3	7.3
Cases requiring								
revision	39	8.8	30	8.7	6	10.3	3	7.3
rABG >20 dB	36		28		5		3	
vertigo	3		2		1		0	

rABG >20 dB and 13 with persistent postoperative vertigo. The results of revision surgery are reported below.

Long-term evaluation

Data from 441 cases evaluated one to 21 years (mean, seven years) after surgery were available.

The rABG was ≤10 dB in 350 cases (79.3%) (Table 1). The mean rABG (in dB) is slightly larger for small stapedotomies (5.2±7.8 dB) than for large stapedotomies (2.9±5.9 dB) and stapedectomies (3.8±6.7 dB), but these differences are not statistically significant.

Revision surgery was scheduled in 39 cases, due to persistent hearing loss in 36 cases and to progressive vertigo in three.

Based on the first and last postoperative audiogram available in these 441 cases, the mean annual hearing loss was calculated. The loss was 0.10 dB (±3.59) per year in the low frequency range (0.5+1+2 kHz) and 0.6 dB (±4.9) in the high frequency (4 kHz).

Revision surgery

In total, 71 (11.7%) of the 604 cases required revision surgery: 57 of the 470 small stapedotomies (12.1%), nine of the 83 large stapedotomies (10.8%), and five of the 51 stapedectomies (9.8%). One revision was necessary in 60 cases, two in nine cases and three in two cases. Indication for revision included lack of hearing improvement in 19 cases, recurrent hearing loss in 36, persistent postoperative vertigo in 13, and late progressive vertigo in three. Most cases of persistent or progressive hearing loss were due to fibrous tissue fixating the prosthesis, or due to erosion of the long process of the incus. Persistent postoperative or progressive vertigo was most frequently due to a prosthesis deeply settled into the oval window, sometimes secondary to retraction of the long process of the incus by fibrous tissue (Table 2). The revision consisted of dissection of the fibrous tissue and repositioning of the prosthesis. In seven cases, the incus was eroded or fixed and, therefore, the piston was attached to the malleus. A Teflon disc was placed around the piston to prevent further development of fibrous tissue. The size of the oval window fenestra was not modified.

The results are shown in Table 3. The 71 cases were seen six weeks after the last (if multiple revisions performed) revision surgery. An rABG ≤10 dB was obtained in 41 cases (57.7%). The mean rABG (10.8±9.7 dB) was significantly larger, and the gain in the high frequency range (14.7±11.9 dB) lower than that observed after primary surgery ($p<0.01$).

A high frequency SNHL >20 dB occurred in nine cases (12.6%). This rate was not significantly different from that observed following primary surgery, but the hearing loss expressed in dB was significantly greater. A low and high frequency SNHL >60 dB occurred in one case, after a second revision.

Table 2. Indications for revision surgery and operative findings according to the size of the perforation. Most cases of persisting or delayed recurrent conductive hearing loss resulted from excessive fibrous tissue or incus erosion, respectively. Vertigo was mainly due to retraction of the incus by fibrous tissue pulling the piston deeply into the vestibule

Revision surgery *Indications for revision*	*Operative findings*	*Small stapedotomies*	*Large stapedotomies*	*Stapedectomies*
Conductive	fibrous tissue	24	4	2
hearing loss	incus erosion	9	2	1
(*n*=55)	loosened loop	5		
	displaced prosthesis	2	1	1
	reobliteration	2		
	fixated malleus	2		
Vertigo	excessively deep			
(*n*=16)	prosthesis	8		
	granuloma	5	1	1
	fibrous tissue		1	

Table 3. Short- and long-term results of revision surgery. The number of cases with an rABG ≤10 dB is significantly lower than after primary surgery

Revision surgery	Short term		Long term	
	n	*%*	*n*	*%*
	71		53	
rABG ≤10 dB	41	57.7	37	69.8
rABG >10 ≤20 dB	18	25.4	8	15.1
rABG >20 dB	11		8	
SNHL >60 dB	1	1.4		
SNHL 4 kHz >20 dB	9	12.7		

Data from 53 cases were available for the long-term evaluation. The functional results were stable (Table 3).

Discussion

This study evaluates the results of 604 operations performed between 1974 and 1997 for stapes fixation caused by otosclerosis. All the operations were performed through an ordinary ear speculum, as described by Schuknecht[7,8]. Local anesthesia was standard, allowing the surgeon to test hearing and to monitor vertigo during the operation. General anesthesia was performed in a few patients, only upon request. All cases were seen six weeks after surgery. An excellent hearing gain with an rABG ≤10 dB was achieved in 78.9% of cases. The rate of success is somewhat lower than that reported by authors calculating the postoperative rABG by subtracting the preoperative bone conduction threshold from the postoperative air conduction threshold[4,6,10-12]. This method tends to artificially improve the result and even to produce overclosure of the postoperative rABG, since the bone threshold improves after surgery[13]. In our series, postoperative bone thresholds were up to 25 dB lower than the preoperative thresholds. In other series, the improvement in bone conduction was even greater[14]. Therefore, our results should be compared to, and are similar to, those reported by authors using the same evaluation criteria[15]. The rate of complications, such as immediate postoperative sensorineural hearing loss, vertigo, persisting or delayed onset conductive hearing loss, is also comparable to that of many other recent reports[12,16-18].

A yearly visit was recommended to all our patients. Long-term evaluation data (one to 21 years; mean, seven years after surgery) were available in 441 cases. The percentage of cases with an rABG ≤10 dB was similar to that observed in the early postoperative period. Therefore, the functional results are stable over time, whatever the size of the oval window fenestration. On the basis of the bone thresholds of the first postoperative and last available audiogram, it was also possible to calculate the annual hearing loss in operated ears. Our findings confirmed previous reports[16,18] showing that the annual hearing deficit was equivalent in patients operated on for otosclerosis, when compared to that observed by Osterhammel in a normal 45- to 65-year-old population, 0.4 dB in the low and 0.8 dB in the high frequency range[19]. Therefore, it seems that neither otosclerosis nor the piston inserted into the inner ear accelerate the physiological hearing loss due to aging.

Since Schuknecht and Applebaum[2] reported their excellent results in 1969, introducing a small diameter Teflon-wire piston through a small fenestra in the footplate, the so-called 'stapedotomy' has become the best corrective procedure for stapes fixation caused by otosclerosis. According to Schuknecht, this technique reduces a number of the many complications of stapedectomy, such as postoperative vertigo, reparative granuloma, and fibrous fixation of the lenticular process to the promontory[8]. In our series, the aim of the surgery was always to create a small (0.8 mm) footplate perforation. But in about one of five cases, a larger stapedotomy or a stapedectomy were performed because of a floating or fractured footplate. The high incidence of larger-than-desirable fenestra reported by authors using CO_2 or argon lasers to perforate the footplate is lower than that observed in our series[20]. Since, for economical reasons, most otologists will not have access to a laser once their residency has been completed, we deliberately chose not to use a laser for the training. To our surprise, the functional results of large stapedotomies or stapedectomies were not obviously worse than those achieved with small stapedotomies and, in contrast to previous studies[8], the rate of complications was not significantly higher! In the low frequency range, the hearing gain of stapedectomies and large stapedotomies was better than that achieved with small stapedotomies while, as in other series[10,21], it was somewhat lower in the high frequency range. We feel that performing a small stapedotomy requires a great deal of surgical skill to perforate the footplate precisely and to position the prosthesis correctly, in order to avoid any parallax that could hinder its movements. This part of the procedure is not easy for otologists in-training. However, stapedotomy can be safely taught to inexperienced surgeons since, in the case of any surgical or anatomical difficulties, the supervising senior otologist can perform a partial or total removal of the footplate and still obtain good functional results, without major complications.

As in other series[10,15,21], the best low frequency hearing gain was achieved in the group of stapedectomies. This finding could be explained by the experimental model of the middle ear developed by Rosowski and Merchant[22], who demonstrated that the gain increases proportionally to the area of movable surface in the oval window. In our series, the piston used for the reconstruction, in nearly all cases, had the same diameter (0.6 mm). However, it is possible that the flexible fatty tissue placed around the piston to seal large oval window fenestra plays a role in the transmission of the sound to the inner ear, by linking to the prosthesis and contributing to an increase in the vibrating surface area.

Revision surgery was necessary in 11.7% of cases, mostly because of persistent or late-onset recurrent conductive hearing loss. Some patients underwent two or three operations before finally obtaining a good hearing gain, which remained stable over time. The operative findings, such as the prosthesis displacement or fixation by fibrous tissue, or incus erosion, were similar to those described by many other authors[23-26]. After revision, an rABG ≤10 dB was achieved in 58% and 70% of the cases at short and long term, respectively. These results are better than those generally reported, which range from 39%[24] to 61%[23]. Most authors are hesitant to reoperate after a first revision procedure. Our series shows that a second or even a third operation is possible if hearing is not restored after the first attempt and that, although the results are not as good as those of primary surgery, they are still encouraging.

References

1. Schuknecht HF, McGee TM, Colman BH: Stapedectomy. Ann Otol Rhinol Laryngol 69:597-609, 1960
2. Schuknecht HF, Applebaum EL: Surgery for hearing loss. N Engl J Med 280:1154-1160, 1969
3. Smyth GDL, Hassard TH: Eighteen years experience in stapedectomy, the case of the small fenestra operation. Ann Otol Rhinol Laryngol 87(Suppl 49):3-33, 1978
4. Somers T, Govaerts P, Marquet T, Offeciers E: Statistical analysis of otosclerosis surgery performed by J. Marquet. Ann Otol Rhinol Laryngol 103:945-951, 1994
5. Strunk CL, Quinn FB, Bailey BJ: Stapedectomy techniques in residency training. Laryngoscope 102:121-124, 1992
6. Vernick DM: Stapedectomy results in a residency training program. Ann Otol Rhinol Laryngol 95:477-479, 1986
7. Schuknecht HF, Bentkover SH: Partial stapedectomy and piston prosthesis. In: Snow JB (ed) Controversy in Otolaryngol, pp 280-291. Philadelphia, PA: Saunders 1980
8. Schuknecht HF: Otosclerosis surgery. In: Nadol JB, Schuknecht HF (eds) Surgery of the Ear and Temporal Bone, pp 223-244. New York, NY: Raven Press 1993
9. Snedecor GW, Cochran WG: Statistical Methods. The Iowa State University Press, Ames (Iowa) (6th edn) 1967
10. Persson P, Harder H, Magnuson B: Hearing results in otosclerosis surgery after partial stapedectomy, total stapectomy and stapedotomy. Arch Otolaryngol (Stockh) 117:94-99, 1997
11. Harkness P, Brown P, Fowler S, Grant H, Topham J: A confidential comparative audit of stapedectomies: results of the Royal College of Surgeons of England comparative audit of ENT surgery 1994. J Laryngol Otol 109:317-319, 1995
12. Ramsay H, Karkkainen J, Palva T: Success in surgery for otosclerosis: hearing improvement and other indicators. Am J Otol 18:23-28, 1997
13. Carhart R: Clinical application of bone conduction audiometry. Arch Otolaryngol 51:798-808, 1950
14. Berliner K, Doyle K, Goldenberg R: Reporting operative hearing results in stapes surgery: does choice of outcome measure make a difference? Am J Otol 17:521-528, 1996
15. Richter E, Mally K, Heger F: Langzeitergebnisse der Stapesplastik mit der Schuknecht-Draht-Teflon-Prothese. Laryngo-Rhino-Otol 73:157-159, 1994
16. Langman A, Jackler R, Sooy F: Stapedectomy: long-term hearing results. Laryngoscope 101:810-814, 1991
17. Kursten R, Schneider B, Zrunek M: Long-term results after stapedectomy versus stapedotomy. Am J Otol 15:804-806, 1994
18. Vartainen E, Karjalainen S: Bone conduction thresholds in patients with otosclerosis. Am J Otol 13(4):234-236, 1992
19. Osterhammel D, Osterhammel P: High frequency audiometry: age and sex variations. Scand Audiol 8:73-78, 1979

20. Lesinski SG, Stein JA: CO2 Laser stapedotomy. Laryngoscope 99:20-24, 1989
21. Sedwick J, Louden C, Cough S: Stapedectomy vs stapedotomy. Do you really need a laser? Arch Otolaryngol Head Neck Surg 123:177-180, 1997
22. Rosowski J, Merchant S: Mechanical an acoustic analysis of middle ear reconstruction. Am J Otol 16:486-497, 1995
23. Langman A, Linderman R: Revision stapedectomy. Laryngoscope 103:954-958, 1993
24. Glasscock ME, McKennan KX, Levine SC: Revision stapedectomy surgery. Otolaryngol Head Neck Surg 96:141-148, 1987
25. Han WW, Armagan I, McKenna MJ: Revision stapedectomy: intraoperative findings, results, and review of the literature. Laryngoscope 107:1185-1192, 1997
26. Pedersen CB: Revision surgery in otosclerosis: operative findings in 186 patients. Clin Otolaryngol 19:446-450, 1994

STAPEDOTOMY PISTON DIAMETER: IS BIGGER BETTER?

Erik Teig and Henrik H. Lindeman

Department of Otolaryngology, Rikshospitalet, University of Oslo, Norway

Abstract

An important question confronting every otosclerosis surgeon is which type of stapes prosthesis should be chosen. A wide variety of prostheses with different shapes, material, and shaft diameters, are commercially available. The present paper addresses the importance of the piston shaft diameter. In the present retrospective study of 225 consecutive stapedotomies performed during the period 1981-1998, prostheses with diameters of 0.4, 0.6, and 0.8 mm were compared. The results show that larger pistons give better hearing results for frequencies up to 2 kHz.

Keywords: stapedotomy, piston shaft diameter, hearing results

Introduction

Stapedectomy and stapedotomy are well-established procedures in the operative treatment of otosclerosis. Over the years, a large variety of stapes prostheses have been developed, and most of these are still commercially available. The question that confronts every otosclerosis surgeon is which prosthesis should he choose, which material should it be made of, how should the attachment to the incus be designed and, for stapes pistons, which piston shaft diameter should be chosen. At present, pistons with shaft diameters of 0.3, 0.4, 0.6, and 0.8 mm are commercially available. So far, there is no general agreement as to the optimal size of the piston shaft diameter. The apparent unimportance of piston size in stapedotomies is surprising, since the surface area (πr^2) of the distal end of the piston is doubled when moving up one size in piston diameter. Everything else remaining unchanged, including piston excursions, this should lead to a similar difference in volume displacement for the various piston sizes, and

Address for correspondence: Erik Teig, MD, PhD, Department of Otolaryngology, Rikshospitalet, NO-0027 Oslo, Norway

The Function and Mechanics of Normal, Diseased and Reconstructed Middle Ears, pp. 281–287
edited by J.J. Rosowski and S.N. Merchant
© *2000 Kugler Publications, The Hague, The Netherlands*

a better hearing result would therefore be expected with a larger piston diameter.

In a recent article, Rosowski and Merchant[1] predicted a postoperative air-bone gap for prostheses of various diameters, based upon model calculations. The model came out clearly in favor of a larger piston diameter. Since, in our clinic, we have used stapes pistons with diameters of 0.4, 0.6, and 0.8 mm, we wished to see whether their predictions were reflected in our patient material. Based upon the postoperative air conduction thresholds, it was found that larger pistons actually gave better hearing thresholds for frequencies up to 2 kHz. For higher frequencies, there was no difference.

Materials and methods

The group studied consists of 225 adult otosclerosis patients consecutively operated on between 1981 and 1998. Two patients who developed severe, sensorineural hearing loss, one due to a postoperative pseudomonas infection, the other for reasons unknown, were not included in the study. All operations were carried out under local anesthesia. The operative procedure utilized a transcanalular approach, as described by Shuknecht and Bentkover[2]. In all cases, a Richards-Smith & Nephew Teflon wire piston was used. The standard choice was a piston with a diameter of 0.6 mm. During the period from 1981-1991, the stapedotomies were performed with a hand drill or an electric microdrill (Skeeter). If the footplate fractured during this procedure, the posterior part of the footplate would be taken out, and a 0.8-mm diameter piston introduced. Since 1991, a CO_2 laser has been used to make the calibrated hole in the footplate. During this period, there have been no fractured footplates. However, since a preliminary study showed that patients with a fractured footplate and a 0.8-mm piston tended to do better than the more perfect operations with a 0.6-mm diameter, it was elected to use the larger piston in patients in whom the oval window niche was judged to be sufficiently wide for a 0.9-mm stapedotomy hole. In most cases, however, a 0.7-mm stapedotomy and a 0.6-mm piston were chosen.

The material consisted of 145 cases with a piston diameter of 0.6 mm and 65 cases with a piston diameter of 0.8 mm. A small series of 14 cases, operated on during 1982 and 1983, with a piston diameter of 0.4 mm, was also included. This group with a small piston diameter also included one case with a very narrow niche and an overhanging facial nerve, in whom a 0.4-mm piston was chosen, bringing the total number of cases receiving a 0.4-mm piston to 15.

All the patients had a preoperative audiogram taken shortly before the operation. The final consultations took place three to four months postoperatively, and the audiograms taken at that time were considered to be the end results. The pure-tone thresholds for the frequencies 250 and 500 Hz, and 1, 2, 3, and 4 kHz were compared in the three piston groups (4, 6, 8), and subjected to a statistical analysis using the Statistical Package for the Social Sciences (SPSS) tool. A one-way analysis of variance (ANOVA) was made using a non-parametric method (the Kruskal-Wallis one-way Anova), since there was a slight skewness in the data, in order to test the significance of any differences between the groups.

Results

The box-and-whisker plots in Figure 1 show the 2.5, 25, 50 (median value), 75, and 97.5 cumulative centile for each of the piston diameter groups for the frequencies in the sample. As the piston size increased, there was a clear tendency

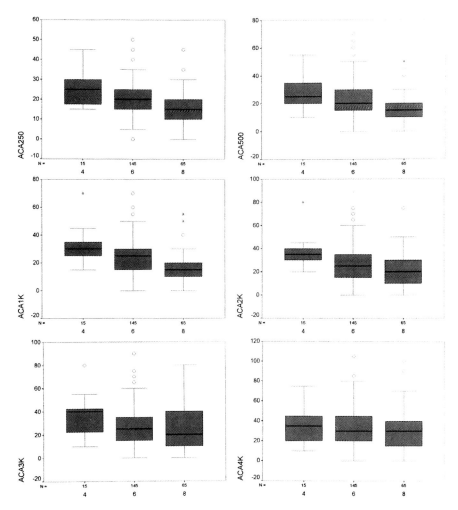

Fig. 1. Air conduction thresholds three to four months after operation (ACA) for the frequencies indicated (abscissa). The box-and-whisker diagrams show the cumulative 2.5, 25, 50 (median value), 75, and 97.5 centile values for the three different piston shaft diameters indicated (values given in 1/10 mm).

for better air conduction thresholds for the frequencies 250 and 500 Hz, and 1 and 2 kHz. For the frequencies 3 and 4 kHz, there was a greater spread in the values, and a possible difference between the groups was less evident. The mean values for each frequency with standard deviation and median values are shown in Table 1. Statistical analyses with the Kruskal-Wallis non-parametric test show p values of less than 0.01 for frequencies between 250 Hz and 2 kHz. For the frequencies 3 and 4 kHz, the difference was not significant.

Since the patients were not randomized prospectively, there was a possibility that the sensory or neural function might differ between the three groups. The preoperative bone conduction thresholds for the frequencies in question in the various piston diameter groups are therefore of interest. Figure 2 shows a box-and-whisker diagram of the preoperative bone conduction thresholds for the various frequencies in the three groups. The median 50 percentile is remarkably similar for all frequencies in the three groups. There was no tendency for patients in the groups that received larger pistons to have had lower bone conduction thresholds before the operation. Similarly, the preoperative air conduction thresholds showed no significant differences in the frequencies tested. However, the average bone conduction thresholds improved after surgery, and there was a tendency for more improvement in the larger piston diameters for the frequencies 1 and 2 kHz (Fig. 3).

Discussion

The present study corroborates Rosowski and Merchant's[1] prediction that air conduction thresholds should improve with increasing piston diameter. How-

Table 1. Postoperative air conduction thresholds

Mean and median values

Prosthesis diameter	Frequency					
	250	500	1 k	2 k	3 k	4 k
0.4 mm (*n*=15)						
mean	26.00	27.33	32.33	36.67	35.00	36.00
SD	(9.85)	(11.93)	(13.34)	(14.92)	(18.52)	(19.74)
median	25	25	30	35	40	35
0.6 mm (*n*=145)						
mean	22.10	22.75	24.69	26.58	27.24	33.86
SD	(10.43)	(12.44)	(12.63)	(13.46)	(16.21)	(20.00)
median	20	20	25	25	25	30
0.8 mm (*n*=65)						
mean	15.07	15.69	17.15	21.46	24.77	30.00
SD	(8.45)	(10.18)	(9.96)	(13.07)	(18.80)	(20.33)
median	15	15	15	20	20	30
One-way Anova	*p*<0.01	*p*<0.01	*p*<0.01	*p*<0.01	n.s.	n.s.

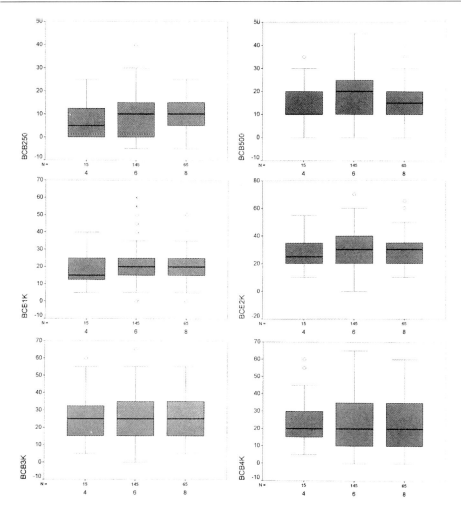

Fig. 2. Bone conduction thresholds before operation (BCB) for the various frequencies. Box-and-whisker diagram parameters as in Figure 1.

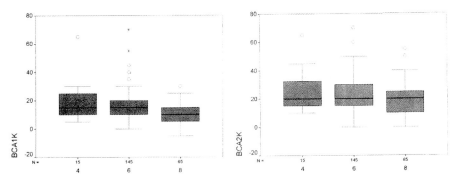

Fig. 3. Bone conduction thresholds three to four months after operation (BCA) for the frequencies 1 and 2 kHz. Box-and-whisker diagram parameters as in Figure 1.

ever, this was true only for frequencies up to 2 kHz. The failure of the present study to show any difference for higher frequencies probably reflects that the sound transmission in stapedotomized ears is dependent upon a number of factors, and that other elements than the piston diameter such as, for example, the coupling between the incus and the stapes prosthesis, might play a more important role for the higher frequencies.

Shuknecht and Bentkover[2] found that, six weeks after surgery, the mean air-bone gap for 500 Hz was 11.31 dB for the 0.6-mm piston compared with 5.32 dB for the 0.8-mm piston. However, there was no statistically significant difference between the two pistons at 1 and 2 kHz. The discrepancy between this and the present findings might be explained by the simultaneous improvement of bone conduction thresholds after stapedotomy, an improvement which, from the present study, appears to be larger as the piston size increases for the frequencies 1 and 2 kHz. These changes in bone conduction responses following alterations in the middle ear system are well known (*e.g.*, Dirks[3]). When Fisch[4] did not find any difference between the results of 0.6 and 0.4 mm stapedotomies, the reason could be that he used the postoperative air-bone gap as the decisive parameter. Grolman *et al.*[5] compared the results with all-Teflon pistons, with shaft diameters of 0.3 and 0.4 mm, in randomly selected patients. They found a statistically significant difference in the gain in air conduction thresholds for frequencies between 125, 250 and 500 Hz, and 1 kHz. In this frequency range, the 0.4-mm piston would give an improvement of 5.3-11.2 dB compared to the 0.3-mm piston. For frequencies 2 kHz and higher, there was no statistical difference. Using gold pistons with diameters of 0.4 and 0.6 mm, Böheim[6] found a statistically significantly better result in the 0.6-mm group for the frequencies 0.5 through 2 kHz (quoted in Schimanski[7]).

When relating the results of the present study, the results of Grolman *et al.*[5], and the calculations of Rosowski and Merchant[1] to the surface area of the distal part of the stapes pistons in question, it would appear that a doubling in the distal surface area leads to an improvement of 5-7 dB in the air conduction thresholds. Thus, a 0.6-mm piston has the potential to improve hearing by 5-7 dB over a 0.4-mm piston, and a 0.8-mm piston the potential to improve hearing by 5-7 dB over a 0.6-mm piston, for frequencies up to 2 kHz.

When earlier studies failed to demonstrate the positive effect of a larger piston shaft diameter, this may have been because the postoperative air-bone gap was used as a basis for the evaluation. When this is used as the sole parameter for comparison, an apparent concomitant improvement of the bone conduction thresholds in important frequencies might blur any actual difference caused by a difference in piston shaft diameter.

Another factor which might influence the end result, is the size of the fenestra. A small piston with a large fenestra diameter will have a larger effective vibrating surface area, and consequently a better hearing result than that of a small piston with a small fenestra diameter. This could be an additional explanation of why some studies did not find a link between differences in piston shaft diameters and hearing results. Thus, Jean Bernard Causse[8] advocates the use of a 0.4-mm piston, but only with a fenestra that is at least 0.6 mm in diameter. In his experience, hearing levels are not as good if the size of the fenestra is smaller than 0.6 when a 0.4-mm piston is used.

References

1. Rosowski JJ, Merchant SN: Mechanical and acoustical analysis of middle ear reconstruction. Am J Otol 16:486-497, 1995
2. Schuknecht HF, Bentkover SH: Partial stapedectomy and piston prosthesis. In: Snow JB Jr (ed) Controversy in Otolaryngology, pp 281-288. Philadelphia/London/Toronto: WB Saunders Co 1980
3. Dirks DD: Bone-conduction testing. In: Katz J (ed) Handbook of Clinical Audiology, 2nd edn, pp 110-116. Baltimore, MD: Williams & Wilkins Co 1978
4. Fisch U: Tympanomplasty, Mastoidectomy, and Stapes Surgery. Stuttgart/New York: Georg Thieme Verlag 1994
5. Grolman W, Tange RA, De Bruijn AJG, Hart AAM, Schouwenburg PF: A retrospective study of the hearing results obtained after stapedotomy by the implantation of two Teflon pistons with a different diameter. Eur Arch Otorhinolaryngol 254:422-424, 1997
6. Böheim K: Ergebnisse mit Goldpistons bei der Stapedektomie mit kleiner Fensterung. Otorhinolaryngol Nova 7:235-240, 1997
7. Schimanski G: Die Steigbügeloperation bei Otosklerose. HNO 46:289-292, 1998
8. Causse JB: Surgical demonstration of stapedectomy at the 10th British Academic Conference in Otolaryngology, Cambridge, July, 1999

MIDDLE-EAR MECHANICS IN RECONSTRUCTED EARS

CHANGES IN EXTERNAL EAR RESONANCE AFTER MASTOIDECTOMY

Open mastoid cavity versus obliterated mastoid cavity

Chul-Ho Jang

Department of Otolaryngology, Wonkwang Medical School, Iksan, Korea

Abstract

The creation of an open mastoid cavity changes the acoustic characteristics of the external ear. The aim of this study was to ascertain the acoustic changes in the external auditory canal occasioned by an open mastoid cavity, and to compare these with mastoid obliteration. External ear resonance (EER) characteristics were measured in 40 normal adult ears, 20 ears with an open mastoid cavity and 40 ears with an obliterated mastoid. The measurement of EER characteristics was performed using a real ear analyzer. An open mastoid cavity changed the mean peak resonant frequency of the external ear from 2.3-2.1 kHz ($p<0.02$), with a mean attenuation of 8 dB SPL at 4 kHz. An obliterated mastoid produced higher resonance frequencies from 2.8-2.5 kHz. The sound pressure gain of an external auditory canal with an open mastoid cavity was higher than with an obliterated mastoid. The author concludes that an open mastoid cavity can affect the resonance frequency, and that this effect is reduced by mastoid obliteration. Therefore, mastoid obliteration results in a more normal ear canal anatomy and function.

Introduction

Canal wall down mastoidectomy is generally more successful in chronic active otitis media with cholesteatoma. Some cavity problems have been lessened by obliteration techniques[1-4]. Obliteration of the cavities has also been performed with cartilage, bone pate, pedicled muscle and alloplastic materials. Because those materials have not been consistently successful, postoperative hollowing has occurred. To prevent hollowing, we have used combined graft materials for mastoid obliteration.

A surgically-created open mastoid cavity could affect the hearing in two ways. Enlarging the volume of the external ear canal alters the resonant characteristics of the external ear, and the ossicular chain may be partially removed in order to enable eradication of the disease[5,6].

Address for correspondence: Chul-Ho Jang, MD, Department of Otolaryngology, Wonkwang Medical School, 570 Iksan, South Korea. *email:* chul@wonnms.wonkwang.ac.kr

The Function and Mechanics of Normal, Diseased and Reconstructed Middle Ears, pp. 291–296
edited by J.J. Rosowski and S.N. Merchant
© 2000 Kugler Publications, The Hague, The Netherlands

Evans *et al.*[7] studied the effect of an open mastoid cavity on resonant properties of the external ear canal in both temporal bones and patients. They found that the open mastoid cavity significantly reduced the resonant frequency of the external ear. This effect, however, was less pronounced in patients compared to that found in temporal bones. The effect of an obliterated mastoid cavity on ear canal resonance properties has seldom been reported. The aim of this study was to investigate the effect of mastoid cavity obliteration, using a combined graft (hydroxyapatite granules, cartilage and inferior-based pedicled muscle), on external ear resonance.

Material and methods

We measured external ear resonance (EER) characteristics in normal adults (40 ears), patients with an open mastoid cavity (20 ears) and patients with an obliterated mastoid (40 ears). The mean age of the subjects was 38 years, with a range of 32-56 years. All patients had a unilateral open mastoid cavity with a normal contralateral ear. The period of observation in all operated cases was a minimum of one year and a maximum of four and a half years. The mastoid obliteration technique using a combined graft is illustrated in Figures 1 and 2.

The measurement of EER characteristics was performed using a real ear analyzer (Fornix 6500-CX with Quick probe II, Frey Inc., USA). The equipment was calibrated prior to each series of measurements. A preliminary experiment was conducted to examine the test/retest reproducibility of the procedure. The patients were seated in a chair, 30 cm from the insertion gain system sound source at 45° azimuth. A speaker position of 45° azimuth and 45° elevation has been found by Killion and Revit[8] to reduce variability associated with

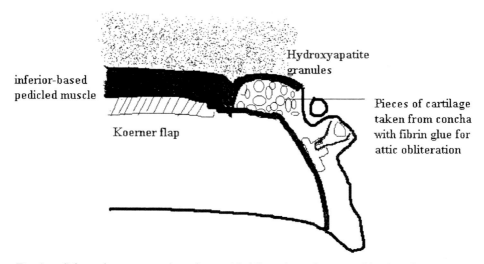

Fig. 1. a. Schematic representation of mastoid obliteration using a combined graft.

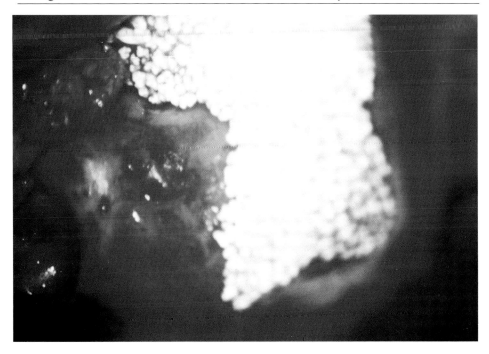

Fig. 1. b. Obliteration using hydroxyapatite granules.

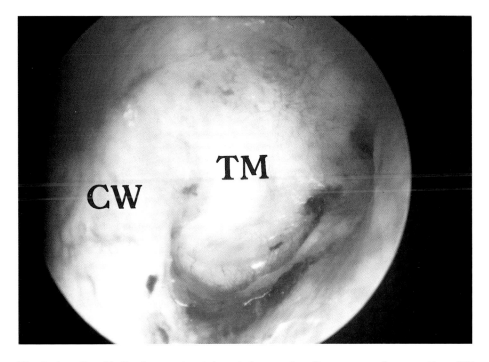

Fig. 2. A well-epithelized reconstructed posterior canal wall, one year after operation. CW: canal wall; TM: tympanic membrane.

probe-tube measurement, and a position of 45° azimuth is recommended in the Fornix manual. Using an otoscope, the probe microphone was positioned within the canal lateral to the eardrum, to a depth of about 17 mm from the canal entrance. The reference microphone was attached to the headband just above the pinna facing forwards.

The sound pressure level was held constant at 70 dB through the frequency sweep from 125 Hz to 8 kHz. Time exposure by noise was two seconds.

Two measurements of external ear resonance were made for both ears of each subject. The probe-tube was completely removed from the ear between measurements. A Mann-Whitney test was used to compare the different groups.

Table 1. Mean and standard deviations of resonance frequency and peak amplitudes for the three groups

	PREq (Hz) (mean SE)		PA (dB) (mean SE)		p value
Normal	2950	107	18.5	2.5	
Open cavity	2350	201	22.5	1.7	**
Obliterated cavity	2750	199	20.5	1.9	

PREq: resonance frequency; PA: peak amplitude; SE: standard error

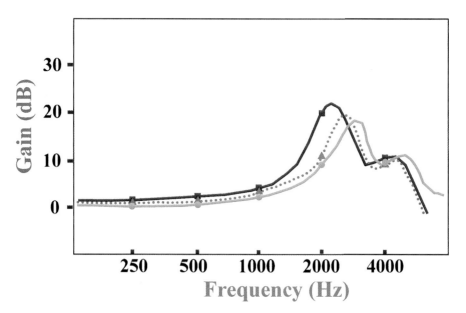

Fig. 3. Response curve of external ear resonance in each of the three groups. Solid line with squares: open mastoid cavity; dashed line with triangles: obliterated mastoid; gray line with circles: normal.

Results

Table 1 and Figure 3 show the mean resonant frequency and amplitude of resonance in an open mastoid cavity, obliterated mastoid and normal ear.

In normal ears, the mean resonant frequency was 2950 ± 107 Hz, and the mean peak amplitude 18.5 ± 2.5 dB. Open mastoid cavities significantly decreased the resonant frequency, 2350 ± 201 Hz (mean $\pm$SD) but increased the peak amplitude 22.5 ± 1.7 dB (mean $\pm$SD), $p<0.01$. Obliterated mastoid cavities increased the resonant frequency 2750 ± 199 (mean $\pm$SD) to close to the normal state and decreased the peak amplitude to 20.5 ± 1.9 dB (mean $\pm$SD). Significant differences ($p<0.05$) were found in resonant frequency and peak amplitude when comparing obliterated mastoid and open mastoid cavities.

Discussion

The external auditory canal has a role in the transfer of sound from the concha to the tympanic membrane. In humans, this has been intensively investigated, all studies demonstrating that the external auditory canal acts as a resonant tube[9]. As a result of this, sound entering the canal can be amplified by as much as 20 dB in the frequency range 2-4 kHz. To some extent, this will help to overcome the middle ear's poorer ability to transfer sound at higher frequencies. This study points out that open cavity mastoidectomy or modified radical mastoidectomy can change the resonant properties of the ear canal. Similar changes have been demonstrated in human temporal bones by Goode et al.[10]

The results from the Goode study showed that an open mastoid cavity significantly decreased resonant frequency without affecting the peak amplitude. This would follow if the major effect of open cavity mastoidectomy was to lengthen the ear canal and, as a consequence, reduce the resonant frequency. Tolley et al.[11] studied the effects of an open mastoid cavity on ear canal resonance. They also attempted to alter resonant properties by obliterating each cavity with silastic foam. No significant differences were found in peak amplitude when comparing normal ears to ears with an open mastoid cavity. Silastic foam obliteration of the mastoid cavity did not produce any significant changes in resonant frequency or amplitude. However, our study shows a significant difference between an open mastoid and an obliterated mastoid.

The difference between Tolley et al.'s and the present results could be the final shape of the ear canal. Minatogawa et al.[12] found that patients who underwent mastoid obliteration using biocompatible materials had a lower incidence of hollowing or retraction of the obliteration when compared with a pedicled muscle flap alone after long-term follow-up (mean, 2.5 years). Hydroxyapatite granules are a good biological material, but protrusion of hydroxyapatite through the external epithelium and exposure of materials, together with the failure of epithelization, are problems. In this study, I covered the hydroxyapatite granules with an inferior-based pedicled muscle flap, which solved the problem. In previous studies, I used bone pate or bone chips, but with poor results since bone pate is very susceptible to infection and bone chips can be absorbed within a few years.

As demonstrated by Gyo et al.[13] and Whittemore et al.[14], canal wall down mastoidectomy also reduces the middle ear air volume. However, the effect of such changes in ear canal resonances is not known. Further studies are required to investigate the correlation between external ear resonance and middle ear volume.

Conclusions

Although canal wall down mastoidectomy changes the acoustics of the external ear canal, this change can be minimized by mastoid obliteration. Mastoid obliteration using hydroxyapatite granules and an inferior-based pedicled muscle flap can give good long-term results.

References

1. Guilford FR: Obliteration of the cavity and reconstruction of the auditory canal in temporal bone surgery. Trans Am Acad Ophthalmol Otolaryngol 65:114-122, 1961
2. Hartwein J, Hormann K: A technique for the reconstruction of the posterior canal wall and mastoid obliteration in radical cavity surgery. Am J Otol 3:169-173, 1990
3. Pou JW: Reconstruction of bony canal wall with autogenous bony graft. Laryngoscope 87:1826-1832, 1977
4. Grote JJ, Van Bitterswijk CA: Reconstruction of the posterior auditory canal wall with a hydroxyapatite prosthesis. Ann Otol Rhinol Laryngol (Suppl) 95:6-9, 1986
5. Browing GG, Gatehouse S: Acoustical characteristics of surgically altered human temporal bones. Clin Otolaryngol 9:87-91, 1984
6. Weiner FM, Ross DA: The pressure distribution in the auditory canal in a progressive sound field. J Acoust Soc Am 18:401-408, 1946
7. Evans RA, Day GA, Browning GG: Open-cavity mastoid surgery: its effect on the acoustics of the external ear canal. Clin Otolaryngol 14:317-321, 1989
8. Killion MC, Revit LJ: Insertion gain repeatability versus loudspeaker location: you want me to put my loudspeaker where? Ear Hear 8(Suppl 5):68S-73S, 1987
9. Djupesland G, Zwislocki JJ: Sound pressure distribution in the outer ear. Acta Otolaryngol (Stockh) 75:350-352, 1973
10. Goode RL, Friedrichs R, Falk S: Effect on hearing thresholds of surgical modification of the external ear. Ann Otol 86:441-450, 1977
11. Tolley NS, Ison K, Mirza A: Experimental studies on the acoustic properties of mastoid cavities. J Laryngol Otol 106:597-599, 1992
12. Minatogawa T, Machizuka H, Kumoi T: Evaluation of mastoid obliteration surgery. Am J Otol 16:99-103, 1995
13. Gyo K, Goode RL, Miller C: Effect of middle ear modification on umbo vibration: human temporal bone experiments with a new vibration measuring system. Arch Otolaryngol Head Neck Surg 112:1262-1268, 1986
14. Whittemore KR Jr, Merchant SN, Rosowski JJ: Acoustic mechanisms: canal wall-up versus canal wall-down mastoidectomy. Otolaryngol Head Neck Surg 118:751-761, 1988

ON THE COUPLING OF PROSTHESES TO THE MIDDLE EAR STRUCTURE AND ITS INFLUENCE ON SOUND TRANSFER

Albrecht Eiber[1], Hans-Georg Freitag[1], Goesta Schimanski[2] and Hans Peter Zenner[3]

[1]Institute B of Mechanics, University of Stuttgart; [2]ENT Department, Hospital Lünen, Lünen; [3]Department of Otolaryngology, University of Tübingen, Germany

Abstract

Sound transfer through a reconstructed middle ear is strongly dependent on the coupling conditions between implant and ossicles. Here, the authors focus on the mechanical description of the coupling to facilitate the improvement of commercial prostheses, to develop new types of passive and active implants and to demonstrate the consequences of different methods of implantation.

The coupling is considered to be a viscoelastic element composed of a spring (stiffness coefficient c) and a damper (damping coefficient d). The authors identified these parameters from measurements on passive prostheses coupled to an artificial stapes. A mathematical model of the observed dynamic behavior was used to simulate the measurements and to determine the mechanical properties of the coupling region. Finally, these parameters and findings are used in a global model of a reconstructed middle ear in order to study dynamic behavior and simulate sound transfer. The coupling parameters strongly depend on the pretension in the coupling region. Only a weak pretension is required for satisfactory sound transmission. A high pretension is necessary to compensate for variations in static pressure in the tympanic cavity and the outer ear canal. This leads to high static load and relaxation of ligaments. Clamping of bell-type prostheses should be avoided because of the risk of dislocation of the stapes. Damping in the coupling region smoothens the transfer function.

Keywords: prostheses, coupling, sound transfer, middle ear models

Introduction

The development and optimization of middle ear implants for ossiculoplasty requires both theoretical and experimental investigations. Theoretical investigations are based on appropriate models of the implant itself and of the recon-

Address for correspondence: Dr.-Ing. Albrecht Eiber, Institute B of Mechanics, Pfaffenwaldring 9, 70550 Stuttgart, Germany. *email:* ae@mechb.uni-stuttgart.de

The Function and Mechanics of Normal, Diseased and Reconstructed Middle Ears, pp. 297–308
edited by J.J. Rosowski and S.N. Merchant
© *2000 Kugler Publications, The Hague, The Netherlands*

structed middle ear. Such models give insight into the dynamic behavior and can be used to study different types of prostheses and different insertion positions and orientations, as well as different coupling conditions.

The sound transfer through the reconstructed middle ear is very sensitive to the point where the prosthesis is coupled to the ossicles, to the spatial direction in which the prosthesis is oriented and, in particular, to the type of coupling between the ossicles and the prosthesis. Moreover, the surgical manipulation of the remaining ossicular chain is of great influence to the dynamic behavior of the reconstructed middle ear.

In this paper, our investigations focus on determining descriptive parameters of the coupling mechanism.

Methods

Models of the middle ear

Classical models often are derived from electrical circuits, *e.g.*, Shaw and Stinson[1], Rosowski *et al.*[2], and Hudde and Weistenhöfer[3]. Such circuits are powerful models for describing the global sound transfer; however, the direct relationship between the parameters of the natural system and the corresponding ones in the model is not always clear. Moreover, the description of three-dimensional motions in such models is generally incomplete. The three-dimensional models used here[4,5] are based on a mechanical description of the ear, and are derived using the well-established approaches of multibody systems, finite element systems and continuous systems[6]. The global multibody system model consists of a full three-dimensional representation of the ossicular chain viscoelastically hinged in the middle ear structure, and includes the air in the outer ear canal, the eardrum and the inner ear as lumped mass systems. The parameters are physical ones like geometrical dimensions, masses, moments of inertia, stiffness and damping coefficients. Similar models have been used elsewhere[7,8]. Pathological situations can be described by changing the parameters or the structure of the model. In order to describe middle ear reconstructions, models of the middle ear structure are extended by adding subsystems describing the implant, as shown in Figure 1. The entire model has 25 degrees of freedom, which are depicted as arrows and symbolic names. The input to the inner ear is given by the translational and rotational motions of the stapes footplate y_S, α_S and γ_S, respectively.

Models of coupling

For reconstructions with either passive or active implants, one of the most critical points in the dynamic behavior is the coupling between the prosthesis and the ossicle. Here, different physical principles of force transduction can be observed, *e.g.*, magnetic force; Van der Waals force; adhesion; friction, sometimes with slip-stick

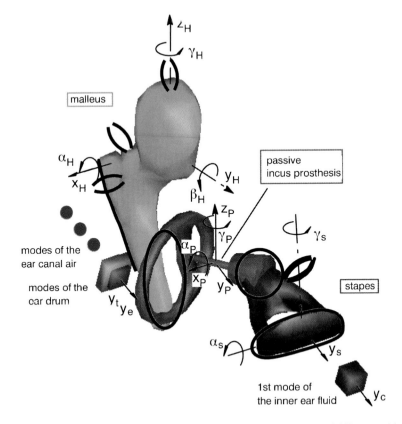

Fig. 1. Three-dimensional multibody system model of a reconstructed middle ear with 25 degrees of freedom.

effects; and contact of material points (form closure).

It is still an open question as to which type of transduction mechanism is dominant in ear reconstructions. The precise transduction mechanism varies with different types of prostheses, and also depends on the particular manner of its insertion into the middle ear.

Mechanically, the coupling can be classified as:

a. force coupling where only forces are acting between the coupled bodies; the motion can then be calculated from the equations of motion;

b. kinematic coupling where the motion is the same for both contact points; the contact forces can then be calculated from the constraint equations.

Such couplings can be *bilateral*, acting in a push and a pull direction, or *unilateral*, acting in one direction only, push or pull, respectively. A specific type of a bilateral coupling is an asymmetrical one with different behavior in push and pull directions. Such asymmetrical or unilateral couplings are nonlinear, and show distortion effects.

The mechanical characteristics of the coupling region have a high influence on the global dynamic behavior, which determines sound transfer through the middle

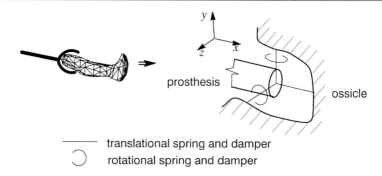

translational spring and damper
rotational spring and damper

Fig. 2. Model of viscoelastic coupling with five degrees of freedom.

ear. The design criteria of an implant should be that all audible frequencies are transmitted in a manner similar to the natural ear, and that the distortion of the transmitted signal should be below a certain limit. These criteria guarantee an effective and safe sound transfer with a good hearing result.

There are lively discussions about the optimal coupling. Mechanically: What is the influence of coupling on kinematics and dynamics? Clinically: How can good sound transfer over a wide range of frequencies be achieved? Which coupling provides safety against impulse loads and stability over a long time? Furthermore, the implant should be biocompatible, and the implant procedure itself simple and practicable even for less trained surgeons.

In this paper, we consider a simplified model of viscoelastic coupling. It consists of five degrees of freedom, one longitudinal, two transversal and two rotational motions perpendicular to the longitudinal direction (Fig. 2). The problem is how to determine the parameters that describe this coupling.

Experiments

The mechanical characteristics of the coupling model were derived from measurements in the laboratory. Here, the stiffness c, the damping d, the nonlinearities and the asymmetries, as well as the maximal transferable forces, are of interest. We concentrated our considerations on the stiffness and damping coefficient corresponding to the longitudinal direction of the prostheses.

Measurements were carried out on the test rig shown in Figure 3. A replica of a stapes made from gold or plastic is mounted on a vibration platform with calibrated dynamic behavior. The platform is considered to be a single degree of freedom vibrator for interpretation of the results. Moving the base of the vibration platform by means of a micromanipulator, the static pretension F_0 in the coupling region can be adjusted.

The prosthesis under investigation is driven by a shaker (Brüel & Kjær 4810). The input signal to the shaker is a multisinusoidal signal of 200 components in the frequency range between 25 Hz and 5 kHz, produced by the computer.

Each measurement is as follows: both the motion of the shaker and of the vibra-

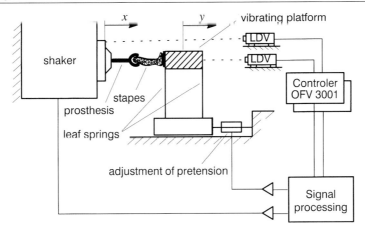

Fig. 3. Test rig for determination of characteristics of coupling between prosthesis and ossicle.

tion platform are measured via laser Doppler vibrometry (Polytec OFV 303 with OFV 3001 controller). From these signals, the transmitted force and the transfer function between the stapes head and prosthesis motion are calculated considering a steady state motion, where the resulting force in the coupling area is

$F(t) = F_0 + \hat{F} \cos \omega t$

with the amplitude $\hat{F}$ and the frequency ω of the harmonic time-dependent part. The resonance peak in the transfer function is used to determine the stiffness c and the damping d of the viscoelastic coupling model. This procedure is carried out for various values of pretension F_0.

Four types of incus prostheses from H. Kurz, Dusslingen are considered:
Partial Ossicular Replacement Prostheses (PORPs)
– a Tübingen-type bell, gold (TAP)
– a Tübingen-type bell, titanium (partial TTP®)
– a Dresden-type bell, gold (DAP)
Total Ossicular Replacement Prosthesis (TORP)
– a Tübingen-type aerial, titanium (total TTP®)
For these prostheses, the following coupling conditions are considered:
– Narrow gap without pretension. The gap between the prosthesis and ossicle is filled with water. The coupling results solely by adhesion.
– Dry contact with high pretension. Direct contact between prosthesis and ossicle, no intermediate material. A small local deformation, due to the very low compliance of material surfaces, takes place. The contact points of the prosthesis and the stapes move together.
– In practice, intermediate layers in the contact zone are used, such as fascia, periosteum, perichondrium, or fat. Here, we used natural fascia and cigarette paper. The paper was found to have similar properties to the materials used in surgery, and yielded reproducible results.
The intermediate layer was placed at the stapes before the prosthesis was brought into contact. In a second case, the contact area was additionally covered with fascia

or cigarette paper after the prosthesis was placed in position. This paper imitates the influence of mucous tissue growing around the coupling. To avoid drying out, the test was carried out in a covered chamber with a built-in humidifier.

Results

The dynamic behavior of isolated passive prostheses was also studied. Measurements carried out on isolated prostheses, and detailed calculations, showed that the structural vibrations of the different prostheses do not play a dominant role in sound transfer.

Measurements

With regard to the coupling region, the following results were achieved:

PORP (bell), not clamped
Extreme values for stiffness occur in the case of a coupling with a water-filled gap and dry contact with high pretension, respectively. The corresponding estimated values are:

$$c_{drop} = 20 \text{ N/m, and}$$
$$c_{dry} = 120\ 000 \text{ N/m.}$$

The damping can be ignored in these cases.

The corresponding stiffness values for contact with intermediate layers of fascia or cigarette paper are within these limits. The results for both materials were similar, and therefore, further experiments were carried out with cigarette paper.

The stiffness coefficient c as a function of pretension F_0 for interposed cigarette paper is shown in Figure 4 as a solid line. In addition to the intermediate layer, the coupling region was covered with strips of wet paper (dashed line in Fig. 4). In the region of positive pretension, the maximum stiffness of about 60 000 N/m was nearly the same as the uncovered estimate. For negative pretension, this coupling shows a stiffness ten times higher than the uncovered version, and contact was maintained up to $F_0 = -0.15$ mN. The estimated damping coefficients were between 0.17 and 0.5 Ns/m for both cases.

TORP (aerial)
Using wet cigarette paper, the maximum stiffness for the uncovered and covered versions was around 100 000 N/m. This coupling is about 50% stiffer than the bell coupling. However, in the negative region of pretension, the situation is quite different: almost no pulling force can be transmitted by the uncovered coupling region. Covering the contact leads to the values shown in Figure 5, which are similar

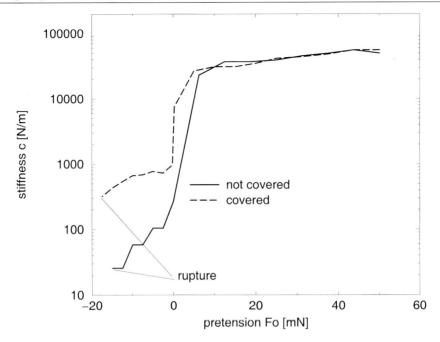

Fig. 4. Stiffness coefficient of a bell-type Tübingen, gold (TAP), depending on the static pre-tension. The intermediate layer is wet cigarette paper. Two cases: in one, the coupling region is uncovered and, in the other, the coupling region is covered with wet cigarette paper.

to the uncovered bell version. The damping coefficients are between 0.8 and 2.2 Ns/m in both cases.

Origin of pretension

A preload of 1 mN corresponds to a static pressure difference between the ear canal and the tympanic cavity of approximately 2 daPa. A comparable dynamic load is a sound pressure level of approximately 120 dB.

The pretension in the reconstructed ear can be generated by a prosthesis longer than the distance between the stapes and eardrum, or by interposing additional slices of cartilage of various thickness. Supposing the stiffness of the eardrum with a prosthesis attached is between 50 and 200 N/m, the corresponding pretension in the prosthesis would be about 5-20 mN for an interposed slice of 0.1 mm thickness. Looking at the available length increments of prostheses of 0.25 mm, the corresponding force increments would be between 12.5 and 50 mN. It should be mentioned that these values are very rough estimations, because other effects, such as shrinking of the healing graft underlying the eardrum, have not been taken into consideration.

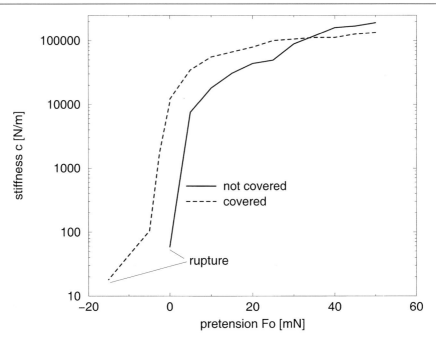

Fig. 5. Stiffness coefficient of an aerial-type Tübingen, titanium depending on the static pretension. The intermediate layer is wet cigarette paper. Two cases: in one, the coupling region is uncovered and, in the other, the coupling region is covered with wet cigarette paper.

Necessary pretension to avoid distortion

Depending on the pretension, the quality of coupling was measured with respect to the sound transfer. A wet cigarette paper was used as the intermediate layer. For various pretensions, the excitation level was increased until the distortion product of the velocity of the platform exceeded a level of 1%. For this specific excitation, the corresponding amplitude of the dynamic part of the coupling force $\hat{F}^{*}$ was calculated and plotted in Figure 6. If the driving force of the implant is below $\hat{F}^{*}$, the transmitted force shows a moderate distortion, above $\hat{F}^{*}$, the amplitudes of the higher harmonics are above 1% of the signal level. As a consequence, it can be seen from Figure 6 that, for a transmission with low distortion, the pretension should be at least five times higher than the transmitted dynamic force.

Simulations

By feeding the measured stiffness and damping coefficients of the coupling into the global model of the reconstructed middle ear, as shown in Figure 1, the motion of the stapes can be calculated. For reconstructed middle ears, the rocking motions of the stapes γ_S and α_S around the minor and major principal axes of the footplate, respectively, may reach a significant level compared to the piston-like motion y_S.

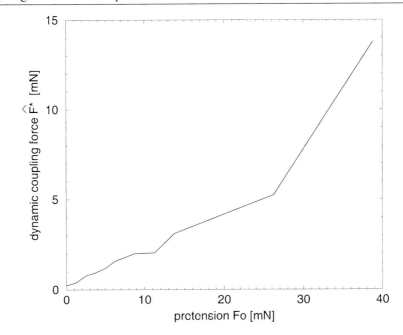

Fig. 6. Measured limit $\hat{F}^*$ of the dynamic part of the coupling force for a distortion of less than 1%, depending on the pretension F_0. Excitation frequency 1 kHz, aerial prosthesis with cigarette paper. Low distortion occurs for $F_0 \geq \approx 5\hat{F}$.

Therefore, excitation of the inner ear is provided by a rocking and piston-like motion. This effect is strongly dependent on the point of attachment and on the orientation of the implant[9].

Nevertheless, only the piston-like motion y_S is considered here to characterize the sound transfer for different coupling conditions. In Figure 7, the velocity of the stapes footplate of a normal ear, due to excitation with a sound pressure level of 60 dB SPL, is plotted.

In the case of a reconstructed ear, a PORP attached to the stapes head and to the lower part of the manubrium is considered. The incus is removed, and all ligaments on the malleus and stapedial muscle are preserved. Two coupling situations with the measured extreme values c_{dry} and c_{drop}, and one with a desirable coupling value c^*, are shown. The velocity v_S of the stapes is compared with the frequency response of the normal ear. This particular reconstruction leads to acceptable hearing results for coupling stiffness c_{dry}. Only 5 dB for frequencies below 1 kHz and around 10 dB for frequencies between 1.5 and 3 kHz are missing, while above 4 kHz there is a gain in hearing. Stiffness values in the magnitude of c^* lead to similar results, except for frequencies above 6 kHz. Such c^* values are delivered by couplings using fascia under moderate pretension of around 5 mN, as can be seen from Figures 4 and 5. It is obvious that the coupling with a very low stiffness limits the sound transfer to a totally unacceptable level. Variations in the pretension, *e.g.*, due

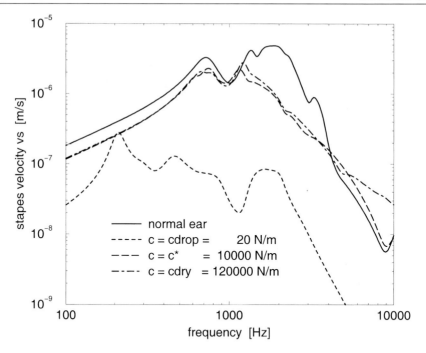

Fig. 7. Simulated stapes velocity for normal and reconstructed ears. Bell-type Tübingen, gold prosthesis (TAP), connected to the stapes head under different coupling conditions.

to static pressure changes, may cause variations in the coupling stiffness in such a broad range. As a consequence, the hearing results vary in a similar range, as shown in Figure 7.

These findings are valid, provided the transmitted forces in the coupling region are not limited or nonlinear due to coupling law or large amplitudes, otherwise distortion occurs. For a certain level and frequency of excitation, the amplitude of the transmitted coupling force $\hat{F}$ can be calculated from the global model. The coupling must be able to transmit this force without distortion, which requires a certain pretension F_0. A very rough estimation of the necessary pretension can be taken from Figure 6 as $F_0 \approx 5\hat{F}$, when the amplitude of coupling force $\hat{F}$ is chosen as $\hat{F} \leq \hat{F}^*$.

To decrease the distortion of sound transfer, the pretension must be increased or, as is possible in the case of active implants, the excitation level must be reduced.

Conclusions

For the sound transfer, sufficient stiffness of the coupling is necessary properly to transmit higher frequencies. Acceptable values could be reached giving a moderate pretension of about 5 mN, in particular in the case of covered coupling regions. There is serious limitation to the quality of sound transfer, due to distortion of the transmitted force. Particularly in the case of active implants with high power, this limitation may be reached, resulting in poor sound discrimination by the patient.

A high pretension of about 50 mN may be desired to maintain the minimum pretension necessary for good hearing quality under various pressure conditions in the tympanic cavity. Too high a level leads to an unphysiological permanent static load, which may cause further damage in the middle ear or creepage in the ligaments, due to long-term relaxation. This may lead to an undesirable reduction of the initially chosen pretension within some months.

The damping coefficient of the coupling does not have much negative influence on the sound transfer. Despite moderate energy dissipation, the damping flattens the dynamic behavior of the coupling. This means that the amplitudes near resonance frequencies are lowered down and, very importantly, amplitudes above the resonance are elevated, due to viscous forces.

During insertion, bell prostheses allow elegant positioning at the stapes head due to the self-centring of the bell. The relatively long thighs of the Dresden-type facilitate this process.

It seems to be an advantage to encompass the stapes head entirely, folding the braces around it. From a macromechanical point of view, this may prevent the prosthesis from total dislocation. Even if the prosthesis is clamped as tight as possible by means of a ring forceps, micromechanically there is still an intermediate

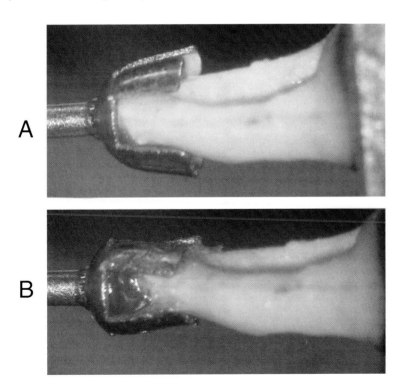

Fig. 8. Bell-type Tübingen connected to the artificial stapes. Dislocation due to clamping the flaps of bell: A. before, and B. after clamping.

gap between the prosthesis and the ossicle, which is mostly filled with fluid, *e.g.*, blood. Therefore, viscoelastic coupling is effective. Furthermore, a totally fixed connection might cause restricted degrees of freedom and the risk of erosion.

Encompassing the stapes with the long branches may provide proper coupling even in the case of negative pretension ($F_0 < 0$), if the prosthesis head plate is able to transmit pulling forces by adhesion, or by placing it between the manubrium and the eardrum. However, a very serious drawback of clamping is the danger of dislocation of the bell from the stapes head, as we noted in our experiments. Figure 8 shows this situation before and after clamping, respectively. This dislocation process could be observed with gold and titanium prostheses, and leads to an undetermined increase of pretension after insertion.

Acknowledgments

This work was partially supported by the German Research Council under grant Nos. Ze 149/7-1 and Schi 119/27-1.

References

1. Shaw EAG, Stinson MR: The human external and middle ear: models and concepts. In: De Boer E, Viergever MA (eds) Mechanics of Hearing, pp 3-10. Delft: University Press 1983
2. Rosowski JJ, Carney LH, Lynch TJ III, Peake WT: The effectiveness of external and middle ears in coupling power into the cochlea. In: Allen JB et al (eds) Peripheral Auditory Mechanics, pp 3-12. Berlin: Springer Verlag 1986
3. Hudde H, Weistenhöfer C: A three-dimensional circuit model of the middle ear. Acustica Acta Acust 83:535-549, 1997
4. Eiber A: Mechanical modeling and dynamical investigation of middle ear. In: Hüttenbrink K-B (ed) Proceedings of the International Workshop on Middle Ear Mechanics in Research and Otosurgery, Dresden. Dresden: Techn Universität 1997
5. Eiber A, Freitag H-G, Burkhardt C, Hemmert W, Maassen M, Rodriguez Jorge J, Zenner H-P: Dynamics of middle ear prostheses: simulations and measurements. Audiol Neuro-Otol 4:178-184, 1999
6. Schiehlen W: Advanced Multibody Systems Dynamics. Dordrecht: Kluwer 1993
7. Beer H-J, Bornitz M, Hardtke H-J, Schmidt R, Hofmann G, Vogel U, Zahnert T, Hüttenbrink K-B: Modelling of components of the human middle ear and simulation of their dynamic behaviour. Audiol Neuro-Otol 4:156-162, 1999
8. Wada H, Koike T, Kobayashi T: Three-dimensional finite-element method (FEM) analysis of the human middle ear. In: Hüttenbrink K-B (ed) Proceedings of the International Workshop on Middle Ear Mechanics in Research and Otosurgery, Dresden. Dresden: Techn Universität 1997
9. Eiber A, Freitag H-G: On simulation models in otology. In: Ambrosio JC, Schiehlen W (eds) Proceedings EUROMECH Coll 404 Lisbon, Portugal. Advances in Computational Multibody Dynamics, pp 729-747. Lisbon: Instituto Superior Técnico 1999

ANALYSIS OF THE FINITE-ELEMENT METHOD OF TRANSFER FUNCTION OF RECONSTRUCTED MIDDLE EARS AND THEIR POSTOPERATIVE CHANGES

Takuji Koike[1], Hiroshi Wada[1] and Toshimitsu Kobayashi[2]

[1]*Department of Mechanical Engineering, Tohoku University, Sendai;* [2]*Department of Otolaryngology, Nagasaki University School of Medicine, Japan*

Abstract

Many middle ear prostheses are available for the reconstruction of missing or damaged ossicles. However, there are few studies that investigate the acoustic properties of these prostheses, and there is no information available that could lead to the design and development of better ossicular replacement prostheses. In this study, three-dimensional finite-element models of a human intact middle ear and reconstructed middle ears using different types of incus replacement prosthesis are established, and an attempt is made to clarify the optimum method for reconstructing the middle ear. Prostheses with a high degree of stiffness, connecting the stapes head to either the malleus manubrium or near to the center of the tympanic membrane, give the best acoustic performance.

Keywords: middle ear, reconstruction, prosthesis, transfer function, finite-element method

Introduction

Numerous techniques have been proposed to reconstruct the ossicular chain, using different prostheses. The best way to select the optimum method would be to compare two or more prostheses in the clinic. However, it is difficult to carry out such trials, and a large number of variables are hard to control. In place of such clinical trials, experiments with ossicular substitution in animals and human temporal bones have been performed[1-4]. However, any knowledge obtained from animal studies cannot be applied directly to humans, due to anatomical differences. Moreover, it is difficult to investigate the effect of postoperative changes on the transfer function of the middle ear using temporal bones. As a result, the acoustic performance of prostheses and their postoperative function has not been well analyzed.

Address for correspondence: Takuji Koike, PhD, Department of Mechanical Engineering, Tohoku University, Aoba-yama 01, Sendai 980-8579, Japan

The Function and Mechanics of Normal, Diseased and Reconstructed Middle Ears, pp. 309–320
edited by J.J. Rosowski and S.N. Merchant
© *2000 Kugler Publications, The Hague, The Netherlands*

Use of the finite-element method (FEM) enables the complicated irregular geometry of biological structures to be modelled easily. The use of FEM also enables the dynamic behavior to be understood in detail without the need for experiments. A few FEM analyses of reconstructed middle ears have already been reported[5-9]. In these studies, the natural frequencies and vibration amplitudes of reconstructed middle ears were examined. However, the sound transmission properties of different prostheses have not been specifically compared. In the present study, three-dimensional FEM models of a human intact middle ear and reconstructed middle ears, using an incus replacement prosthesis (IRP), have been established. The effects of the material, the shape and contact point of the IRP, and the postoperative changes in the stiffness and shape of the tympanic membrane (TM) on middle ear transfer function are analyzed.

The finite-element method model

Figure 1(a) shows a FEM model of an intact human right middle ear. The geometry of this model was based on the dimensions obtained from the study of Kirikae[10]. Two hundred and thirty-two flat triangular plate elements were used to model the TM. In this model, both the pars tensa and pars flaccida were considered, and Young's modulus of the pars flaccida was taken to be one-third that of the pars tensa. The boundary condition at the tympanic ring consists of linear (K_L) and torsional (K_T) springs. Eighty-two hexahedral elements were used to model the ossicles. The functions of the anterior malleal ligament, posterior incudal ligament, tensor tympani tendon, stapedial annular ligament, and stapedial tendon were taken into account.

Young's modulus and the density of the TM were determined, based on the values obtained in the study of Wada and Kobayashi[11]. Poisson's ratio of the TM was 0.3. Young's modulus of the ossicles was assumed to be uniform, and was taken to be 1.2×10^{10} N/m^2. The density of each ossicle was determined based on the values obtained in Kirikae's study[10]. The stiffness of the tympanic ring and Young's moduli of the ligaments and tendons were unknown. In this study, their mechanical properties were determined by comparison between the numerical results obtained from the FEM analysis and the results of measurement of the manipulated temporal bones, which were obtained by the sweep frequency impedance meter (SFI), developed by our group[11].

The cochlear impedance was estimated to be damping dominant[12-16]. Therefore, in this study, the loading of the cochlea on the stapes footplate was expressed by the damping D_C. The damping, except for that of the cochlea, was expressed by

$$C = \alpha M + \beta K \tag{1}$$

where C, M and K were the damping, mass and stiffness matrices, respectively, and α and β were the damping parameters.

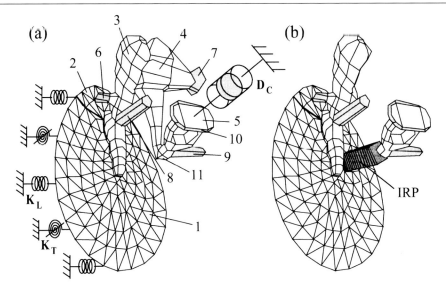

Fig. 1. FEM model of a human right middle ear. *(a)* Intact middle ear. Boundary condition at the tympanic ring consists of linear (K_L) and torsional (K_T) springs, and loading of the cochlea on the stapes footplate is expressed by damping (D_C). 1. TM (pars tensa); 2. TM (pars flaccida); 3. malleus; 4. incus; 5. stapes; 6. anterior malleal ligament; 7. posterior incudal ligament; 8. tensor tympani tendon; 9. stapedial tendon; 10. annular ligament; 11. incudostapedial joint. *(b)* An example of a reconstructed middle ear model. The incus is replaced by an incus replacement prosthesis (IRP) connecting between the stapes head and near to the center of the TM. The cross-sectional area is 1.0 mm².

Figure 1(b) shows an example of a reconstructed middle ear model. In this case, the incus was replaced by an IRP, connecting between the stapes head and near to the center of the TM. The cross-sectional area of the IRP was 1.0 mm².

Numerical results

In order to evaluate the transfer function of the middle ear, transmission factor (TF = P_C/P_T) was defined as the ratio of the intracochlear pressure P_C in the scala vestibule close to the stapes to the stimulus pressure P_T in front of the TM. A high TF means high efficiency of the sound pressure transmission of the middle ear. The effects of the material, shape, and contact point of the prosthesis on the transfer function of the middle ear were examined, based on the TF.

Effect of the materials

The effect on the transmission factor of the materials used for the IRPs was analyzed. Figure 2 shows numerically obtained TFs of an intact and the recon-

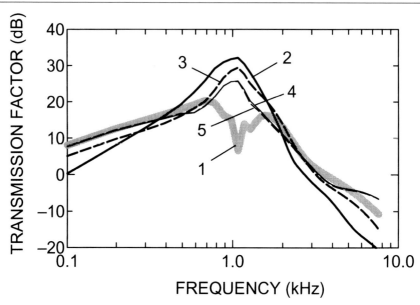

Fig. 2. Transmission factors of four different materials used for IRPs. The incus has been re-placed by the IRP between the head of the stapes and near to the center of the TM, as shown in Figure 1(b). The cross-sectional area of the IRP is 1.0 mm². 1. Intact ear; 2. tragal cartilage; 3. conchal cartilage; 4. incus; 5. hydroxyapatite.

structed middle ear displayed in Figure 1(b), *i.e.*, the incus was replaced by an IRP connecting between the stapes head and near to the center of the TM, and the cross-sectional area of the IRP was 1.0 mm². IRPs made of four different materials, *i.e.*, tragal cartilage, conchal cartilage, incus, and hydroxyapatite, were analyzed. The mechanical properties of these materials are shown in Table 1. The TFs of IRPs made of incus and hydroxyapatite were nearly the same as that of the intact ear, except at the frequency around 1.0 kHz. However, the IRP made of tragal cartilage had a relatively low TF at both low and high frequencies compared to the intact ear. The TF of the IRP made of conchal cartilage showed a medium value between those of tragal cartilage and hy-droxyapatite.

Table 1. Mechanical properties of the materials used for the prostheses

	Density (g/cm³)	Young's modulus (N/m²)
Tragal cartilage	1.1	4.0×10^6
Conchal cartilage	1.1	1.7×10^7
Incus	2.2	3.7×10^8
Hydroxyapatite	3.1	1.55×10^{11}

Effect of the shape

The TFs of the reconstructed middle ears were calculated using the three IRPs with the same attachment as that of the IRP to the posterior part of the TM, but a different cross-sectional area. The mechanical properties of the tragal cartilage were used to constrain the elements of the IRPs. The shapes of the IRPs are shown in Figure 3, and the TFs obtained using these models in Figure 4. The IRP with a 16.0 mm^2 cross-sectional area gave the best performance of the three types of IRPs, particularly in the high frequency region.

Effect of the contact point

The effect of the contact point of the IRP on the TF was analyzed. An intact and four different reconstructed middle ear models are shown in Figure 5. The contact points of the IRP were near to the center, posterior, and inferior points

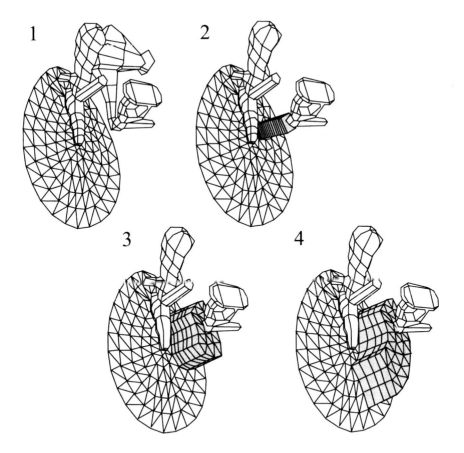

Fig. 3. Intact and reconstructed middle ear models. The IRPs are attached to the posterior part of the TM. 1. Intact ear; 2. the cross-sectional area of the IRP is 1.0 mm^2; 3. 16.0 mm^2; 4. 24.0 mm^2.

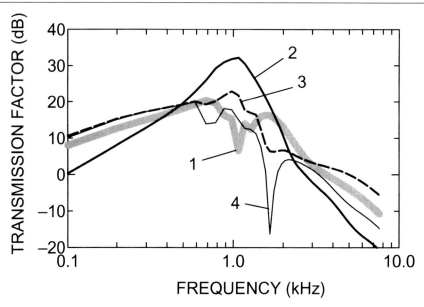

Fig. 4. Effect of the shape of the IRP on the transmission factor. Transmission factors were obtained from the models shown in Figure 3. 1. Intact ear; 2. the cross-sectional area of the IRP is 1.0 mm^2; 3. 16.0 mm^2; 4. 24.0 mm^2.

of the TM, and the midpoint of the malleus manubrium. In these models, all the IRPs were made of hydroxyapatite and their cross-sectional area was 1.0 mm^2. Figure 6 shows the TFs obtained from these models. The IRP connecting between the head of the stapes and the malleus manubrium provided a high TF, particularly at frequencies above 1.5 kHz, whereas the contact point of the IRP at the inferior portion gave the worst performance at frequencies ranging from 0.8-2.5 kHz.

Effects of the stiffness and shape of the tympanic membrane

The stiffness of the TM changes after surgery. Therefore, the effects of the stiffness on the transfer function of reconstructed middle ears were examined. Figure 7 shows the TFs when the stiffness of the TM had changed. The incus was replaced by the IRP connecting between the head of the stapes and near to the center of the TM, shown in Figure 1b. The IRP was made of hydroxyapatite and its cross-sectional area was 1.0 mm^2. The frequency with the largest TF shifted to high, and the TF decreased at frequencies below 0.5 kHz and increased above 1.5 kHz with an increase in the stiffness of the TM.

The shape of the TM is changed by the surgery. The effect on the TF was analyzed. Figure 8 shows the reconstructed middle ear models with the TM extended in a superior or posterior direction. The incus was replaced by the IRP made of hydroxyapatite connecting between the head of the stapes and near to the center of the TM. The cross-sectional area of the IRP was 1.0 mm^2.

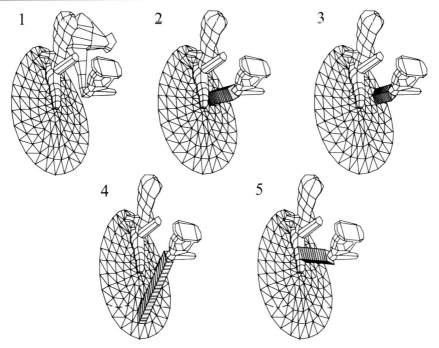

Fig. 5. An intact and four different reconstructed middle ear models. 1. Intact ear; 2. near to the center point of the TM; 3. posterior point of the TM; 4. inferior point of the TM; 5. the midpoint of the malleus manubrium.

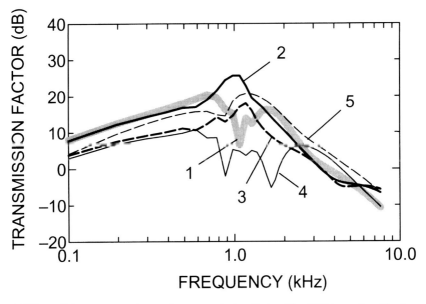

Fig. 6. Effect of the contact point on the transmission factor. The IRP is made of hydroxyapatite, its cross-sectional area is 1.0 mm^2. Transmission factors are obtained from the models shown in Figure 5. 1. Intact ear; 2. near to the center point of the TM; 3. posterior point of the TM; 4. inferior point of the TM; 5. the midpoint of the malleus manubrium.

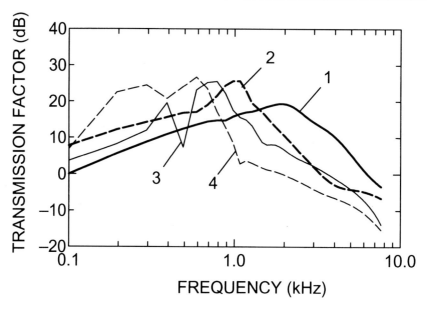

Fig. 7. Effect of the stiffness of the TM on the transmission factor. The incus is replaced by the IRP connecting between the head of the stapes and near to the center of the TM, as shown in Figure 1(b). The IRP is made of hydroxyapatite, its cross-sectional area is 1.0 mm². 1. Young's modulus of the TM is 3.34×10^8 N/m²; 2. 3.34×10^7 N/m² (normal value); 3. 3.34×10^6 N/m²; 4. 3.34×10^5 N/m².

At low frequencies, the TF increased proportionally in the area of the TM (Fig. 9). However, the effect of the shape of the TM was small in the mid- and high frequencies.

Discussion

A prosthesis with a high transfer function at the broad frequency region is desirable in the majority of patients with a pure conductive hearing loss. As shown in Figure 2, the TF curve of the IRP tended to peak at the frequency around 1.0 kHz. This peak was caused by the resonance of the reconstructed middle ear. In contrast, the TF curve of the intact middle ear had several small peaks at frequencies around 1.0 kHz, because the intact middle ear had a complicated vibration mode at these frequencies[17].

The IRPs made of incus and hydroxyapatite had a relatively high TF over a broad frequency region. However, the TF of the IRP made of tragal cartilage was lower over the entire frequency region, except at around 1.0 kHz. This difference was caused by the stiffness of the IRPs. When tragal cartilage was used for the IRP, as its Young's modulus was relatively small, it vibrated with bending movements. This is why the IRP made of tragal cartilage had a lower TF at both low and high frequencies. Figure 2 suggests that an IRP with a high

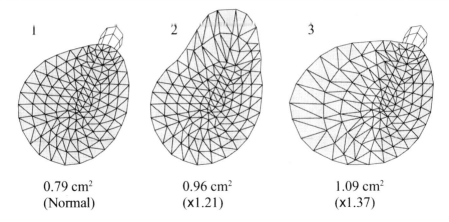

0.79 cm²   0.96 cm²   1.09 cm²
(Normal)   (×1.21)   (×1.37)

Fig. 8. The shape of the TM viewed from the external auditory meatus. 1. Normal shape; 2. the TM extended in a superior direction; 3. the TM extended in a posterior direction.

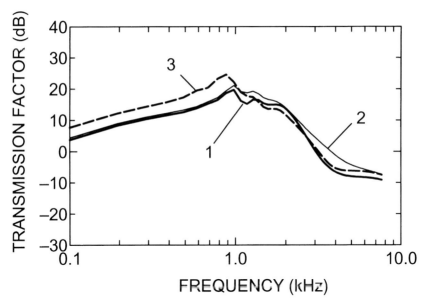

Fig. 9. Effect of the shape of the TM on the transmission factor. The incus is replaced by connecting the IRP between the head of the stapes and near to the center of the TM. The IRP is made of hydroxyapatite, its cross-sectional area is 1.0 mm². The numbers correspond to those in Figure 8.

degree of stiffness is recommended. When the IRP made of tragal cartilage was used, because of its advantages of good affinity with the living body and easy shaping, as shown in Figure 4, it is necessary to use a prosthesis with a relatively large cross-sectional area in order to increase its stiffness. However, if the cross-sectional area is too large, the TF is low at high frequencies, due to the large mass.

As shown in Figure 6, the TF varied with the contact point of the IRP. This

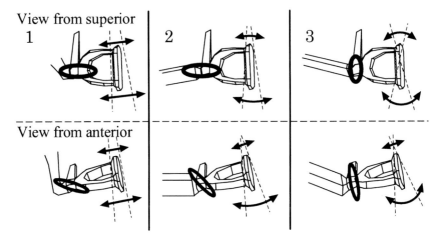

Fig. 10. Vibration mode of the stapes at the frequency 1.0 kHz. The IRP is made of hydroxya-patite, its cross-sectional area is 1.0 mm². The numbers correspond to those in Figure 5. The direction of the movement of the stapes footplate and the locus of the stapes head are shown by arrows and ellipses, respectively.

variance was derived from the difference in the vibration mode of the stapes. Figure 10 shows the vibration modes of the stapes of the intact and recon-structed middle ear models at 1000 Hz using the IRP attachments near to the center and to the posterior point of the TM, which were displayed in Figures 5(1), 2 and 3. The IRP was made of hydroxyapatite and its cross-sectional area was 1.0 mm². The direction of the movement of the stapes footplate and the locus of the stapes head are shown by arrows and ellipses, respectively. The stapes of the intact ear had a hinge-like, as well as a piston-like, movement, and the stapes head had an elliptical locus stretched along the direction from the external auditory meatus to the cochlea. When the IRP was attached near to the center of the TM, the vibration mode of the stapes was almost the same as that of the intact ear. In contrast, when the IRP was attached to the posterior point of the TM, the long axis of the elliptical locus of the stapes head was perpendicular to that of the intact ear, and the stapes showed a rocking motion. Due to the difference in these vibration modes, the TF of the IRP attached near to the center of the TM was larger than that attached to the posterior point.

As shown in Figure 7, the stiffness of the TM affected the TF of the recon-structed middle ear. This implies that the hearing level improves in the high frequency region, but becomes worse in the low frequency region, if the stiff-ness of the TM increases. Figure 9 suggests that the prognostic hearing level is only affected at low frequencies, and that the effects are small at mid- and high frequencies, if the shape of the TM is changed due to surgery.

The following conclusions can be drawn:

1. The high degree of stiffness of the IRP increases the sound power transmit-ted to the cochlea at both low and high frequencies.

2. The transfer function varies considerably, according to the cross-sectional area of the IRP made of tragal cartilage. There is an optimum value for the area that shows the best transfer function over the entire frequency region.
3. Better transfer function is shown when the IRP is attached to the malleus manubrium or near to the center of the TM than when the IRP is attached to the posterior point. In contrast, the worst transfer function is shown when the IRP is attached to the inferior point.
4. With increasing stiffness of the TM, the transmission factor decreases at low frequencies and increases at high ones. In addition, the transfer function increases proportionally with an increase in the area of the TM at low frequencies, while the TM area effect on the transfer function is small at mid- and high frequencies.

References

1. Elbrond O, Elpern BS: Reconstruction of ossicular chain. Arch Otolaryngol 84:490-494, 1966
2. Vlaming MSMG, Feenstra L: Studies on the mechanics of the reconstructed human middle ear. Clin Otolaryngol 11:411-422, 1986
3. Nishihara S, Goode RL: Experimental study of the acoustic properties of incus replacement prostheses in a human temporal bone model. Am J Otol 15:485-494, 1994
4. Asai M, Huber AM, Goode RL: Analysis of the best site on the stapes footplate for ossicular chain reconstruction. Acta Otolaryngol (Stockh) 119:356-361, 1999
5. Williams KR, Blayney AW, Lesser THJ: A 3-D finite element analysis of the natural frequencies of vibration of a stapes prosthesis replacement reconstruction of the middle ear. Clin Otolaryngol 20:36-44, 1995
6. Ladak HM, Funnell WRJ: Finite-element modeling of the normal and surgically repaired cat middle ear. J Acoust Soc Am 100:933-944, 1996
7. Blayney AW, Williams KR, Rice HJ: A dynamic and harmonic damped finite element analysis model of stapedotomy. Acta Otolaryngol (Stockh) 117:269-273, 1997
8. Eiber A, Freitag HG, Burkhardt C, Hemmert W, Maassen M, Jorge JR, Zenner HP: Dynamics of middle ear prostheses-simulations and measurements. Audiol Neurootol 4:178-184, 1999
9. Prendergast PJ, Ferris P, Rice HJ, Blayney AW: Vibro-acoustic modeling of the outer and middle ear using the finite-element method. Audiol Neurootol 4:185-191, 1999
10. Kirikae I: The Structure and Function of the Middle Ear, pp 38-63. Tokyo: University of Tokyo Press 1960
11. Wada H, Kobayashi T: Dynamical behavior of middle ear: theoretical study corresponding to measurement results obtained by a newly developed measuring apparatus. J Acoust Soc Am 87:237-245, 1990
12. Møller AR: An experimental study of the middle ear and it transmission properties. Acta Otolaryngol (Stockh) 60:129-149, 1965
13. Lynch TJ III, Nedzelnitski V, Peake WT: Input impedance of the cochlea in cat. J Acoust Soc Am 72:108-130, 1982
14. Aritomo H, Goode RL: Cochlear input impedance in fresh human temporal bones. Otolaryngology – Head & Neck Surgery 97:136-152, 1989
15. Zwislocki J: Analysis of some auditory characteristics. In: Luce RD, Bush RR, Galanter E (eds) Handbook of Mathematical Psychology III, p 66. New York, NY: John Wiley 1965

16. Merchant SN, Ravicz ME, Rosowski JJ: Acoustic input impedance of the stapes and cochlea in human temporal bones. Hearing Res 97:30-45, 1996
17. Wada H, Koike T, Kobayashi T: Three-dimensional finite-element method (FEM) analysis of the human middle ear. In: Hüttenbrink KB (ed) International Workshop on Middle Ear Mechanics in Research and Otosurgery. Dresden, Bibliothek der HNO-Universitätsklinik, pp 76-81, 1997

ASSESSMENT OF VIBRATION CHARACTERISTICS OF DIFFERENT CARTILAGE RECONSTRUCTION TECHNIQUES FOR THE TYMPANIC MEMBRANE USING SCANNING LASER VIBROMETRY

D. Mürbe, Th. Zahnert, M. Bornitz and K.-B. Hüttenbrink

Department of Otorhinolaryngology, Medical Faculty, Technical University, Dresden, Germany

Abstract

The sound transmission properties and resulting hearing improvement of reconstruction of the tympanic membrane are strongly influenced by the material and geometry of the transplants used. Combining mechanical stability and biocompatibility cartilage is a widely-used reconstruction material in tympanoplasties. However, different reconstruction techniques use different shapes and positions of cartilage slices, *e.g.*, cartilage plate, palisade technique, and island technique. The aim of the present study was to investigate the sound transmission properties of different reconstruction techniques. Therefore, vibrational amplitudes of the various transplants were measured by means of scanning laser vibrometry using an ear canal-tympanic membrane model. When exposed to a defined acoustic sound excitation, different frequency response functions were found for different reconstruction techniques. The results demonstrated that, apart from material characteristics, the sound transmission properties of the reconstructed tympanic membrane were strongly influenced by the reconstruction technique.

Keywords: middle ear reconstruction

Introduction

Successful reconstruction of the tympanic membrane always brings with it the major challenges of complete and permanent closure of the defective membrane and optimal hearing improvement. From a mechanical point of view, both demands are mainly effected by the transplant material and its shape and position within the reconstructed membrane. Apart from temporalis fascia and perichondrium, cartilage transplants from the cavum conchae or tragus are used for reconstruction of the tympanic membrane. While the insertion of membranous materials such as fascia and perichondrium results in successful closure

Address for correspondence: Dirk Mürbe, MD, Department of Otorhinolaryngology, Technical University, Fetscherstrasse 74, D-01307 Dresden, Germany

The Function and Mechanics of Normal, Diseased and Reconstructed Middle Ears, pp. 321–329
edited by J.J. Rosowski and S.N. Merchant
© *2000 Kugler Publications, The Hague, The Netherlands*

of the tympanic membrane in 95% of normal ventilated middle ears, in cases of tubal dysfunction, adhesive processes, tympanic fibrosis, and defects of the entire tympanic membrane, healing has a much poorer prognosis[1,2]. In these cases, cartilage has a better prognosis than fascia or perichondrium, the effect probably being the result of its higher mechanical stability under negative pressure changes in the middle ear[3-5]. However, the increasing mass and stiffness of the reconstructed tympanic membrane due to the use of cartilage transplants, leads to raised acoustic impedance, which alters the acoustic transfer characteristics[6]. The extent of this change strongly depends on the material properties of the graft, as seen by its mass density and Young's modulus. The latter parameter, and the thickness of the cartilage, determine the stiffness of the transplant. Furthermore, it can be assumed that the sound transmission properties of the reconstructed membrane are influenced by the shape and location of the graft within the tympanic membrane, thus reflecting a specific surgical technique.

The surgeon aims to optimize the acoustic quality of the reconstructed tympanic membrane. Reduced thickness of the cartilage transplant is one approach to improving its sound transmission properties, respecting demands on mechanical stability. This has been investigated in an earlier part of this study[7]. The aim of the present investigation was to assess the effect of different, commonly used, cartilage reconstruction techniques on the sound transmission properties of reconstructed tympanic membranes using characteristic shape and positioning of the cartilage graft, such as the palisade technique and the cartilage island technique[4].

Material and methods

The sound-induced vibrational amplitudes of different cartilage specimens were measured using an auditory ear canal-tympanic membrane model (Fig. 1). Two aluminium plates of varying size (60×60×6 and 30×30×6 mm, respectively) with a central hole (diameter, 8 mm), were pressed together by two fixation springs. The various grafts being investigated were clamped between the plates for simulation of the tympanic membrane suspension. To represent the external auditory canal, a plastic tube (length, 2 cm) with an inner diameter of 8 mm was attached on one side of the aluminium plates. A sound source (DH68-Praecitronic, Germany) was coupled to the free end of the tube and delivered the excitation signal. After calibration of the sound generator, acoustic stimulation was performed with a periodic chirp signal (SPL 90 dB). A probe microphone (KE4, Sennheiser, Germany) monitored the sound-pressure level 2 mm in front of the specimen. The vibrations of the cartilage grafts were measured by scanning laser vibrometry (Polytec PSV-200) at the back of the specimen (measuring points, $n=133$). Signal processing and Fast Fourier Transformation were performed by a signal analyzer in the frequency range from 200 Hz to 4 kHz.

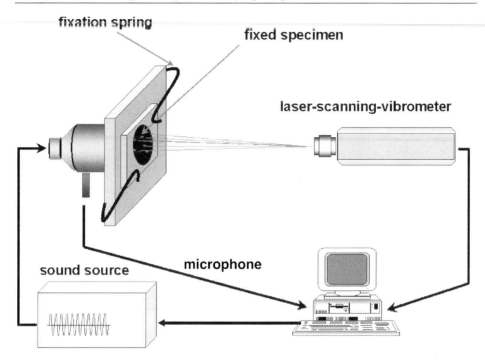

Fig. 1. External auditory canal-tympanic membrane model for measurement of vibrational amplitudes of cartilage transplants by scanning laser vibrometry. For simulation of the tympanic membrane suspension, the grafts were clamped between two aluminium plates with a central hole. A plastic tube (inner diameter, 8 mm) was attached on one side of the aluminium plates to represent the external auditory canal. Acoustic stimulation was performed with a periodic chirp signal (SPL 90 dB) at the free end of the tube, and monitored by a probe microphone.

Cartilage specimens from the cavum conchae, obtained from human bodies within 48 hours' postmortem, were investigated immediately after collection. Throughout all measurements, a perichondrium graft was clamped between the aluminium plates and moistened frequently. The use of a permanent membrane underlying the cartilage grafts permitted the investigation of cartilage chips that were too small to be fixed by our model's suspension. After determination of the cartilage thickness by light microscopy (1 mm), a cartilage plate of about 1 cm^2 was cut, sufficient in size to be clamped between the aluminium plates of our model. After vibration measurement, the cartilage plate was sliced into parallel strips (width, 2 mm; length, 10 mm), which were positioned in either a flat or on-edge position, hereafter called flat palisade and upright palisade. Furthermore, 4-mm and 7-mm diameter cartilage discs (thickness, 1 mm) were cut and positioned centrally on the perichondrium, hereafter called small island and large island (Fig. 2). The cartilage plate and strips were long enough be held within the two layers of our spring-clamped support system; the cartilage discs simply rested on the clamped perichondrial graft.

Frequency response functions (displacement versus sound pressure) averaging

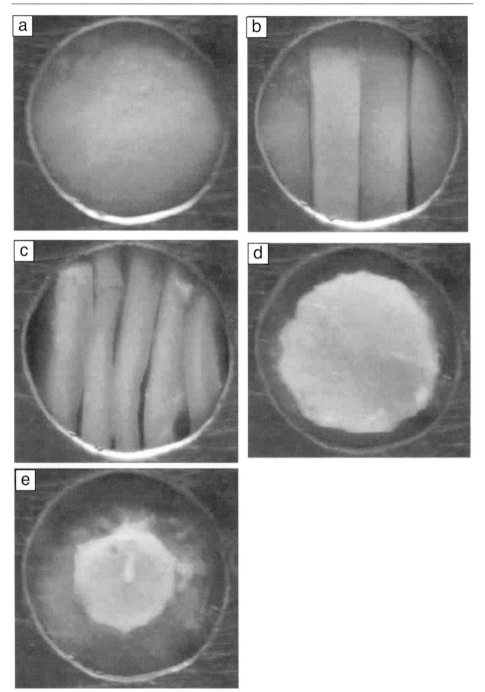

Fig. 2. Illustration of the five different tympanic membrane reconstruction techniques of the study: *a.* cartilage plate; *b.* flat palisade; *c.* upright palisade; *d.* large island; and *e.* small island transplant (view of the specimens from behind).

vibrational amplitudes of all measured points were displayed for the different grafts. This gave an equivalent of the volume displacement of the specimen. To describe the sound transmission properties of different reconstruction techniques, the frequency and amplitude of the first mode (first resonance) were determined from the frequency response functions.

Results

Fresh cartilage specimens, obtained from cavum conchae only and with a thickness of 1.0 mm, were used in order to standardize the effects of Young's modulus and thickness throughout the measurements of the different reconstruction techniques.

At the first mode, where transplants typically show a peak in motion, vibrational amplitudes were estimated, as seen in Figures 3 and 4, for flat palisade and small island transplants. As expected, reduced stiffness due to slicing the plate into palisades decreased the first resonance frequency and increased its amplitude, reflecting improved sound transmission properties of the transplant. This change was greater when the palisades were inserted in a flat rather than an upright position. Cutting island transplants from a cartilage plate showed similar effects, the reason being the reduced size and mass of the island grafts. The small island transplant revealed better acoustic transfer characteristics than

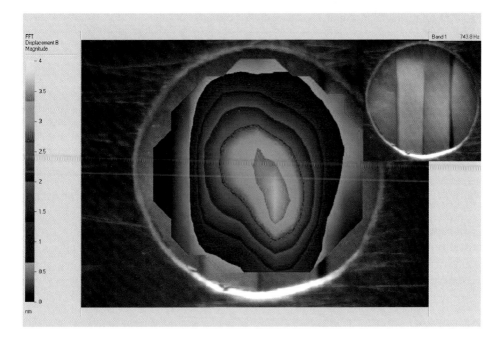

Fig. 3. Vibrational amplitudes (displacement) of the flat palisade transplant at its first mode (744 Hz).

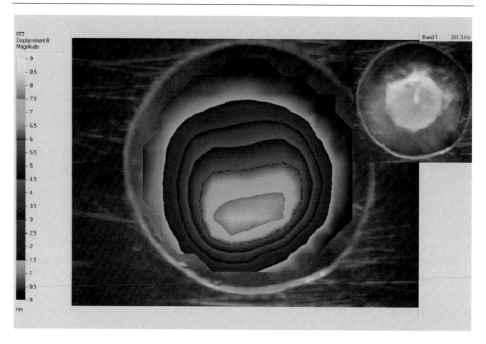

Fig. 4. Vibrational amplitudes (displacement) of the small island transplant at its first mode (281 Hz).

Table 1. First resonance frequency (Hz) and amplitude of first resonance frequency (nm) for the different tympanic membrane reconstruction techniques

Reconstruction technique	First resonance frequency (Hz)	Amplitude of first resonance frequency (nm)
Plate	1186	0.5
Upright palisade	993	1.6
Flat palisade	744	3.8
Large island	337	4.7
Small island	281	8.9

the large island graft. The gain in acoustic quality of both island transplants appeared to be much more prominent compared to the palisades (Table 1).

Frequency response functions of the different tympanic membrane reconstruction techniques are displayed in Figure 5. By and large, the effects on the sound transmission properties described at the first mode (Table 1) are representative of transmission in the entire frequency range from 0.2-4 kHz.

Discussion

The use of cartilage for reconstruction of the tympanic membrane has been established, particularly in cases of chronic tubal dysfunction, adhesive

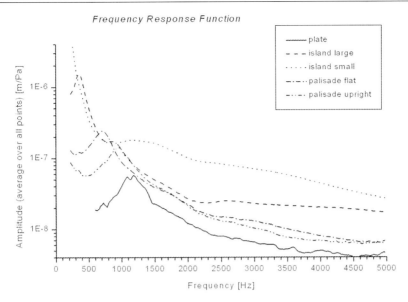

Fig. 5. Frequency response function (spatially averaged displacement per sound pressure) for the cartilage plate, flat palisade, upright palisade, large island and small island transplants.

processes, and total or recurrent defects of the tympanic membrane[3-5]. In these cases, cartilage has a better prognosis for permanent closure compared to temporalis fascia and perichondrium, which are predominantly used for tympanic membrane reconstruction in normal ventilated middle ears[1,2]. Since increased mass and stiffness of the cartilage reconstructed eardrum might adversely affect its transfer characteristics, the choice of material should also consider the acoustic consequences of the transplanted material.

Clinical studies, comparing results of pure-tone audiometry after tympanic membrane reconstruction with fascia, perichondrium and cartilage, show contradictory results[8-10]. However, clinical results may be misleading, due to confounding variables such as middle ear inflammation or persistent tubal dysfunction with effusion, etc. In order to exclude these factors, we developed an experimental set-up with an auditory canal-tympanic membrane model. This model offers the advantage of reproducible test conditions, in contrast to a temporal bone model in which reproducible placement and fixation of the various cartilage transplants cannot be ensured[6].

Various factors are likely to influence the sound transmission characteristics of the transplant. Material properties such as the transplant's mass density and Young's modulus, as well as the stiffness, determine the acoustic quality, the latter also depending on the thickness of the grafted tissue. Further, the surgical processing of the cartilage could affect the acoustic properties of the transplant, the shape and position of the transplant within the tympanic membrane being decisive factors in this alteration[8,11,12].

In a previous part of this study, Young's modulus of cartilage from the cavum conchae and tragus was investigated, yielding average values of 3.4 and 2.8 N/mm² , respectively, but this difference was not significant. Furthermore, an improvement in the acoustic transfer qualities of the transplants was found after reduction of the thickness of the cartilage layer. Cartilage plates with a layer thickness of about 500 µm were considered an acceptable compromise between appropriate acoustic properties and sufficient mechanical stability against static middle ear pressure changes[7].

The aim of the present study was to focus on the influence of various surgical techniques on the sound transmission properties of the transplant. Cartilage can be inserted as a large plate, or in the form of several parallel full-thickness strips (the palisade technique), or as a small piece that 'floats' on the remainder of the tympanic membrane (the island technique). Furthermore, the insertion can be modified by using combined tragal-perichondrium transplants[3,4,10,13,14].

In the present study, frequency response functions (displacement versus sound pressure) from 0.2-4 kHz were estimated. An averaged function (equivalent to the volume displacement of the specimen) was calculated from 133 points which were measured by scanning laser vibrometry. Frequency and amplitude of the first mode were determined to assess the sound transmission properties of the tested reconstruction techniques because both represent characteristic parameters such as the mass and stiffness of the transplant. Reduced stiffness due to slicing the cartilage plate into palisades decreased the first resonance frequency and increased its amplitude, both effects reflecting improved sound transmission properties of the transplant. This change was more prominent when the palisades were positioned flat rather than upright, reflecting the influence of the thickness of the cartilage reconstruction on its sound transmission properties. Both island transplants showed lower frequency and higher amplitude values at the first mode compared to plate and palisades, the reason for this being the reduced size and mass of the island grafts. Consequently, the small island transplant revealed better acoustic transfer characteristics than the large island graft. However, the gain in acoustic quality of both island transplants appeared to be much more prominent compared to the palisades. This reflects the determining factor of suspension of the transplant in the osseous annular rim, as simulated by the aluminium plates, in our investigation. If the transplant is suspended in the osseous annular rim, the acoustic transfer characteristics of the reconstructed tympanic membrane are determined by the stiffness. However, a cartilage island with a regular tympanic membrane surrounding it mainly influences the vibrational characteristics by its mass, as the stiffness of the membrane is determined by the surrounding tympanic membrane remnant. In principle, it can be assumed that small cartilage transplants, embedded in a normally vibrating tympanic membrane, will only influence the vibration pattern of the tympanic membrane in a definite frequency, if the cartilage is in a region of maximum amplitude. However, larger cartilage plates may influence the transfer behavior of the entire frequency range, since the bending strength of the entire tympanic membrane increases with the size of the implanted cartilage pieces.

In conclusion, our experimental results suggest that cartilage palisade as well as cartilage island transplants improve the sound transmission properties of reconstructed tympanic membranes, compared to a 1-mm thick cartilage plate. In cases of adequate surrounding tympanic membrane remnants, the otosurgeon should try to create a cartilage island reconstruction, since the suspension of cartilage palisades in the osseous annular rim is likely to increase the acoustic transfer loss of the reconstructed membrane. Furthermore, a small cartilage island underneath the tympanic membrane, placed on top of total ossicular replacement prosthesis (TORP) or partial ossicular replacement prosthesis (PORP) implants, may only affect the transfer characteristics slightly, while protecting the tympanic membrane. In cases of chronic tubal dysfunction, suspension of the cartilage transplant in the osseous annular rim is necessary in order to achieve a stiffer reconstruction. A future study will investigate which of a palisade technique or a thinned cartilage plate will provide better sound transmission properties of the reconstructed membrane.

References

1. Hüttenbrink KB: Die operative Behandlung der chronischen Otitis media (I-III). HNO 42:582-593, 648-657, 701-718, 1994
2. Palva P: Surgical treatment of chronic middle ear disease. Acta Otolaryngol (Stockh) 104:279-284, 1987
3. Goodhill V: Tragal perichondrium and cartilage in tympanoplasty. Arch Otolaryngol 85:480-491, 1967
4. Heermann HJ, Heermann H, Kopstein E: Fascia and cartilage palisade tympanoplasty: nine years experience. Arch Otolaryngol 91:229-240, 1970
5. Hildmann H, Luckhaupt H, Schmelzer A: Die Verwendung von Knorpel in der Mittelohrchirurgie. HNO 44:597-603, 1996
6. Schöttke H, Hartwein H, Pau HW: Einfluss unterschiedlicher Transplantatmaterialien bei der Tympanoplastik Typ 1 auf den Schalldruckpegel im Gehörgang. Otolaryngol Nova 2:318-320, 1992
7. Zahnert T, Hüttenbrink KB, Mürbe D, Bornitz M: Experimental investigations of the use of cartilage in tympanic membrane reconstruction. Am J Otol 21:322-328, 2000
8. Adkins WY: Composite autograft for tympanoplasty and tympanomastoid surgery. Laryngoscope 100:244-247, 1990
9. Dornhoffer JL: Hearing results with cartilage tympanoplasty. Laryngoscope 107:1094-1099, 1997
10. Milewski C: Composite graft tympanoplasty in the treatment of ears with advanced middle ear pathology. Laryngoscope 103:1352-1356, 1993
11. Hüttenbrink KB: Mechanical aspects of middle ear reconstruction. In: Hüttenbrink KB (ed) Middle Ear Mechanics in Research and Otosurgery, pp 165-169. Dresden: Department of Oto-Rhino-Laryngology. Dresden University of Technology, 1997
12. Williams KR, Blayney AW, Lesser THJ: Mode shapes of a damaged and repaired tympanic membrane as analysed by the finite element method. Clin Otolaryngol 22:126-131, 1997
13. Glasscock ME, Jackson CG, Nissen AJ et al: Postauricular undersurface tympanic membrane grafting: a follow-up report. Laryngoscope 92:718-727, 1982
14. Tolsdorff P: Tympanoplastik mit Tragusknorpeltransplantat: 'Knorpeldeckel-Plastik'. Laryngol Rhinol Otol 62:97-102, 1983

PHYSIOLOGICAL INCUS REPLACEMENT WITH AN 'INCUS REPLICA' PROSTHESIS

Clinical and laboratory evaluation

Robert P. Mills[1], Eric Abel[2] and Richard Lord[2]

[1]Department of Otolaryngology, Lauriston Building, Royal Infirmary, Edinburgh; [2]Department of Biomedical Engineering, University of Dundee, Dundee; UK

Abstract

An ossicular prosthesis produced by making a mold from a cadaveric incus and injecting ionomeric cement into it was cemented to the malleus head and stapes head and evaluated *in vivo* and *in vitro*. An initial study was carried out on three patients with absence of the incus due to chronic suppurative otitis media. The performance of the prosthesis was further evaluated in fresh human temporal bones using a laser vibrometer. Two patients obtained good hearing results and have been followed for three years. In the third case, the hearing did not improve and at revision surgery it was found that the incudo-stapedial joint reconstruction had failed. The results of the *in vitro* experiments indicate that the prosthesis performs almost as well as the intact ossicular chain and that cementing the incudo-stapedial joint, as well as the incudomalleolar joint, enhances sound transmission rather than making it worse. A physiological incus replacement prosthesis is likely to provide hearing results superior to those obtained with a conventional prosthesis.

Keywords: ossiculoplasty, laser vibrometer

Introduction

Reconstruction of defects of the ossicular chain generally involves making a link between the malleus handle or tympanic membrane and the stapes head or footplate. This creates an ossicular assembly which has more in common with avian middle ear anatomy than the mammalian three-ossicle pattern. However, there are significant differences between the avian and reconstructed human middle ears[1]. While some ossiculoplasty operations produce satisfactory hearing results, others do not. This is, in part, due to other aspects of the pathology

Address for correspondence: Robert P. Mills, MS, MPhil, FRCS, Department of Otolaryngology, Lauriston Building, Royal Infirmary, Edinburgh EH3 9EN, Scotland, UK

The Function and Mechanics of Normal, Diseased and Reconstructed Middle Ears, pp. 331–337
edited by J.J. Rosowski and S.N. Merchant
© *2000 Kugler Publications, The Hague, The Netherlands*

of chronic ear disease, but some failures may be attributed to the limitations of conventional surgical techniques.

The ideal reconstruction would be one in which the ossicular defect was repaired with restoration of the mammalian three-ossicle pattern. Relatively crude attempts to achieve this using the 'sleeve' technique[2] or the Apelbaum and Plester prostheses have produced encouraging results[3]. Small incus defects have also been repaired successfully using ionomeric cement[3,4]. None of these techniques is applicable when the entire incus long process or the whole incus is missing. In addition, the bulk of the incus is increased and this can result in fixation to surrounding structures. In order to overcome these limitations, we have developed an incus-like prosthesis which connects the malleus head to the stapes head.

Material and methods

The 'incus replica prosthesis' (IRP) was made from ionomeric cement. At first 'Ionocap' cement (IONOS) was used, but following the withdrawal of this material from the market, we switched to 'Biocem' (Corinthian Medical). Molds were made from Coltene light body dental impression material using cadaveric in-cudes. The cement was injected into the molds and allowed to set. The result-ing IRP was finished using a diamond burr.

Patient study

In order to determine the feasibility of using the IRP in the clinical setting, three operations were carried out on patients with absent incudes. All had had conventional ossicular reconstructions which had failed to produce satisfactory hearing results and were prepared to accept a novel approach to their problem. Two of the three had had a previous cortical mastoidectomy and, in the third, this was carried out as part of the surgery. Bone removal was extended antero-superiorly to expose the malleus head in the attic. The middle ear was opened via the external auditory meatus. The prosthesis was introduced via the attic and cemented to the malleus head using ionomeric cement. In the first case, the incudo-stapedial joint was not cemented, but in the other two, more cement was used to attach the lower end of the prosthesis to the stapes head. In the first case, an incudostapedial joint splint made from a Paparella grommet was in-serted. Mean air-bone gaps, mean residual hearing losses and mean hearing changes were calculated using the frequencies 500, 1000 and 2000 Hz.

Laboratory study

The performance of the IRP was further evaluated in fresh human temporal bones using a laser Doppler vibrometer (Polytec CLV). A cortical mastoidec-tomy with a posterior tympanotomy was carried out to provide access to the ossicular chain. The vestibule was approached via the internal auditory meatus to expose the undersurface of the stapes footplate. A small spot of retroreflective paint was applied to the medial side of the stapes footplate to ensure that consistent recordings could be obtained. The mass of the paint applied was insignificant compared to the mass of the stapes. A hole was drilled in the posterior wall of the external auditory meatus close to the tympanic membrane, and a piece of polythene tubing was introduced and fixed in place with epoxy resin. This was connected to a microphone so that the sound pressure level at the level of the tympanic membrane could be recorded. A larger piece of polythene tubing was inserted into the external auditory meatus and similarly fixed with epoxy resin. This was connected to a loudspeaker so that sound could be introduced directly into the ear canal. The temporal bone specimen was fixed in a holder mounted on an adjustable platform which could be used to adjust its position with precision (Fig. 1). Sound of known frequency and loudness was introduced via the external auditory meatus and stapes velocity was measured using the laser vibrometer, and footplate displacement was calculated by numerical integration of the velocity data. Measurements were made using frequencies from 125-8000 Hz and sound pressure levels of 90-110 dB. An initial series of measurements was made with the ossicular chain intact. The incus was then removed and a further series of results recorded. The IRP was then introduced and cemented to the malleus head. Its lower end was applied to the head of the stapes, but not cemented. Following the completion of a further series of recordings, the lower end of the prosthesis was cemented to the stapes head and a final set of results recorded. The experiment was carried out on five temporal bone specimens. All measurements were made within a six-hour period, as existing data indicate that no changes in middle ear performance occur over this period[5].

Results

Patient study

Two of the three patients reported subjective hearing improvement and commented favorably on the quality of their hearing. Following the third operation, in which both joints were cemented, the hearing did not improve. This ear was re-explored 15 months later, and it was found the lower end of the prosthesis was not attached to the stapes head. The hearing results for all three cases are summarized in Figure 2 using the Glasgow Benefit Plot[6].

Laboratory study

A representative set of recordings is presented in Figure 3. There were some variations between experiments in the pattern of responses at different frequencies, but these were consistent for measurements made on the same specimen.

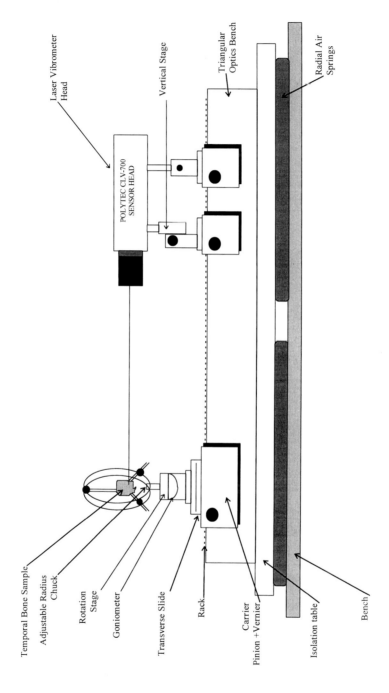

Fig. 1. Diagram showing the set-up for the laboratory experiments.

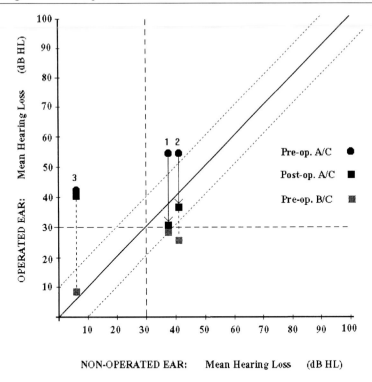

Fig. 2. Hearing results for the clinical study presented using the Glasgow Benefit Plot.

The performance of the IRP was comparable with that of the intact ossicular chain, and cementing of the prosthesis to the stapes head improved sound transmission rather than diminishing it.

Discussion

Our results indicate the technical feasibility of introducing a prosthesis which connects the malleus head to the stapes head, and suggest that such a reconstruction might be expected to perform almost as well as an intact ossicular chain. This, in turn, suggests that better results might be expected with such a prosthesis than are obtainable with conventional columella-type devices, and an approach of this type merits further study. We have subsequently compared a conventional partial ossicular replacement prosthesis with the IRP using the same experimental protocol, and have shown that the IRP is superior.

The results of the laboratory investigation must be interpreted with some caution because they were recorded from essentially 'healthy' middle ear spaces, lacking the other pathology associated with chronic suppurative otitis media. However, since the prosthesis has been found to compare favorably with the intact ossicular chain which must be considered the 'gold standard' for ossicu-

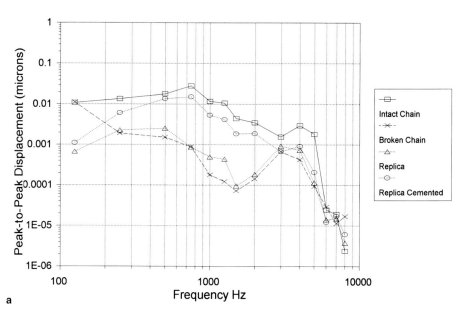

a

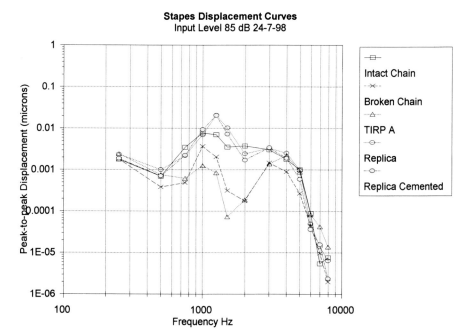

b

Fig. 3. Graphs showing stapes displacements at different frequencies. Data set showing: *(a).* Poor transmission of sound with the incudo-stapedial joint uncemented and good transmission following cementing. *(b).* Equally good transmission with the incudo-stapedial joint cemented and uncemented.

lar function, it seems likely that improved hearing results could be expected. This view is supported by the findings in the first two surgical cases. The three cases selected must be considered poor candidates for successful ossicular reconstruction because of their middle ear pathology and previous surgical failure.

Examination of the graphs presented in Figure 3 indicates that the removal of the incus resulted in less reduction of stapes displacement than might have been expected. We believe that this is due to removal of cochlear impedance, which results from our surgical approach to the vestibule. We are currently carrying out further experiments to investigate this possibility and others.

In the surgical cases, the middle ear was opened via the external auditory meatus by raising a tympano-meatal flap. The experience from the temporal bone experiments indicates that the IRP could be introduced via a posterior tympanotomy without disturbing the tympanic membrane. Given that a common cause of failure is lateralization of the ossicular graft as result of changes in drum position during healing[7], this could be a significant advantage.

The IRP would be an ideal prosthesis for use in ears that have undergone a previous intact canal wall mastoidectomy. In other cases, at least a cortical mastoidectomy, and ideally a posterior tympanotomy, would have to be carried out. This would increase the time required for surgery and the risk of facial nerve trauma. However, in expert hands, neither of these differences would be significant, and the more extensive surgery would be justified if better hearing resulted.

Acknowledgments

The laboratory work was supported by a grant from the Scottish Hospitals Endowment Research Trust.

References

1. Mills RP: Applied comparative anatomy of the avian middle ear. J Roy Soc Med 87:155-156, 1994
2. Mills RP: Physiological reconstruction of the incus long process. Clin Otol 21:499-503, 1996
3. Maassen MM, Zenner HP: Tympanoplasty type 11 with ionomeric cement and titanium gold angle prosthesis. Am J Otolaryngol 19:693-699, 1998
4. Babighlan G: Use of glass ionomer cement in otological surgery: a preliminary report. J Laryngol Otol 106:954-959, 1992
5. Vlaming MSMG, Feenstra L: Studies on the mechanics of the normal human middle ear. Clin Otolaryngol 11:353-363, 1986
6. Browning GG, Gatehouse S, Swan IRC: The Glasgow Benefit Plot: A new method for reporting benefits from middle ear surgery. Laryngoscope 101(2):180-185, 1991
7. Mills RP: Anatomical and mechanical aspects of ossiculoplasty. Thesis, London University, 1994

NEW AREAS OF RESEARCH:
ACTIVE MIDDLE-EAR IMPLANTS & MEASUREMENTS
OF MIDDLE-EAR MECHANICS

DIRECT SOUND DETECTION FROM THE OSSICULAR CHAIN

Iain L. Grant[1] and Kai Kroll[2]

[1]Department of Otolaryngology, The Ohio State University, Columbus, OH; [2]St Croix Medical, Minneapolis, MN, USA

Abstract

Successful implantation of a totally implantable cochlear implant or active middle ear implant is contingent upon a functional sound input stage. A piezoelectric bimorph placed on the malleus head provides a viable alternative to a subcutaneously implanted microphone as the input stage for such a device. A bimorph detecting malleus motion would benefit from the inherent gain in the external auditory canal and low power consumption characteristics of piezoelectric sensors. This cadaver temporal bone study documents frequency response, ossicular tracking, and minimum sensitivity of such a sensor. Results indicate a dynamic range of 80 dB, nominal sensitivity of 382 mV/Pa at 1000 Hz, minimum sensitivity of around 26 dB SPL, and precise ossicular tracking out to 4 kHz. Alteration of the mechanical characteristics of the sensor could improve these figures further. In the tested implementation, the piezoelectric bimorph positioned on the malleus head provides a viable sound input stage for a totally implantable active middle ear or cochlear implant.

Introduction

The current generation of cochlear implants and active middle ear implants are partially implantable. They comprise an externally mounted input stage consisting of microphone and transcutaneous transmission coil. Input is electrically coupled to the internally mounted receiver coil and output stage. In the case of a cochlear implant, the output is the electrode, whereas in an active middle ear implant, the output consists of a piezoelectric or electromagnetic vibrating element. With miniaturization, decreasing power requirements and improvements in battery technology, totally implantable hearing devices are becoming possible. Although in their infancy, such devices offer very real potential to patients with moderate to severe sensorineural hearing losses. Although conventional hearing aids have made formidable strides within the last

Address for correspondence: Iain L. Grant, MD, Department of Otolaryngology, The Ohio State University, 456 West 10th Avenue, Columbus, OH 43210, USA. *email:* ilgrant@compuserve.com

The Function and Mechanics of Normal, Diseased and Reconstructed Middle Ears, pp. 341–352
edited by J.J. Rosowski and S.N. Merchant
© 2000 Kugler Publications, The Hague, The Netherlands

decade, patients with moderate to severe sensorineural losses are still poorly served. The high gains necessary to treat sensorineural losses are difficult to achieve without feedback, and the hair cell loss results in speech discrimination impairments can only be overcome by direct electrical stimulation of the cochlear nerve.

Any totally implantable hearing device, whether it be cochlear implant or active middle ear implant, requires an input stage. Currently, this stage is in the form of a conventional microphone. Implantation of such microphones is technically difficult. Optimal sensitivity considerations require that the diaphragm be close to the skin surface, risking the possibility of extrusion[1]. The internal environment of the body necessitates that the device is sealed and protected, however, this impairs sensitivity.

An alternative to a microphone was first outlined by Gyo *et al.* in 1984[2]. This consists of a piezoelectric element placed against the lateral surface of the malleus head in the disarticulated ossicular chain (Fig. 1). The ceramic element consists of a bilayer of oppositely polarized sheets of PZT5A, separated by a thin layer of platinum paste. This material has the property of reversible electromechanical transduction. Displacement of the tip of the rigidly fixed bimorph generates a voltage. Alternatively, a voltage applied to the transducer generates motion at the tip. Such transducers are used extensively in industry for detection of low amplitude vibrations and nanopositioning.

The use of piezoelectric ceramic materials as components in hearing devices is not new. In 1984, the Japanese, under the direction of Professor Yanagihara,

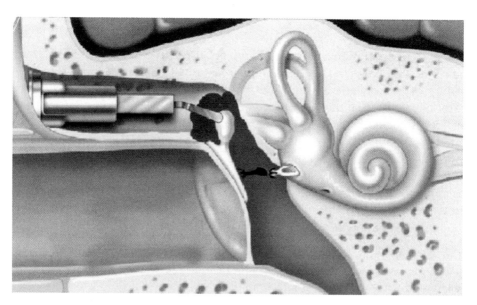

Fig. 1. Piezoelectric sensing concept. The piezo sensor is positioned on the lateral surface of the malleus head in the disarticulated ossicular chain. In this drawing, a second bimorph can be seen driving the stapes. The sensor is equally appropriate for driving a cochlear implant passing through the round window.

developed and implanted a partially implantable hearing device consisting of an external conventional microphone and implanted piezoelectric driver transducer. Although only 90 such devices were implanted, many still continue to function up to 15 years after implantation, attesting to the longevity of the piezo material used[3-5]. Considerable improvements in ceramic materials have occurred in the interim.

Experimental method

Fresh temporal bones were harvested within 24 hours of death. Specimens were mounted in a temporal bone holder and a was mastoidectomy performed. The ossicular chain was identified and the facial recess opened so as to obtain a good view of the stapes footplate. The external auditory canal was drilled down to within 3 mm of the tympanic membrane and a 2-ml coupler assembly bonded to the canal remnant.

A probe microphone ER7c and insert earphone ER2 (Etymotic Research, Elk Grove Village, IL, USA) were placed in the coupler with the probe tip 3 mm from the tympanic membrane. An HP35670A dynamic signal analyzer (DSA) (Hewlett Packard, Palo Alto, CA, USA) was used to generate the stimulus and record the data. The beam of a Polytec QFV 303 laser Doppler vibrometer (LDV) (Polytec, Tustin, CA, USA) was directed at the structure of interest. The output of the DSA was connected via an IEEE 1394 interface to a personal computer. 'BoneWerks', a purpose-written software program, integrated the laser velocity signal to compute displacement and normalized sensor voltage and displacement results to 100 dB SPL. Voltage generated from the microphone was converted to sound pressure level by dividing by a factor of 50 mVrms per Pascal. Prior to commencing the experiment, the microphone had been calibrated against an ER10 microphone of known performance. An experimental schematic is seen in Figure 2.

The ear was stimulated acoustically with a swept sine acoustic stimulus at nominally 100 dB SPL, and measurements made of stapes footplate motion.

The ossicular chain was disarticulated and the sensor placed on the malleus head 1 mm below the insertion of the superior malleolar ligament. The contact was optimized by varying the bimorph load against the malleus, stimulating the ear with a 100 dB SPL acoustic stimulus, and determining maximum sensor output voltage at 1000 Hz.

The sensor was stimulated acoustically and the sensor voltage, laser velocity, and tympanic membrane sound pressure level were measured simultaneously. The acoustic stimulus was then progressively lowered and sensor voltage measured to determine the minimum sensitivity of the system.

The following experiments were designed to determine the useful bandwidth and range of system function:
1. Measurement of intact chain footplate displacement at 100 dB SPL. The ear

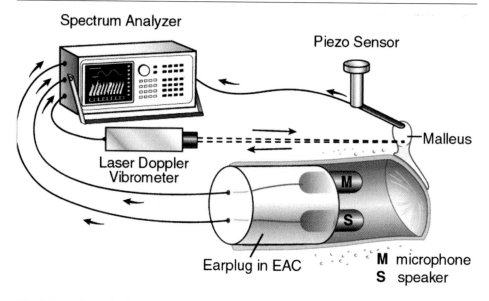

Fig. 2. Experimental schematic drawing showing the temporal bone preparation with sensor on the malleus head, probe microphone and speaker in the external auditory canal, and measurement equipment.

was stimulated acoustically with a 100 dB SPL swept sine stimulus from 100 Hz to 10 kHz, and stapes footplate displacement was recorded.

2. Measurement of sensor voltage at 100 dB SPL. With the sensor optimized on the lateral surface of the malleus head, the above stimulus was applied and sensor voltage was recorded across frequency.

3. *Ossicular tracking.* The LDV was directed at the sensor tip during a swept sine sweep. The LDV was then directed to a point immediately adjacent to the sensor on the malleus head and the sweep repeated. Phase relative to the sound source was determined during both sweeps, and the phase of the sensor tip relative to the malleus head determined.

4. *Minimum sensitivity.* Starting at 100 dB SPL, the sensor voltage was recorded across frequency. The acoustic stimulus was progressively reduced in 6-dB decrements, and the sweeps repeated until the noise floor of the measurement system had been reached. Sensor voltage and sound pressure level at the tympanic membrane were recorded.

The tests were performed on eight temporal bones. Temporal bone specimens were harvested fresh, and the majority of measurements completed within 24 hours of harvest. Specimen details included a mean age of 59 years (35-83 years), five female, three male. A view of the sensor in position on the lateral surface of the malleus head is seen in Figure 3. In this right cadaver specimen, the surgeon is looking through the mastoid towards the middle ear. Anterior is towards the upper edge of the photograph and superior to the left margin. The facial recess has been widely opened and the incus removed. The sensor tip is

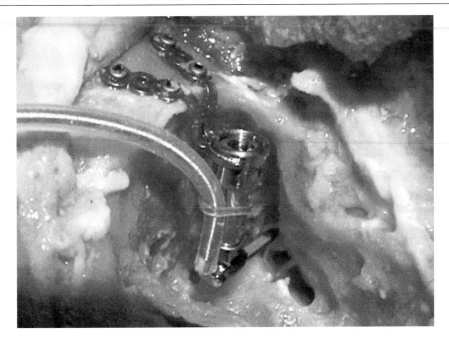

Fig. 3. Surgical view in right cadaver specimen. The view is taken looking through the mastoid towards the middle ear. Anterior is to the upper margin of the photograph, and superior is to the left. The facial recess has been opened and the incus removed. The sensor is positioned on the lateral surface of the malleus head. The stapes is visible in the depth of the facial recess.

seen resting on the lateral surface of the malleus head. The stapes is visible in the depths of the facial recess.

Results

Figure 4 shows the mean stapes footplate displacement in the intact ossicular chain at 100 dB SPL. Results are based on 68 measurements in eight temporal bone specimens. Displacements have been corrected for an estimated 30° cosine error inherent in directing the LDV through the facial recess. Results of two other series are plotted for comparison[6,7]. Mean footplate displacement is 85 nm at 1000 Hz. Stapes displacement is relatively flat out to 1 kHz, and rolls off smoothly at 36 dB per decade out to 10 kHz. Stapes footplate displacement recorded in this series compares favorably with other published series, and gives an indication of the malleus roll-off required for the sensor to function as the input stage in a totally implantable hearing device.

Figure 5 shows the mean sensor voltage at 100 dB SPL. The fine lines indicate the mean ± two standard deviations either side of the mean. Measurements were taken with the sensor optimally coupled on the malleus head. Mean out-

Stapes Displacement at 100 dB SPL

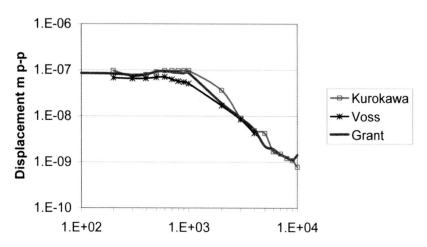

Fig. 4. Mean intact chain stapes footplate displacement at 100 dB SPL. Two other published series are plotted for comparison.

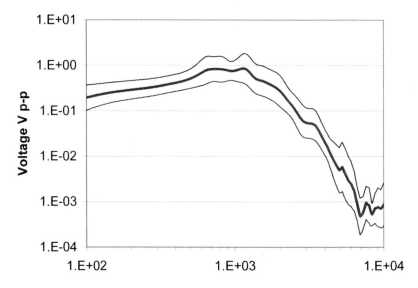

Fig. 5. Mean sensor voltage at 100 dB SPL. The fine lines indicate mean ± two standard deviations.

put at 1 kHz is 764 mV, giving a nominal sensitivity of 382 mV/Pa. Sensor signal commences at 200 mV at 100 Hz, and gently increases 10 dB to reach a system resonant peak at 1200 Hz. Beyond this frequency, the system rolls off at a rate of 37 dB per decade out to 3 kHz, and then accelerates. The noise floor of the measurement system is 100 μV. Calculations of the noise floor of the sensor alone suggest it is around 20 μV.

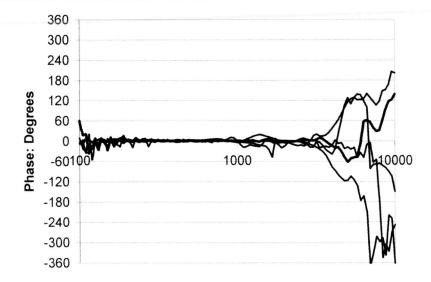

Fig. 6. Phase of sensor tip relative to motion of the malleus head at 100 dB SPL.

Figure 6 shows the phase of the sensor tip relative to the malleus head at 100 dB SPL. This measurement was made in five temporal bone specimens. The sensor is seen to track malleus motion out to 4 kHz. Sensor malleus motion briefly moves out of phase around the resonant frequency of the system (1200 Hz). Above 4 kHz, the tracking relationship becomes erratic.

Figures 7 and 8 show the sensor output voltage and corresponding sound pressure levels as the acoustic driving stimulus is progressively reduced in 6-dB decrements. Results have not been normalized. By a curve matching process, the minimum sensitivity can be determined. Figure 8 shows the tympanic membrane sound pressure level progressively decreasing in a linear manner. As levels approach 50 dB SPL, the microphone signal becomes erratic and, by 40 dB SPL, the ER7c microphone is functioning at a level just above the noise floor of the microphone preamplifier. However, the corresponding sensor output voltage traces remain robust at this level. The electrical source level commenced at 1 Vrms and was reduced 60 dB to 1 mVrms. This was the minimum drive that the HP35670A could provide to the ER2 speaker. As can be seen in Figure 7, even at this minimum generated sound pressure level, which corresponds to around 40 dB SPL, good sensor signal is evident out to 2500 Hz. Although only a single representative plot of minimum sensitivity is recorded here, similar results were seen on implanting the sensor in all eight temporal bones.

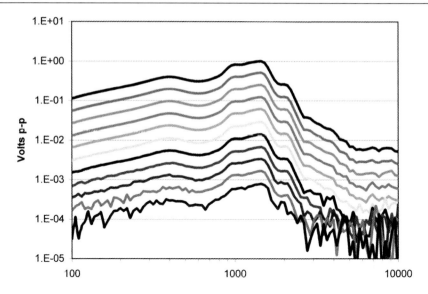

Fig. 7. Sensor voltage at progressively decreasing acoustic stimulus presentation levels. Corresponding sound pressure levels are seen in Figure 8. In this study, the nominal driving voltage to the ER2 starts at 1 Vrms. This corresponds to 97 dB SPL (at 1000 Hz), but varies across frequency as a result of external canal acoustics. The voltage is progressively decreased in 6-dB decrements.

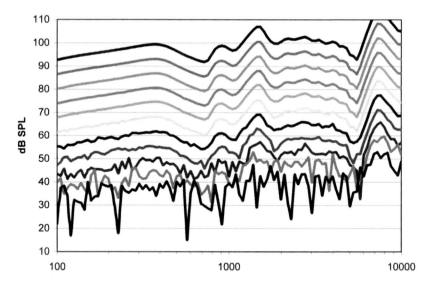

Fig. 8. Sound present levels corresponding to sensor voltage levels in Figure 7.

Discussion

This series of experiments attempts to quantify the nominal sensitivity, frequency response, and minimum sound pressure level over which a piezoelectric sensor positioned against the malleus head can function usefully. A sensor used in this manner is essentially emulating the function of a microphone, however, the dynamics of a microphone diaphragm are totally different from the ossicular chain, and hence a direct comparison of sensitivity and roll-off is not valid.

A piezoelectric sensor, such as the one used in this study, has three advantages. Firstly, as the sensor is placed at the medial end of the external auditory canal, it benefits from the frequency dependent amplification of the external canal. This peaks at 3 kHz with a gain of 22 dB and assists in localizing the direction of a sound[8]. Secondly, a piezoelectric sensor has an extremely low current draw. This is of the order of 5 microAmps, including the impedance matching amplifier. Such low current draw would significantly prolong battery life in a totally implantable hearing device or cochlear implant. Thirdly, scanning laser Doppler vibrometry studies have shown motion of the tympanic membrane to break into a complex series of modes above 2 kHz. The dense adherence of the tympanic membrane to the malleus handle acts as a signal averager[9,10]. This concept, outlined by Khanna and Decraemer[9], results in the malleus averaging the complex displacement modes for transmission along the ossicular chain. A sensor positioned on the malleus head can benefit from this anatomical signal averaging process.

Figure 5 shows sensor output at 100 dB SPL. Nominal sensitivity is 382 mV/ Pa at 1000 Hz. This is a nominal sensitivity figure. As malleus displacement varies across frequency, so does the sensitivity of such a measurement system. This sensitivity is 50 dB greater than the 1.1 mV/Pa at 1000 Hz reported by Gyo et al.[2]. Several reasons account for this difference. Firstly, the sensors in this study have incorporated an impedance matching amplifier within the bimorph. This serves to electrically match the high impedance sensor with a low impedance sound processor input. In addition, it provides 20 dB of gain. The remaining 30 dB can be accounted for by the following factors:

1. *Ceramic element.* The ceramic material used in this study was PZT5A. Displacement sensitivity measured in the temporal bone is 4×10^6 Vm^{-1} compared with 8×10^5 Vm^{-1} used by Gyo et al. This would account for a further 14 dB.

2. *Bimorph length.* Sensors used in this study had a cantilever length of 8.5 mm compared with 7 mm (3 dB).

3. Use of fresh temporal bones compared with the preserved bones used in the earlier study.

4. Optimization of the sensor on the malleus head.

The greater voltage achieved in this study is of considerable consequence. The noise floor of the measurement system used in this study is 100 µV. Calculations of noise originating from the sensor suggest that the sensor noise is around 20 µV. This is 85 dB below 382 mV, suggesting that the sensor has a very wide dynamic range, as will be seen later in the discussion.

Figure 4 demonstrates stapes roll-off in the intact chain to be 36 dB per decade. Other investigators have also confirmed similar roll-off rates[6,11]. Ideally, this roll-off must be matched by any system directly driving the ossicular chain. The sensor in this study was demonstrated to roll-off at 37 dB per decade out to 3 kHz, and accelerate beyond 3 kHz. This matches stapes roll-off very well in the speech frequencies. Additionally, optimizing the mechanical impedance of the sensor relative to the chain is likely to result in a closer match to the normal stapes roll-off at high frequencies.

For a sensor to faithfully reproduce sound detected at the ossicular chain, it needs to follow the precise motion of the chain. Figure 6 shows the sensor to follow the motion of the chain well out to 4 kHz. A slight loss of tracking occurs at 1200 Hz, due to the resonance of the middle ear and the bimorph. The sensors used in this study were not optimized for resonant characteristics, nor were they impedance-matched to the mechanical impedance of the ossicular chain. Such modifications are likely to improve ossicular tracking and high frequency sensor response. In the tested implementation, useful signal is generated at a range well beyond the speech frequencies. Some of the tracking loss above 4 kHz could be artifactual. In this study, adequate reflection necessary for use of the LDV was obtained by using adhesive reflective paper. Adherence of this material to moist biological tissues is poor and it is possible that reflector motion does not truly represent motion of the ossicular chain and hence introduces phase related errors. These would be more evident at high frequencies.

Loss of ossicular tracking may also be an issue with inequality of air pressure across the tympanic membrane. Static motions of the tympanic membrane associated with failure to open the eustachian tube may affect the ability of the sensor to track the motion of the malleus. Ossicular tracking at high frequency and with middle ear pressure differentials could be improved by fixing the sensor into the head of the malleus. This is the subject of a further paper currently under preparation.

For such a sensor to function well as an alternative to a microphone, it must function at sound pressure levels significantly below that of conversational speech (60 dB SPL). Figures 6 and 7 show the sensor voltage and sound pressure level simultaneously measured at the tympanic membrane. By a process of curve matching, the minimum sensitivity of the sensor can be determined.

Figure 7 demonstrates the sensor output to decrease linearly with decreasing sound pressure level. From Figure 8 it is apparent that the noise floor of the ER7c probe microphone is being approached around 40 dB SPL. The corresponding sensor voltage at this level is still robust in the speech frequencies, indicating good sensor function at this level. Due to a limitation in the source of the signal analyzer used in this study, the minimum driving voltage to the ER2 was 1 mVrms. Again, this does not appear to be limiting the sensor. Calculated minimum sensitivity appears to be limited by resistor thermal noise in the impedance matching amplifier. This occurs at a level of 26 dB SPL. Although the minimum sensitivity does not confirm sensor function at this level, the robust sensor signal at 40 dB suggests that there is reserve in the sensor and that the minimum sensitivity of 26 dB SPL is possible. In a separate series of experiments, the upper limit of sensor function before clipping of the imped-ance matching amplifier occurred was 106 dB SPL[12]. Hence, the dynamic range of the sensor is 80 dB.

Conclusions

This series of experiments examines the use of a piezoelectric bimorph posi-tioned against the malleus head as an alternative to a microphone. Nominal sensitivity is 382 mV/Pa at 1000 Hz. The sensor bandwidth extends from 100 Hz out to 7 kHz, with accurate tracking of ossicular motion to 4 kHz. Minimum sensitivity is certainly better than 40 dB SPL and is probably around 26 dB SPL. The dynamic range is 80 dB. Modifications of the mechanical impedance and fixation of the sensor into the malleus head would likely improve on these performance statistics. The low current draw and relative simplicity of such a system make the concept of a piezoelectric sensor positioned against the malleus head a viable alternative to a conventional microphone in a totally implantable hearing device, or perhaps with even greater application in the totally implant-able cochlear implant.

Acknowledgments

The authors acknowledge St Croix Medical for providing funding for this study. They also wish to acknowledge Christine Gralapp for her assistance with the artwork.

References

1. Deddens AE, Wilson EP, Lesser TH, Fredrickson JM: Totally implantable hearing aids: the effects of skin thickness on microphone function. Am J Otolaryngol 11(1):1-4, 1990
2. Gyo K, Yanagihara N, Araki H: Sound pickup utilizing an implantable piezoelectric ce-ramic bimorph element: application to the cochlear implant. Am J Otol 5:273-276, 1984
3. Yanagihara N, Gyo K, Hinohira Y: Partially implantable hearing aid using piezoelectric ceramic ossicular vibrator. Otolaryngol Clin N Am 1:85-99, 1995
4. Suzuki JI, Kodera K, Nagai K et al: Partially implantable piezoelectric middle ear hearing device: long term results.. Otolaryngol Clin N Am 1:99-106, 1995
5. Gyo K: Update on the Ehime middle ear implant. Oral presentation at the Second Interna-tional Symposium on Middle Ear Mechanics in Research and Otosurgery. Harvard Medical School, Boston, MA, 1999
6. Kurokawa H, Goode RL: Sound pressure gain produced by the human middle ear. Otol HNS 113:349-355, 1995
7. Voss SE: Effect of tympanic membrane perforations on middle ear sound transmission: measurements, mechanisms and models. PhD Thesis Harvard University, 1998

8. Shaw EAG, Stinson MR: The human external and middle ear: models and concepts. In: Wright D (ed) Scott Brown's Otolaryngology, p 53. London: Butterworth Heineman 1987

9. Khanna SM, Decraemer WF: Vibration modes and the middle ear function. In: Hüttenbrink KB (ed) Middle Ear Mechanics in Research in Otosurgery. Proceedings of the International Workshop on Middle Ear Mechanics in Research and Otosurgery. Dresden University of Technology, Dresden, Germany, 1996

10. Ball GR, Huber A, Goode RL: Scanning laser Doppler vibrometry of the middle ear ossicles. ENT J 76(4):213-222, 1997

11. Goode RL, Ball GR, Nishihara S et al: Laser Doppler vibrometer (LDV): A new clinical tool for the otologist. Am J Otol 17:813-822, 1996

12. Grant IL, Kroll K: The piezoelectric ossicular sensor: a microphone alternative in a totally implantable hearing device. Am J Otol (in press)

MIDDLE EAR ELECTROMAGNETIC IMPLANTABLE HEARING DEVICE

Initial clinical results

J.V.D. Hough[1], R. Kent Dyer, Jr[1], Kenneth J. Dormer[1,2], Pamela Matthews[1], Rong Z. Gan[1,3] and Mark W. Wood[1]

[1]Hough Ear Institute, Oklahoma City; [2]University of Oklahoma Health Sciences Center, Oklahoma City; [3]University of Oklahoma, Norman, OK, USA

Abstract

This article describes the authors' recent experiences with electromagnetic middle ear hearing devices and introduces a new device, the SOUNDTEC™ Direct Drive Hearing System (DDHS). A description of the device, details of the surgical procedure and results of a five-subject Food and Drug Administration (FDA) feasibility study are included. The system is composed of two elements: an neodymium iron boron (NdFeBo) magnet implant encased in a titanium laser-welded cylinder, and an external portion composed of a behind the ear (BTE) sound processor/coil assembly. The implant is secured around the incudo-stapedial joint via a titanium wireform. Outcome measures six months postoperatively were compared to preoperative baseline data in four subjects. Significant improvements in high frequency functional gain (16 dB increase for high frequency warble tone average (HFWTA)), speech discrimination (18.5% increase), functional absence of acoustic feedback, reduced occlusive effect, as well as significant improvement in subjective measures of patient satisfaction, were noted with the SOUNDTEC DDHS when compared to results achieved with a well-fitted hearing aid.

Keywords: sensorineural hearing loss, electromagnetic implantable hearing device, neodymium iron boron

Introduction

There have been many dramatic advances in the area of microscopic ear surgery in recent decades, which have given relief to individuals with profound deafness as well as to those with conductive hearing loss. However, the largest group of individuals with hearing impairment, those with moderate to severe sensorineural hearing loss (SNHL), are often disappointed to find that amplifi-

Address for correspondence: R. Kent Dyer, Jr, MD, Hough Ear Institute, 3400 NW 56th Street, Oklahoma City, OK 73112-4466, USA

The Function and Mechanics of Normal, Diseased and Reconstructed Middle Ears, pp. 353–366
edited by J.J. Rosowski and S.N. Merchant
© 2000 Kugler Publications, The Hague, The Netherlands

cation with external hearing aids is the only treatment option available. Despite the many improvements in hearing aid technology, conventional hearing aids continue to have significant limitations, such as: discomfort, occlusive effects, cosmetic factors, limited functional gain, poor sound quality, difficulty hearing in noise, and presence of feedback. These limitations of conventional hearing aids have led to increasing interest in implantable hearing devices.

Historical background

The search for methods of transmitting amplified sound into the inner ear by direct vibration of an implant attached to the ossicular chain involves two basic technologies: electromagnetic and piezoelectric coupling. Wilska[1] first evaluated electromagnetic induction by placing a 10-mg iron prosthesis onto the tympanic membrane of a normal hearing individual. The electromagnetic field generated by a coil placed into the ear canal created a reciprocal vibration of the prosthesis and was perceived by the subject as a clear tone. In recent years, others[2-8] have placed magnets on the tympanic membrane, as well as on various locations within the middle ear and mastoid, in order to drive the ossicular chain directly via electromagnetic coupling.

The piezoelectric crystal was first investigated as a middle ear driver by Vernon *et al.*[9] Subsequently, Hough and Vernon (unpublished observations, 1980) investigated the use of piezoelectric crystals temporarily placed onto the ossicular chain of volunteers undergoing routine middle ear surgery. This coupling produced excellent amplification of sound, but challenges related to attachment of the crystal and maintaining electrical insulation prevented further development of this concept.

In the early 1980s, our team began investigating the use of rare earth permanent implantable magnets attached to the ossicular chain in various locations[10]. Three different implant configurations were developed: a donut-shaped magnet designed to fit around the incudo-stapedial joint; a design which was interposed between the malleus handle and promontory; and one between the stapedial head and the malleus. All neodymium iron boron magnets were electroplated with gold, and hermetically sealed with Parylene C (Union Carbide).

In 1988, the first long-term study in five volunteers with moderate SNHL was accomplished using an implant at the incudo-stapedial joint[11]. After initially noting good hearing results, oxidation of the magnetic material occurred secondary to moisture penetration. This caused loss of magnetic strength and necessitated explantation of all implants.

A samarium-cobalt rare earth (Sm-Co) magnet was chosen to replace neodymium iron boron for the second-generation implant. However, due to its lesser magnetic strength, the Sm-Co magnets were necessarily heavier (63 mg) than the previous design. Three of the original five patients were re-implanted with these Sm-Co magnets in 1990[12]. Initial aided hearing results in all three patients were encouraging. However, unaided residual hearing thresholds measured six months postoperatively were significantly poorer in the high frequencies compared to pre-implant thresholds. This threshold shift necessitated removal of the implants.

Progress in technology between 1990 and 1996 provided many key answers. In 1996, the problem of water penetration was solved by encasing the implant in a laser-welded titanium canister which could then be attached to the incudo-stapedial joint by titanium wireform. A more powerful NdFeBo magnet was chosen to reduce implant size and weight. Finally, the prosthesis itself was re-designed as a cylinder, which brought the magnet into co-axial alignment with the ear canal coil and closer to the undersurface of the tympanic membrane in order to provide better magnetic coupling.

This implant has been clinically tested, and a revised design using a stronger NdFeBo magnet is now being manufactured under the name SOUNDTEC™ Direct Drive Hearing System (DDHS). An initial feasibility study involving the first five patients was approved by the FDA in April 1998. Presently, a Phase II multi-center clinical study of 100 subjects involving five co-investigators at various locations in the USA is under way. The device has been placed in 15 subjects to date, four of whom have been wearing the implant over one year with excellent results.

Principle of the operation

The present SOUNDTEC DDHS operates on the basic principle that sound can be conveyed to the middle ear ossicles through non-acoustic transmission using electromagnetic-permanent magnet coupling. Acoustic signals are received by the microphone of the sound processor and transformed into electrical signals. These signals are then amplified, programmed, and sent to the coil in the ear canal. Interaction between the alternating electromagnetic field of the coil and the implant magnet results in attractive and repulsive forces, which drive the ossicles directly, producing amplified sound perception (Fig. 1).

Material and methods

Description of the device

The present SOUNDTEC DDHS consists of two components: the portion implanted inside the middle ear cavity, and an external device consisting of a behind the ear sound processor and an electromagnetic coil incorporated into a custom-deep ear canal mold.

Implant portion
Based on anatomical and mechanical principles, the optimal location for magnet attachment is the incudo-stapedial joint. This position on the ossicular chain was chosen for mechanical performance, implant safety, and stability. Vibra-

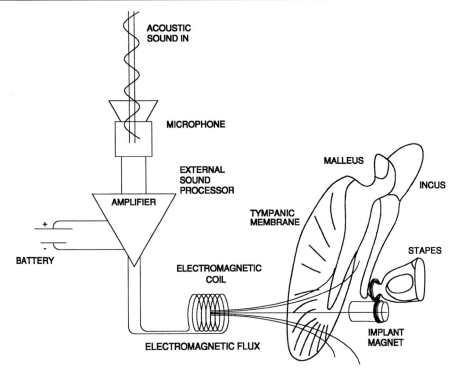

Fig. 1. Schematic of the SOUNDTEC DDHS principle of operation.

tory transmission into the inner ear is enhanced by co-axial alignment of the implant and coil. Since the strength of an electromagnetic field varies with the cube of the distance between coil and magnet, the distance between coil and magnet is designed to be minimal.

The NeFeBo magnet (magnetized along its long axis) is coated with Parylene C and hermetically sealed in a laser-welded titanium cylinder. A titanium alloy wireform attachment ring provides a method of securing the implant around the incudo-stapedial joint (Fig. 2). The wireform is provided in two anatomical orientations to accommodate either the right or left ear. The attachment ring is placed off center along the long axis of the cylinder to bring the implant close to the undersurface of the tympanic membrane and away from the promontory. The implant design used in the FDA feasibility study weighed 37.5 mg. The current NdFeBo implant design being utilized in phase II clinical trials is even smaller, weighing only 27 mg.

External portion
Presently, the external device includes an analogue BTE sound processor to allow easy accessibility for upgrading the amplifier electronics. In-the-ear and in-the-canal prototypes are being developed, and will soon be implemented. The electromagnetic coil is encased in a custom deep ear canal mold that brings the coil tip to within approximately 4 mm of the implant (Fig. 2).

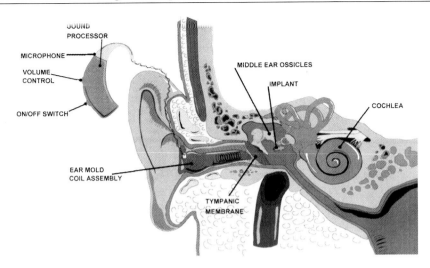

Fig. 2. Diagram of the SOUNDTEC DDHS sound processor, earmold/coil assembly and implant.

The present BTE sound processor of the SOUNDTEC DDHS consists of a microphone, a pre-amplifier, and a power amplifier. The processor employs a dual channel wide-dynamic-range input compression system. The class D power amplifier has an excellent (600-hour) battery life which equates to two to four weeks of full time use.

Description of the procedure

The surgical technique is a straightforward well-known transcanal approach, making it possible to perform surgery either in an outpatient surgery center or an office procedure room environment. Surgery is performed under local anesthesia utilizing standard transcanal stapedectomy techniques familiar to most otolaryngologists, and can be completed in less than 45 minutes.

A Rosen incision is made in the posterior canal wall and a standard stapedectomy tympanomeatal flap is elevated to expose the posterior one half of the tympanic cavity. Bone from the posterior-superior canal wall may need to be removed in order to adequately visualize the stapes superstructure. The incudostapedial joint capsule mucosa is delicately incised with an extremely fine sickle joint knife. The long process of the incus is then elevated just enough to allow insertion of the attachment ring into the joint space. This elevation of the incus is accomplished either by using a specially-designed suture sling technique or with a SOUNDTEC right angle hook. Insertion of the implant is accomplished either with a suction-operated SOUNDTEC insertion instrument (Fig. 3) or with an open-mouthed cylinder-holding forceps. Only specially-designed non-magnetic instruments and specula should be used during the implant insertion process to expedite implant positioning. Following insertion of the wireform

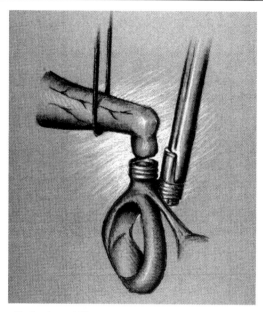

Fig. 3. The implant cylinder is stabilized by the SOUNDTEC insertion instrument while the wireform attachment ring is placed around the head of the stapes.

attachment ring, the lenticular process is allowed to reappose with the stapes capitulum through the ring. A fibrous union will form during the healing process to re-establish incudo-stapedial joint continuity.

Placement of the attachment ring is adjusted so that the magnet cylinder is axially aligned with the ear canal, and a Gelfoam™ 'cast' is placed into the middle ear to stabilize the implant at the conclusion of the procedure (Fig. 4). Special care is taken to ensure that the promontory, posterior canal wall, and undersurface of the tympanic membrane do not come into contact with the implant, since this increases the risk of synechia formation. If there is close apposition with adjacent middle ear structures, small discs of Gelfilm™ sheeting can be inserted. Finally, the tympanomeatal flap is returned to its original position at the conclusion of surgery.

Postoperative fitting

Following completion of surgery, an eight-week healing period is allowed prior to fitting of the external sound processor. After healing is completed, a specially-designed electromagnetic search coil is introduced into the ear canal at the time of processor fitting in order to locate the position of the implant beneath the tympanic membrane surface. During the mapping procedure, the subject is asked to indicate when the audible tone produced by the search coil is perceived to be loudest, while the search coil is moved to various locations near the tympanic membrane surface. The alignment between coil and implant

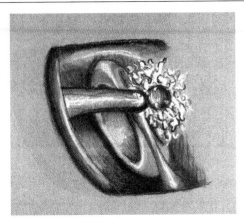

Fig. 4. The implant cylinder is axially aligned with the ear canal and supported by a temporary Gelfoam cast.

associated with greatest loudness perception represents the optimal coil position for that individual. This coil location and orientation will later be approximated when the custom-deep ear canal mold is fabricated by the audiologist.

Patient selection criteria

Inclusion criteria for implant candidacy are as follows:
1. Bilateral symmetrical SNHL
2. Mild-moderate to moderately severe SNHL (Fig. 5)
3. Bone thresholds within 10 dB of air threshold
4. High frequency pure tone average (PTA) of 1 K, 2 K, and 4 kHz between 35-70 dBHL
5. Patients with discrimination scores greater than 60% (NU-6)
6. Duration of hearing loss at least two years without fluctuation
7. At least six months of recent hearing-aid experience and use of well-fitted hearing aid (as defined by the study guidelines) in the ear to be implanted for at least three months
8. Age 21-80 years

Additional requirements include the following: *(1)* no history of chronic otitis externa/media or history suggestive of retrocochlear pathology; *(2)* subjects must have significant cognitive skills and motivation; *(3)* the ear canal size must be adequate to accept the deep earmold/coil assembly; *(4)* dissatisfied hearing-aid user.

Description of the study

The five subject FDA feasibility study investigational device exemption (IDE) was completed in April, 1998. Outcome measures obtained six months postop-

AIR CONDUCTION THRESHOLDS

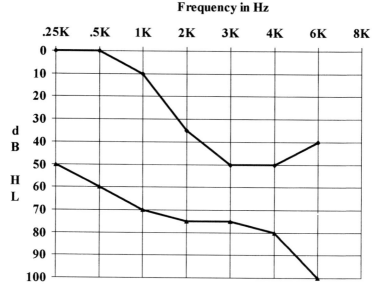

Fig. 5. Audiometric criteria of candidates for SOUNDTEC DDHS (pure-tone air conduction thresholds). Upper and lower air conduction threshold boundaries are included.

eratively were compared to the preoperative baseline data. The results of this study are the primary subject of this report. One of the five subjects was classified as an adverse event, and was not included in this analysis. The middle ear of this subject was explored and binding cicatricial adhesions released. This individual now reports good functional gain with the DDHS and is awaiting audiometric testing.

All subjects in this study had been 'well-fitted' with a conventional hearing aid that met the National Acoustic Laboratories' (NAL)-R criteria[13] for at least three months prior to implantation. Pass criteria of subject's hearing aid frequency response are ±5 dB for 500 through 2000 Hz and ±12 dB for 3000 and 4000 Hz for NAL-R target, using real ear measurements. The NAL-R criteria recommend a 30-50% improvement in aided thresholds over unaided soundfield measurements.

Results

Objective findings

Residual hearing
Figure 6 illustrates the effect of loading on residual hearing. An average of 12 dB residual hearing loss was noted following placement of a 37.5-mg im-

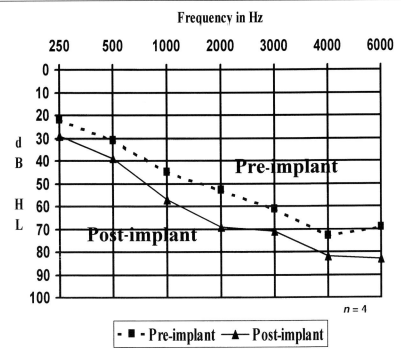

Fig. 6. Residual hearing loss associated with loading of the ossicular chain by a 37.5-mg implant. Preoperative and postoperative pure-tone air conduction thresholds are shown.

plant onto the ossicular chain. The hearing loss was slightly greater in the higher frequencies. Fortunately, due to the moderately severe hearing loss present prior to implantation, this loss was not perceived by the subjects as being remarkable. Furthermore, the excellent functional gain achieved overshadowed this threshold shift.

Functional gain
Functional gain for the hearing aid condition in this study was calculated by comparing the subjects' pre-implant unaided soundfield thresholds with the aided thresholds achieved using well-fitted hearing aids. Functional gain achieved for the SOUNDTEC DDHS condition was obtained by comparing the subjects' postoperative unaided thresholds to aided thresholds achieved with the DDHS.

Figure 7 illustrates average functional gain increase observed between 500 and 4000 Hz with SOUNDTEC compared to hearing aid. An average increased gain of 14.8 dB is noted with SOUNDTEC beyond the gain achieved with a well-fitted hearing aid over this frequency range. In general, the subjects preferred more mid and high frequency gain with SOUNDTEC than the amount prescribed by NAL-R.

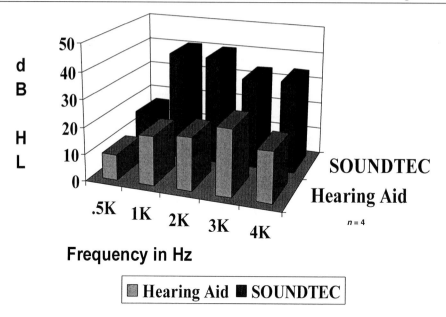

Fig. 7. Average functional gain with SOUNDTEC DDHS compared to well-fitted hearing aid. The soundfield thresholds were performed in 2-dB increments.

Soundfield threshold comparison
Aided soundfield thresholds with SOUNDTEC compared to aided soundfield thresholds achieved with the subjects' previously worn hearing aids are shown in Figure 8.

Increase in high frequency gain
An average increased functional gain of 16 dB across speech frequencies for high frequency warble tone average (2000, 4000, 6000 Hz) was observed compared with the subject's previous hearing aid performance.

Speech discrimination
Table 1 shows that speech discrimination scores using NU-6 average showed

Table 1. Speech discrimination scores with 63 dB presentation level in soundfield

Subject no.	NU-6 score (50) in quiet (soundfield)	
	Previous hearing aid (%)	*SOUNDTEC (%)*
1	80	92
2	64	92
3	50	86
4	88	86
Average scores	70.5	89

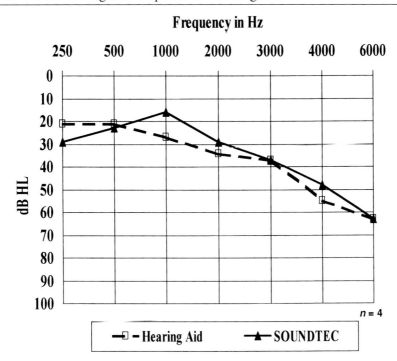

Fig. 8. Aided soundfield thresholds with SOUNDTEC compared to aided soundfield thresholds achieved with the subjects' previously-worn hearing aids.

an average increase of 18.5% with SOUNDTEC compared with the subjects' previously-worn hearing aids.

Subjective measures

Subjective measures of patient benefit and satisfaction were evaluated, including the abbreviated profile of hearing aid benefit (APHAB) and the Hough Ear Institute profile (HEIP) (Table 2). Compared with a well-fitted hearing aid, ease of communication increased 15.8 points, benefit in background noise increased by 19 points, and benefit in reverberant conditions improved by 15 points with the SOUNDTEC DDHS, as demonstrated with the APHAB. In general, a ten-point or greater improvement in APHAB score is considered to be significant. For the group as a whole, the HEIP self-assessment questionnaires showed a 19% increase in satisfaction and a 36% improvement in sound quality when compared to their previously-worn hearing aid. All patients noted reduction of occlusive effects and functional absence of feedback with the SOUNDTEC DDHS.

Perhaps the most compelling evidence of subjective satisfaction with the SOUNDTEC DDHS is that all four patients have worn their device successfully and comfortably for the past year, and all have spontaneously asked, "When can I have my other ear done?"

Table 2. Measures of benefit (APHAB) and satisfaction (HEIP) with SOUNDTEC DDHS versus hearing aid

Abbreviated Profile of Hearing Aid Benefit (APHAB)			Hough Ear Institute Profile (HEIP)		
Ease of communication	Benefit in reverberation	Benefit in background noise	Increase in satisfaction (%)	Presence of feedback	Quality of speech (%)
+15.4	+15	+19	+19	Functional absence of feedback	+36
(n=4)					

Discussion

Performance factors in implantable hearing devices

There are several critical questions that must be asked when evaluating the potential benefit of any implantable hearing device (IHD). First and foremost, does the IHD perform significantly better than the best hearing aid technology presently available? Secondly, does the hearing benefit outweigh the potential risks of the surgical procedure? Thirdly, in this era of cost containment and third party reimbursement challenges, does the hearing benefit to the patient outweigh the costs associated with the procedure? Finally, can the sound processor be upgraded in the future without further surgery?

Benefits of SOUNDTEC DDHS

Based on both objective and subjective measures of hearing enhancement, results of the feasibility study indicate that the SOUNDTEC DDHS is clearly superior to a well-fitted hearing aid among the subjects studied. Specific advantages include: better high fidelity hearing, a dramatic improvement in functional gain (16 dB for HFWTA), functional absence of acoustic feedback with the present BTE design, lack of an occlusive effect and greater comfort due to the presence of an open ear mold, as well as better overall speech discrimination (18.5%). Since this is an electromagnetic system, there is no need for a receiver, which is a primary source of sound distortion in conventional hearing aid circuits. Consequently, sound is perceived as being more natural and pleasing with the SOUNDTEC DDHS than is possible with conventional hearing aids. Since sound is transferred into the middle ear through electromagnetic induction, there is no need for implanted electronics or wire connections within the temporal bone. Lastly, the patient may wear a conventional hearing aid in the opposite ear, or a hearing aid may be used in the surgical ear, if necessary (for example, if a sound processor is damaged or being repaired).

Surgical advantages of SOUNDTEC DDHS

One of the advantages of the SOUNDTEC DDHS relates to its simplicity. The transcanal technique is a well-known surgical approach which is routinely utilized in otology and can be performed under local anesthesia as an outpatient procedure. The technique is not difficult for a trained otolaryngologist to perform and is a relatively quick procedure, requiring less than 45 minutes. The ossicular chain is not destroyed, making the procedure readily reversible if the implant should need to be removed. Recovery is rapid facilitating an early return to work. Since the sound processor is presently located externally, no surgery is required to repair or upgrade the electronics.

Risks of the procedure

The risks of surgery are the same as those to be expected in a routine tympanotomy for stapedectomy, but without opening the oval window. Since the labyrinth is not entered, the chance of total hearing loss is extremely remote.

The laws of physics dictate that mass loading of the ossicular chain will inevitably occur when any middle ear prosthesis is placed upon it. Loading of the ossicular chain has been observed to shift the resonance frequency of the middle ear transformer downwards, thereby diminishing the capacity to provide high frequency gain. The degree of residual hearing loss seen will be directly related to the mass load applied to the system and to the location of placement in the middle ear[14]. The goal is to minimize the loading effect, while simultaneously maximizing functional gain in order to overshadow the hearing loss that occurs with mass loading. In the feasibility study, our subjects experienced an average of 12 dB residual hearing loss, primarily due to loading effects.

In order to reduce the amount of loading, we have changed the size and weight of the implant and are now using an implant that is 30% lighter (22.7 mg) and one-third shorter. This new implant design is now being used in the ongoing Phase II clinical trials. Preliminary results show an approximately 50% reduction in the residual hearing loss with the upgraded implant compared with the feasibility study results (unpublished observations, 1999). With this improvement, we expect an even greater functional gain and subjective improvement.

Conclusions

Recent technological advances in the area of biomedical engineering have made possible the development of several implantable hearing devices, which promise to bring greatly-improved hearing to individuals suffering from sensorineural hearing loss. The SOUNDTEC DDHS offers many significant advantages to those individuals with mild to moderately severe SNHL who are dissatisfied with conventional hearing aids, as demonstrated in this feasibility study. The significant improvements noted in functional gain, speech discrimination, the functional absence of acoustic feedback, as well as subjective measures of satisfaction with the SOUNDTEC DDHS, make it an attractive alternative to conventional hearing aids in individuals with mild to moderately severe sensorineural hearing impairment.

Acknowledgments

The authors would like to thank Don Nakmali, BSEE, Gordon Richard, PE, Anita Montgomery, and Karen Koehn, for their substantial support and professional contribution.

References

1. Wilska A: Eine Methode zur Bestimmung der Horschwellenamplituden des Trummelfells bei verschiedenen Frequenzen. Skand Arch Physiol 72:161-165, 1935
2. Hough J, Vernon J, Johnson B, Dormer K, Himelick T: Experiences with implantable hearing devices and a presentation of a new device. Ann Otol Rhinol Laryngol 97:60-65, 1986
3. Fredrickson JM, Tomlinson D, Davis ER, Odkuist LM: Evaluation of an electromagnetic implantable hearing aid. Can J Otolaryngol 2:53-62, 1973
4. Rutschmann J: Magnetic audition-auditory stimulation by means of alternating magnetic fields acting on a permanent magnet fixed to the eardrum. IRE Trans Med Electron 6:22-23, 1959
5. Glorig A, Moushegian G, Bringewald R, Rupert AL, Gerken GM: Magnetically coupled stimulation of the ossicular chain: measures in kangaroo rat and man. J Acoust Soc Am 2:694-696, 1972
6. Goode R, Glattle T: Audition via electromagnetic induction. Arch Otoloaryngol 98:23-26, 1973
7. Maniglia A, Ko W, Rosenbaum M, Zhang RX, Dolgin SR, Montague FW: Electromagnetic implantable middle ear hearing device of the ossicular-stimulating type: principles, designs, and experiments. Ann Otol Rhin Laryngol 136:3-16, 1988
8. Kartush JM, Tos M: Electromagnetic ossicular augmentation device. Otol Clin N Am 28:155-172, 1995
9. Vernon J, Brummetr R, Denniston R, Doyle P: Evaluation of an implantable type hearing aid by means of cochlear potentials. Volta Rev 1:20-29, 1972
10. Dormer K, Phillips M: Auditory prosthesis: implantable and vibrotactile devices. IEEE Eng Med Biol Magazine June:36-41, 1987
11. Hough J, Dormer K, Meikle M, Baker S, Himelick T: Middle ear implantable hearing device: ongoing animal and human evaluation. Ann Otol Rhinol Laryngol 97:650-658, 1988
12. Baker S, Wood M, Hough J: The implantable hearing device for sensorineural hearing impairment. Otol Clin N Am 28:147-153, 1995
13. Byrne D, Dillon H: The National Acoustic Laboratories' (NAL) new procedure for selecting the gain and frequency response of a hearing aid. Ear Hear 7:257-265, 1986
14. Goode R, Nishihara S: Experimental study of the acoustic properties of incus replacement prostheses in a human temporal bone model. Am J Otol 15:485-494, 1994

CLINICAL MEASUREMENTS OF TYMPANIC MEMBRANE VELOCITY USING LASER DOPPLER VIBROMETRY

Preliminary results, methodological issues and potential applications

Saumil N. Merchant[1,2,3], Kenneth R. Whittemore[1,2], Becky Poon[3], C.-Y. Lee[1,2] and John J. Rosowski[1,2,3]

[1]Department of Otology and Laryngology, Harvard Medical School, Boston; [2]Department of Otolaryngology and Eaton-Peabody Laboratory, Massachusetts Eye & Ear Infirmary, Boston; [3]Speech and Hearing Sciences Program, Harvard – MIT Division of Health Sciences & Technology, MIT, Cambridge, MA, USA

Abstract

Traditional methods of investigating the mechanics of middle ear function in patients with conductive hearing loss and middle ear disease include audiometry and tympanometry. These methods cannot reliably differentiate among ossicular pathologies, especially when the tympanic membrane is intact or when there has been previous middle ear surgery. Laser Doppler vibrometry has been proposed as a method to improve the diagnosis of middle ear lesions. Recently-introduced laser Doppler vibrometry devices with improved demodulators make it possible to measure tympanic membrane velocity in a non-invasive manner in the span of a few minutes. In this paper, the authors present their preliminary measurements of tympanic membrane velocity using laser vibrometry and discuss the potential applications and some methodological issues related to clinical laser vibrometry measurements.

Keywords: middle ear, conductive hearing loss

Introduction

The assessment of middle ear function in a clinical setting usually involves otoscopy, audiometry, and tympanometry. While these techniques are useful, they cannot reliably differentiate among ossicular pathologies, especially when

Address for correspondence: Saumil N. Merchant, MD, Department of Otolaryngology, Massachusetts Eye & Ear Infirmary, 243 Charles Street, Boston, MA 02114, USA. email: snm@epl.meei.harvard.edu

The Function and Mechanics of Normal, Diseased and Reconstructed Middle Ears, pp. 367–381
edited by J.J. Rosowski and S.N. Merchant
© 2000 Kugler Publications, The Hague, The Netherlands

the tympanic membrane (TM) is intact, or when there has been previous middle ear surgery. Recently, laser Doppler vibrometry (LDV) has been demonstrated to be a sensitive measure of middle ear function[1-3], with finer spatial resolution than audiometry and tympanometry. While the latter traditional measures are sensitive to the function of the entire TM and middle ear, LDV employs a 100-μm diameter laser spot that can be focused at various locations on the TM and malleus, thus allowing measurement of the velocity of that location on the TM or malleus. Furthermore, unlike tympanometry, laser vibrometry is relatively unaffected by the ear canal. We believe that LDV measurements, together with audiometric data, may be useful in the more precise diagnosis of conductive hearing loss and determination of some of the structural bases for failed tympanoplasties. In this paper, we will present preliminary measurements that we have made in normal ears, and use those data to discuss the promise and some potential pitfalls of clinical LDV measurements.

Methods

Subjects

Our study population consisted of 22 normal ears from 17 subjects, with ages ranging from 22 to 50 years; eight of the subjects were female. The ears were otoscopically normal with no history of chronic ear disease, with audiometric thresholds no greater than 20 dB HL at all frequencies, and no discernible air-bone gap.

Equipment

Each subject lay on his or her back on an examination table, without any constraints, with the ear to be examined turned up. A speculum coupled to a closed sound-delivery system was inserted into the subject's ear canal (Fig. 1). The sound level produced in the ear canal at maximum signal input was near 1 pascal peak (91 dB SPL) over the 300-4000 Hz range, with lower output outside that band. The system had a glass back that allowed us to focus the beam of the LDV through the speculum onto the TM. Because no reflective beads were used, the measurements were restricted to the area of the triangular 'light reflex', a naturally reflective region near the umbo of the malleus in the center of the tympanic membrane (Fig. 2). The laser spot was focused on locations with reasonable reflectivity that were as close as possible to the umbo, generally within 1 mm.

Sound stimulus and measured velocity

The stimulus delivered by the ER3-A earphone was a combination of nine simultaneous tones, ranging from 300 Hz to 6 kHz. The overall sound level

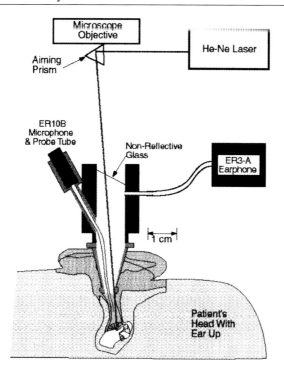

Fig. 1. The laser Doppler vibrometry measurement system (Polytec HLV 1000). A glass-backed speculum with an integrated Etymotic ER3A earphone and ER10B microphone with probe tube is placed in the ear canal with the probe-tube tip within 4-8 mm of the tympanic membrane. The laser, attached to the arm of the operating microscope, sent a beam to a joystick-controlled aiming prism that was mounted under the microscope's objective. The laser and the microscope were confocal. The examiner aimed the beam at a spot of high reflectivity near the umbo.

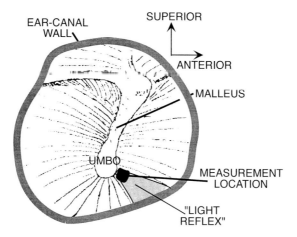

Fig. 2. Schematic of the portion of the TM visible through the LDV speculum. The anterior-inferior quadrant is hidden by the ear canal wall. The area of the light reflex is in light gray, while the measurement location is marked in dark gray.

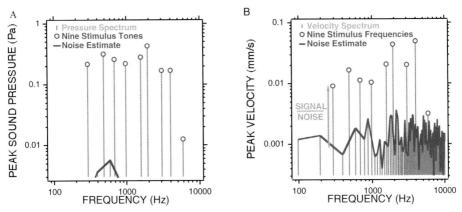

Fig. 3. A. Spectra of the sound stimulus. *B.* A velocity response from a human tympanic membrane. The spectral lines at stimulus frequencies are marked by circles. The thick dark line connects the lines at non-stimulus frequencies and is an estimate of the noise in the spectra.

varied between 70 and 90 dB SPL. The duration of the stimulus was three to five seconds. Figure 3 gives an example of the spectrum of the sound stimulus (left) and the spectrum of the measured velocities (right). The gray spectral lines at the stimulus frequencies (whose peaks are marked with open circles) show the sound pressure and velocity signal at each stimulus frequency. The transfer functions included in the results are ratios of the measured velocity and sound pressure at each stimulus frequency.

The spectral lines at non-stimulus frequencies (joined by the thick dark line) are estimates of the noise in the stimulus and response. The noise in the laser signal depends on the level of the reflected light and on the stability of the patient, microscope, and laser. Poor reflectivity or small motions of the subject or laser produce bursts of noise out of the demodulator that result in an increase in the wideband noise spectrum. The simultaneous determination of the signal and noise around each frequency allowed us to quantify the signal-to-noise ratio of the velocity measurements. The gray line with double arrows in Figure 3B defines a signal-to-noise ratio of a factor of ten (20 dB). In general, all the data we accepted as reliable met a 20-dB signal-to-noise criterion. In Figure 3B, all the stimulus frequency results meet this criterion except for the 6000 Hz data point which is within a factor of two of the noise floor.

Results

Measurement of the velocity/sound pressure transfer function

The velocity per sound pressure transfer function results from 22 individual ears are illustrated in Figure 4. The magnitude of the transfer function describes the growth of velocity with sound pressure, while the angle describes the relative phases of the velocity and pressure. In general, the transfer function magnitude was lowest at 300 Hz and increased with frequency until near 800 Hz, where there was a peak or inflection in the magnitude. At frequencies below 800 Hz, the angle of the transfer function suggested that velocity led pressure by between 0.20 and 0 periods. This behavior is consistent with a stiffness-controlled system.

Between 800 and 3000 Hz, the magnitude was roughly constant and the angle decreased toward about –0.25 periods. At higher frequencies, the magnitude tended to increase, while the angle continued to become more negative. The range of the transfer function magnitude at any one frequency was about an order of magnitude (20 dB), while the standard deviation was a factor of two (6 dB).

A comparison of the mean and standard error in our population and the median of Goode et al.'s[2] measurements in 64 normal ears is made in Figure 5. At frequencies of 4000 Hz and below, the magnitude of the mean velocity measured in our ears was nearly identical to that measured in the other study. The significant difference at 6000 Hz may be due to differences in methods that will be discussed later.

Linearity

The effect of stimulus level on TM velocity measurements needs investigation because the duration of the stimuli (three to five seconds) is long enough, and

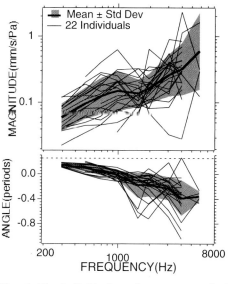

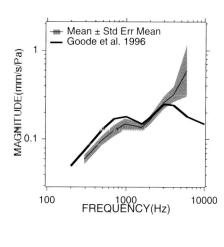

Fig. 4. The individuals and mean ± standard deviation of the magnitude and angle of the velocity transfer function from the light reflex near the umbo in 22 normal ears.

Fig. 5. A comparison of our preliminary mean ± the standard error of the mean from 22 normal ears with the published mean of Goode et al.[2].

the stimulus level (70-90 dB SPL) high enough to evoke the acoustic reflex in some subjects. Measurements made at several stimulus levels in subjects (*e.g.*, Fig. 6) demonstrated that the measured transfer function was essentially independent of stimulus level, even when the stimulus level was above the audiometrically determined reflex threshold (80 dB in the subject in Fig. 6). The observed linearity indicates that the acoustic reflex did not affect our measured responses, a result that may be specific for the stimulus levels and durations we used, and may not be generalizable to other stimulus paradigms.

Repeatability

The repeatability of any clinical measurements is an important concern. We estimated the minute-to-minute repeatability in individual subjects (Fig. 7A) by making measurements before and after removing and repositioning the speculum, sound source and laser. The factor of 1.5 or less variations observed in these measurements may be due to a small change in the measurement location, or a change in the angle between the laser beam and the TM.

Long-term repeatability was determined by measurements in individual subjects made over weeks (Fig. 7B). These measurements varied by a factor of

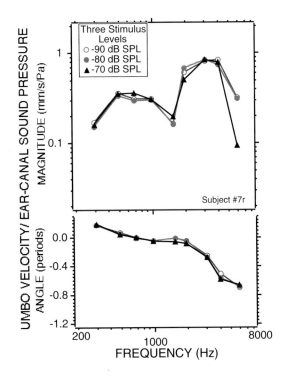

Fig. 6. Measurements of the tympanic-membrane velocity/sound pressure transfer function in one ear at three different stimulus levels (70, 80 and 90 dB SPL). The similarity of the magnitude and the phase response at the three levels is indicative of a 'level-independent' linear response.

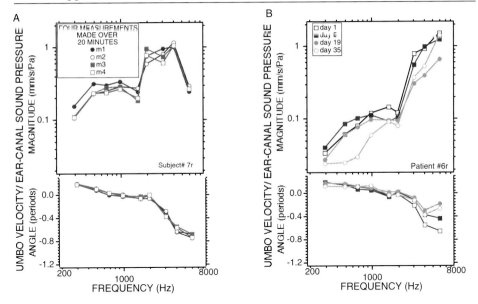

Fig. 7. A. Four transfer function measurements made over a 20-minute period in a single subject. The speculum was removed from the ear canal between these measurements. *B.* Four transfer function measurements made over a period of 34 days in a single subject.

three to four. We suspect that some of these changes resulted from *a.* variations in the measurement location related to larger variations in the relative position of the head and laser, and *b.* changes in the condition of the middle ear that result from alterations in middle ear static pressure.

The latter mechanism was investigated in another ear (Fig. 8) by asking the subject to manipulate his middle ear pressure by swallowing and Valsalva maneuvers. The middle ear pressure was monitored by tympanometry (226 Hz). A middle ear pressure of +8 cm H_2O (+80 daPa) reduced the low-frequency velocity response by 30% (about 3 dB). The effect of middle ear static pressures on the velocity at higher frequencies was less consistent.

A preliminary result from an abnormal ear

Figure 9 compares TM velocity measured from the light reflex near the umbo in a patient's ear with the mean and standard deviation of our normal population. The patient had a 20-dB air-bone gap, an intact and normal-appearing TM, and normal tympanograms at 226 Hz. The patient's TM near the umbo was observed to move with velocities that were as much as an order of magnitude (20 dB) larger than our mean velocity magnitude, especially at low frequencies. This increased velocity is significantly larger than our normal mean. The phase of the measured velocity in the patient was similar to that of the mean, except that it reached a value of 0 at a lower frequency than normal. This decreased zero-crossing frequency and the peaked low-frequency magnitude

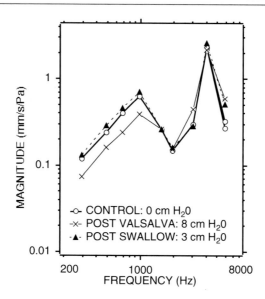

Fig. 8. Three measurements of the velocity/sound pressure transfer function in a single subject, made before and after changes in middle ear static pressure. The first measurement (control) was made after the subject swallowed and had a middle ear pressure of 0 cm H_2O. The second measurement (Xs) was made after a Valsalva manoeuver generated a 8-cm H_2O positive pressure in the middle ear. The third measurement (triangles) was made after swallowing returned the pressure to near-static conditions.

are consistent with a lower middle ear resonance. At subsequent exploratory middle ear surgery, this patient was found to have an erosion of the long process of the incus, with only a fibrous band of tissue connecting the incus and stapes head. The observed pathology is consistent with the hyper-mobile TM velocity of Figure 9, and illustrates the potential diagnostic utility of laser vibrometry.

Discussion

Laser Doppler vibrometry has been used for several years to measure motion of the TM and ossicles in animals and cadaveric human temporal bones (*e.g.*, Buunen and Vlaming[4], Vlaming and Feenstra[5], Kurokawa and Goode[6]). Recently, LDV devices with improved demodulators have made it possible to measure TM and malleal velocity in live subjects, in whom it has been demonstrated to be a sensitive measure of middle ear function with finer spatial resolution than clinical tympanometry and other acoustic-admittance based tests[1-3,7]. Laser vibrometry is based on a class II, FDA approved laser, with less than 1 mW of output power (class II lasers do not cause tissue or eye damage on brief exposure). Our own studies and those of others[1-3,7] indicate that accurate, safe and non-invasive measurements of TM and malleal motion can be

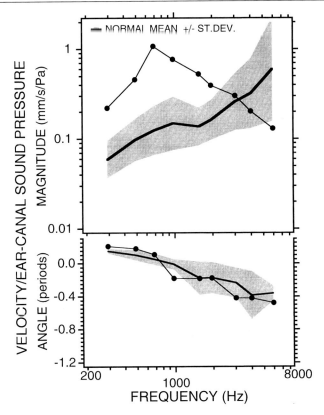

Fig. 9. A measurement of the velocity of the tympanic membrane near the umbo of a patient with a fibrous union of the incus and stapes (circles). The thicker line and shaded region is the mean ± standard deviation of our normal subjects. The patient had a 20-dB air-bone gap and normal tympanograms.

made in normal subjects with moderate sound stimulus levels. A set of measurements takes 15-20 minutes per ear. It is pertinent to consider several methodological issues and potential limitations, as well as potential applications of laser vibrometry. An understanding of these issues is necessary for the proper interpretation of measurements made using laser vibrometry.

Methodological issues and potential limitations of laser vibrometry

Signal-to-noise ratio
In general, we have used a 20-dB signal-to-noise criterion in order to determine what data we will accept as being reliable using laser vibrometry. The intensity of the sound stimulus can be adjusted by a manual attenuator on the Polytec HLV 1000 instrument, but cannot be made more than 90 dB SPL. Figure 10, which shows a typical frequency response of the earphone and sound coupler in our system, demonstrates that our stimulus signal has a range of 300 Hz to

6 kHz. The response drops off at low frequencies below 300 Hz as a result of acoustic leaks (it is difficult to obtain good seals in the ear canal, especially in ears with canal wall-down mastoid cavities that have enlarged ear canals). The response also drops off at high frequencies greater than 5-6 kHz because of low sound output from the earphone.

The noise in the laser signal depends on the amount of reflected light, and the stability of the patient, the microscope and the laser. Poor light reflectivity from the surface of the TM, or small motions of the laser or the subject, produce bursts of noise from the demodulator that result in an increase in the noise level in the measurements. In our experience, the light reflex (which is an area of the TM in the anterior-inferior quadrant that is generally perpendicular to the line of sight), is an area of good natural reflectivity. For other areas of the TM, and especially in post-surgical ears, we have found that it necessary to place reflectors in order to increase the level of reflected laser signal. Also, variations in anatomy, such as narrow or tortuous canals, exostoses of the canal and stenosis of the ear canal (*e.g.*, from chronic external otitis), can all impede access to the TM for laser measurements.

Level dependence of measurements: linearity
It is important to investigate the effects of stimulus level. This is necessary because normal subjects have intact acoustic reflexes, and the three to five seconds of stimulus duration is long enough, and the stimulus level (60-90 dB) is high enough, to evoke a reflex contraction in some subjects. In preliminary testing of 4 subjects, using stimulus levels from 70-90 dB SPL, we found that the TM velocity response from near the umbo was linear (Fig. 6). The observed linearity indicates that the acoustic reflex did not affect our measured responses, a result that may be specific for the stimulus levels and durations we used, and may not be generalizable to other stimulus paradigms. Additional measurements are necessary to investigate this issue.

Accuracy of sound pressure measurements in the ear canal at high frequencies
The transfer function of TM velocity per ear canal sound pressure depends on the location where the ear canal sound pressure is measured. Variations in sound pressure within the ear canal, as a function of distance, can become significant at frequencies greater than 2 kHz[3]. Hence, at these high frequencies, accurate measurement of ear canal sound pressure as close as possible to the TM becomes necessary. In our measurements, the tip of the probe tube measuring ear canal pressure was placed within 4-8 mm of the TM. We believe that our data are accurate up to 5-6 kHz.

Intra-subject variability
The repeatability of laser vibrometry measurements needs to be established. In our preliminary study, we found that, for a given subject, short-term (minute-to-minute) variability was a factor of 1.5 (~3 dB) and longer term (week-to-

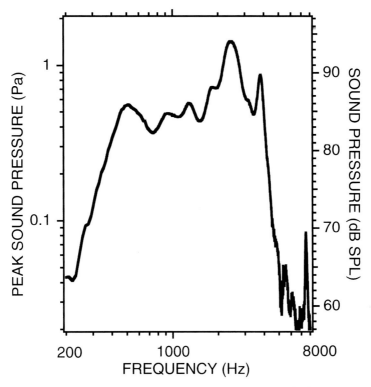

Fig. 10. Typical frequency response of the earphone and sound coupler in our system.

week variability) was a factor of three to four (~10-12 dB) (Figs. 7A and B). We suspect that there are several sources of the variability in the observed responses: as shown in Figure 8, our data suggest that changes in middle ear static pressure can affect the measured laser velocity of the TM at low frequencies. Some of this variability can be alleviated by requiring the subject or patient to equalize the middle ear pressure by swallowing several times before making measurements. While varied middle ear pressures can produce factors of two to three variations in the low frequency response, they cannot explain some of the variability observed in the high frequency response. The high frequency variability was less when we made repeated measurements in the same subject over a span of minutes versus a span of weeks (Fig. 7). We believe that removing the coupler and repositioning the laser can lead to fairly reproducible measurements, as long as the relative positions of the subject's head and the microscope do not change (as was the case in our minute-to-minute measurements). We hypothesize that larger differences in the relative position of the patient and the laser led to variations in the location of the light reflex, and therefore, variations in the measurement location in our longer term, week-to-week measurements. Our hypothesis is also supported by the high degree of repeatability in studies where reflectors were placed on the umbo[2]. The Goode et al.[2] measurements made with a reflector placed on the umbo were always from the same location and would not be affected by variations in the TM's reflectivity.

The difference between measurements from a reflector on the umbo and measuring from the light reflex area *near* the umbo might also explain the high-frequency differences between our and the Goode *et al.*[2] mean seen in Figure 5. Khanna and Tonndorf[8] demonstrated spatial variations in the motion of the TM that were most variable at high frequencies, and they also noted that the umbo moved less than some other areas on the TM. Decraemer *et al.*[9] also noted large variations in the velocity and phase response of different TM locations to high-frequency sound. We hypothesize that the areas of the TM within the light reflex and just anterior to the umbo move more at high frequencies than the umbo itself does. Since our data and those of Goode *et al.*[2] were both made by measuring ear canal sound pressure at about the same distance from the TM, we do not believe that variations in ear-canal sound pressure can explain the differences between the two data sets at high frequencies.

Inter-subject variability
As shown in Figures 4 and 5, our measurements in 22 normal ears, as well as those of Goode *et al.*[2], show a 20-dB range of umbo velocity magnitudes with a standard deviation of ±6 dB. The standard deviation in angle is ±0.15 periods at 1000 Hz and lower frequencies, and increases to 0.4 periods at 6 kHz. This moderately large variability will complicate efforts to use laser vibrometry as an *independent* objective measure of hearing loss. Indeed, as is the case in Figure 9, some conductive impairments can actually increase the velocity of TM motion. Attempts to use LDV as a clinical tool will need to bear this variability in mind, and will require determinations of both the sensitivity and selectivity of LDV in specific diagnostic decisions.

Potential applications of laser vibrometry

There are several potential applications of clinical LDV measurements in normal subjects and in patients with diseased ears.

Normal ears: to understand normal motion of the TM and malleus
To date, site-specific measurements of TM and malleal motion could only be made in cadaveric ears using laser Doppler vibrometry or other more complicated methods, such as time-averaged holography (*e.g.*, Tonndorf and Khanna[10]). Laser vibrometry now offers a non-invasive clinical tool for measuring site-specific TM and malleal motion in live subjects relatively quickly. Malleal velocity is a direct determination of the input to the ossicular chain. Measurements made in normal ears will be useful in refining human models of TM and malleal function. For example, such data can be used to investigate the axis of rotation of the malleus, the relative velocity of different quadrants of the TM, and correlations between measurements of velocity and measurements of acoustic impedance and reflectance at the level of the TM.

Diseased middle ears: differential diagnosis of ossicular lesions
The current battery of tests using audiometry and tympanometry cannot reliably differentiate ossicular pathology in patients who have conductive hearing losses and intact TMs[11,12]. For example, fixation of the malleus can be particularly difficult to diagnose both pre- and intra-operatively. We believe that a combination of laser vibrometry and audiometry offers the potential to improve our ability to diagnose specific ossicular causes of conductive hearing loss in patients with aerated middle ears and normal TMs. We hypothesize that: *(i) malleus fixation* will lead to a conductive loss and decrease in malleal velocity that are of similar magnitude; *(ii) stapes fixation* will result in a conductive loss that is much larger than the decrease in malleal velocity; and *(iii)* partial or complete *ossicular discontinuity* will result in a conductive loss with an increase in malleal velocity. The data from Figure 9 are consistent with the hypothesis put forward in *(iii)*.

Reconstructed middle ears
1. Tympanic membrane reconstruction: After repair and replacement of the TM for chronic otitis media, there can be a persistent conductive hearing loss, even when the ossicular chain is intact and mobile, and the middle ear is aerated. For example, Figure 11 shows postoperative air-bone gap data from 18 ears that had total drum replacement with temporalis fascia, as part of a type I tympanoplasty procedure. In all these patients, the middle ear became aerated after surgery and the ossicular chain was intact and mobile. The canal wall was kept intact in all these patients. There is a wide 0-35 dB range in the air-bone gap. We hypothesize that variations in the structural properties of the reconstructed TM are responsible for the 0-35 dB range of air-bone gaps. We predict that TM velocities similar to those in our normal subjects should be associated with near-perfect surgical results (air-bone gap <10 dB). As long as the middle ear is aerated at normal static pressure and there is no ossicular fixation, air-bone gaps of 10-35 dB should result from too thick, too stiff or too loose a TM graft. Laser vibrometry offers the potential of being able to determine TM motion at specific locations on the reconstructed drum and, by correlating vibrometry results with structural features of the TM, it may be possible to better understand the anatomical basis for good and poor hearing results.

2. Ossicular reconstructions and other tympanoplasties: There is a wide 0-60 dB range of postoperative air-bone gaps after tympanoplasty procedures that require reconstruction of the ossicular chain[11]. There are three major structural parameters that determine postoperative air-bone gaps after such procedures: aeration of the middle ear, mobility of the ossicular prosthesis (or graft), and coupling between the TM and the ossicular prosthesis. Problems in any one of the parameters can lead to large 40-60 dB air-bone gaps. It is sometimes difficult to differentiate between the three parameters by otoscopy or tympanometry alone. The addition of laser vibrometry may provide clues to the differential

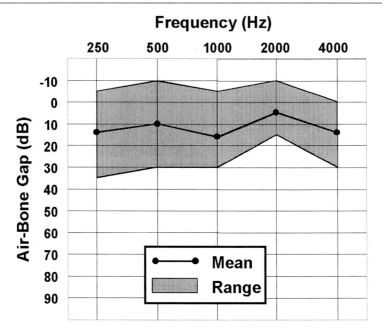

Fig. 11. Mean and range of postoperative air-bone gap data from 18 ears that had total drum replacement with temporalis fascia. The 18 ears were otherwise similar in that the canal wall was kept intact, all three ossicles were present and mobile, and the middle ear became aerated after surgery.

diagnosis of cases with large, 40-60 dB conductive losses after ossicular (or combined ossicular and TM) reconstructions. For example, non-aeration of the middle ear due to fibrosis or fluid would result in poor velocities at multiple locations on the reconstructed TM; fixation of an ossicular prosthesis in an aerated ear would result in poor velocities of the TM over the prosthesis, with larger velocities at other locations; and poor coupling between the TM and prosthesis in an aerated ear would result in large velocities in all areas of the TM, including over the prosthesis.

Acknowledgments

This work was supported by grants from the National Institutes of Health (NIH). We also acknowledge the generous financial gift of Monte and Anne Wallace, which helped finance the purchase of the laser Doppler vibrometer.

References

1. Stasche N, Foth HJ, Baler A, Huthoff C: Middle ear transmission disorder: Tympanic membrane vibration analysis by laser-Doppler vibrometry. Acta Otolaryngol (Stockh) 114:59-63, 1994
2. Goode RL, Ball G, Nishihara S, Nakamura K: Laser Doppler vibrometer (LDV) a new clinical tool for the otologist. Am J Otol 17:813-822, 1996
3. Rodriguez Jorge J, Zenner HP, Hemmert W, Burkhardt C, Gummer AW: Laservibrometrie: ein Mittelohr- und Kochelaanalysator zur nicht-invasiven Untersuchung von Mittel-und Innenohrfunktionsstörungen. HNO 45:997-1007, 1997
4. Buunen TJF, Vlaming MSMG: Laser-Doppler velocity meter applied to tympanic membrane vibrations in cat. J Acoust Soc Am 69:744-750, 1981
5. Vlaming MSMG, Feenstra L: Studies of the mechanics of the normal human middle ear. Clin Otolaryngol 11:353-363, 1986
6. Kurokawa H, Goode RL: Sound pressure gain produced by the human middle ear. Otolaryngol Head Neck Surg 113:349-355, 1995
7. Goode RL, Ball G, Nishihara S: Measurements of umbo motion in human subjects: methods and possible clinical applications. Am J Otol 14:247-251, 1993
8. Khanna SM, Tonndorf J: Tympanic membrane vibrations in cats studied by time-averaged holography. J Acoust Soc Am 51:1904-1920, 1972
9. Decraemer WF, Khanna SM, Funnel WRJ: Interferometric measurement of the amplitude and phase of tympanic membrane vibrations in cat. Hearing Res 38:1-18, 1989
10. Tonndorf J, Khanna SM: Tympanic-membrane vibrations in human cadaver ears studied by time-averaged holography. J Acoust Soc Am 52:1221-1233, 1972
11. Nadol JB, Schuknecht HF: Surgery of the Ear and Temporal Bone. New York, NY: Raven Press 1993
12. Hall JW, Chandler D: Tympanometry in clinical audiology. In: Katz J (ed) Handbook of Clinical Audiology, 4th edn, pp 283-299. Baltimore, MD: Williams & Wilkins 1994

THE HEARING LASER VIBROMETER
Initial clinical results

R. Kent Dyer, Jr[1], Kenneth J. Dormer[1,2], Mario Pineda[3], Kerri Conley[1], James Saunders[2] and Michael Dennis[2]

[1]Hough Ear Institute, Oklahoma City, OK; [2]University of Oklahoma Health Sciences Center, Oklahoma City, OK; [3]Polytec PI, Inc., Tustin, CA, USA

Abstract

A modified laser Doppler interferometer, the hearing laser vibrometer (HLV), was utilized to examine both normal and diseased ears in the clinic and in the operating room. HLV measurements were performed on 80 ears, including those with normal hearing (n=12), sensorineural hearing loss (SNHL, n=33), conductive loss (n=4), and mixed loss (n=31). HLV measurements obtained from the umbo included velocity and coherence. Data acquisitions required less than five minutes per ear. Normal ears showed a nearly flat transfer function with a coherence approximately equal to 1.0, between 500 and 5000 Hz. Individuals with conductive and mixed hearing losses and no history of surgery showed a significant correlation between normalized stapes velocity and degree of conductive hearing loss. Intraoperative HLV measurements quantitatively documented, for the first time, an improved ossicular mobility following corrective stapedectomy.

Keywords: middle ear mechanics, stapedectomy, air-bone gap, laser Doppler interferometry, umbo displacement, tympanic membrane vibration

Introduction

The utility of laser Doppler interferometry (LDI) as a tool for making accurate displacement and velocity measurements in temporal bone research is well recognized[1-4]. Currently, LDI is becoming an objective standard for measuring middle ear implantable hearing device performance in mechanical and temporal bone models[5]. The need for a more rapid and accurate method of measuring middle ear function in a clinical setting prompted the consideration of LDI as a tool for otological and audiological evaluations.

The purpose of this study was to determine if a laser Doppler interferometer

Address for correspondence: R. Kent Dyer, Jr, MD, Hough Ear Institute, 3400 NW 56th Street, Oklahoma City, OK 73112-4466, USA

The Function and Mechanics of Normal, Diseased and Reconstructed Middle Ears, pp. 383–397
edited by J.J. Rosowski and S.N. Merchant
© 2000 Kugler Publications, The Hague, The Netherlands

could be adapted to perform mechanical analyses of normal and hearing-impaired ears in the clinic and diseased ears in the operating room.

We had suggested to a commercial laser company (Polytec GmbH, Waldbronn, Germany) that a laser Doppler interferometer be coupled to an operating microscope with calibrated sound source and digitizing data acquisition system for *in vivo* middle ear mechanical analyses. A customized prototype interferometer, the hearing laser vibrometer (HLV-1000, Polytec PI, Tustin, CA), was developed and tested in this study to evaluate tympanic membrane vibration at the umbo on a series of normal hearing individuals, as well as on subjects with varying degrees of conductive and sensorineural hearing loss. The results of this beta testing study show that LDI (or vibrometry) is a potentially objective and efficient method for evaluating tympanic membrane vibration in a clinical setting. Also, for the first time, correlation has been shown between the audiometric air-bone gap and the umbo velocity transfer function. A potential application of hearing laser vibrometry in the surgical management of individuals with middle ear pathology has been recognized but additional studies are necessary for validation of the methodology and improvement of the hearing laser vibrometer (HLV).

Material and methods

Device description

It is well documented that heterodyne Doppler interferometry provides high-resolution velocity and displacement measures with a nanometer and sub-nanometer noise floor (in displacement) above 1 kHz[6,7]. A schematic of the HLV system (Fig. 1) depicts such an interferometer with a carrier frequency, modulated at 35 mHz, used as the system sensor. A helium-neon laser with an associated joy-stick-controlled aiming prism was coupled to an operating microscope (Zeiss, Model OPMI-1FC). The HLV provided velocity resolution of 0.1×10^{-6} m/sec at 1 $\sqrt{Hz}$ spectral bandwidth with a frequency range of 0.5 Hz to 50 kHz.

A hand-held speculum adapter (HLV-Z-010) contained an earphone and probe microphone (ER-2 and ER-7, Etymotic Research, Elk Grove IL) for delivery of a calibrated acoustic signal to the tympanic membrane, while maintaining nearly constant ear pressure levels at the tympanic membrane surface. The speculum adaptor, a closed chamber when inserted in the ear canal, contained a window for observation of the laser beam. The probe microphone, with a flat response between 250 Hz and 10 000 Hz, monitored the input sound pressure level (SPL) and provided this information to the computer controller. The distal end of the probe microphone tubing was positioned in the speculum adapter to within 4 mm of the tympanic membrane surface. A Bruening speculum was used to couple the adapter to the subject's ear and was positioned by the operator's hand during all measurements (Fig. 2).

Acoustic signals originated from a waveform generator (Model HP-33120A, Hewlett Packard, Palo Alto, CA) and were controlled by the HLV workstation and data acquisition system. Dynamic signal acquisition was accomplished by a digital signal processor which acquired two-channel time domain traces from velocity (HLV sensor) and sound pressure level (ER-7) measurements near the drum coupling region (DCR) described by Hudde and Engel[8]. A quiet, but not sound attenuated, procedure room or operating room was used for all measurements.

Signal analysis was performed using a two-channel fast Fourier transform (FFT) acquisition board (PCI-4451, National Instruments, Austin, TX). Two different software programs were used in this study for digital signal processing. An initial data set (117 ears) was acquired using HLV version 1.0 software, which presents a multi-tone random phase multi-frequency acoustic stimulation. A second data set (80 ears) was tested with the VibSoft version 1.1 software, which presents a log sweep 'chirp' excitation signal from 250 Hz to 10 kHz over a 160-msec duration. The VibSoft software utilizes velocity information to derive coherence, displacement, acceleration, phase relationships and H_1 transfer function derived as:

$$H_1 = FFT(velocity)/FFT^*(reference) \times FFT^2(reference)$$

This velocity transfer function (H_1) is a measure of umbo velocity as it relates to the input voltage of the earphone, an analog of sound pressure level expressed in Pascals. The H_1 is unique for each ear but allows for normalization

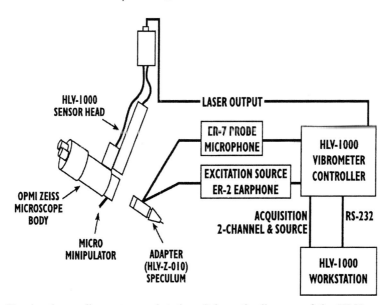

Fig. 1. Hearing laser vibrometer workstation. Schematic diagram of the HLV, a computer-controlled, automated data acquisition and sound delivery system integrated with a laser Doppler interferometer and operating microscope.

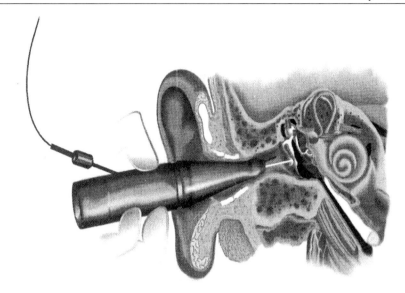

Fig. 2. Speculum adapter assembly. A Bruening pneumatic speculum and adapter assembly is shown being stabilized in the ear canal by the clinician during HLV data acquisition, requiring only about five seconds.

of the input signal, and is therefore an accurate measure of mechanical performance.

Subjects

The Hough Ear Institute, in collaboration with the University of Oklahoma, invited adult volunteers from their respective clinical otolaryngology practices to participate in this study. The subjects were divided into four study groups, based on audiometric evaluations. The first group (12 ears) was designated as normal controls. These subjects had normal hearing sensitivity between 250 and 8000 Hz with word recognition scores greater than 90% and no known history of ear pathology. All normal control subjects had normal otoacoustic emission testing, normal tympanograms and acoustic reflexes.

The second group (33 ears) included subjects with varying degrees of sensorineural hearing loss relative to speech reception threshold. The third group (four ears) consisted of patients with purely conductive hearing loss and normal cochlear function. The degree of conductive hearing loss was determined by averaging the conductive losses at 250, 500 and 1000 Hz. The fourth group (31 ears) included subjects with mixed hearing loss defined as a bone conduction speech reception threshold greater than 15 dB HL and conductive hearing loss average greater than 15 dB HL.

Institutional review board approval was granted at each participating institution, and informed consent was obtained from all volunteers at the outset of the study. Inclusion criteria were as follows: *(1)* age >18 years; *(2)* normal external ear canal anatomy; and *(3)* normal umbo landmarks. Individuals with abnormalities of the malleus handle or excessive motion-induced HLV artifact, as indicated by 'dropouts' in coherence and velocity data, were excluded from the study. Individuals who had previously undergone otological surgery were accepted if the other inclusion criteria were met.

Subject testing

All subjects underwent a standard audiological evaluation within 28 days of HLV data acquisition. Evaluation included pure-tone speech and imittance audiometry, and otoacoustic emissions. The appearance of the tympanic membrane, as well as any pertinent history of prior ear surgery or middle ear pathology, was also noted.

For HLV assessment, subjects were placed in a supine position on a standard examination table with their face directed away from the investigator.

Three separate measurements were performed on each subject. The reliability of velocity data being acquired was assessed in real time by observing the time domain signal on the computer screen and watching for HLV signal dropouts. A dropout is an instance of zero backscattered light to the HLV photodetectors and contains no Doppler shift (velocity) information. Time domain data blocks with dropouts were rejected. The total time required for making three independent HLV measurements was less than five minutes per subject.

The correlation between H_1 transfer function and audiometric air-bone gap was determined using the Pearson rank correlation one tailed test and a commercial statistics software package (Prism, GraphPad, Inc.). Significance was established at $p<0.05$.

Results

A composite graph depicting umbo displacement as a function of frequency in ears with normal hearing, sensorineural loss, and conductive/mixed hearing loss is shown in Figure 3. Umbo displacement, heretofore, has been a principle standard for evaluating middle ear mechanics. Although it is easily comprehended in terms of mechanical analyses, its fidelity as a measurement is critically dependent on replicable and controlled sound pressure level at the tympanic membrane for all frequencies measured. An 80 dB SPL was not always precisely deliverable at the tympanic membrane due to variability of probe tube position and ear canal volume between individuals. Thus, the value of the transfer function, which normalizes the input signal, was demonstrated.

Umbo Displacement and Hearing Levels

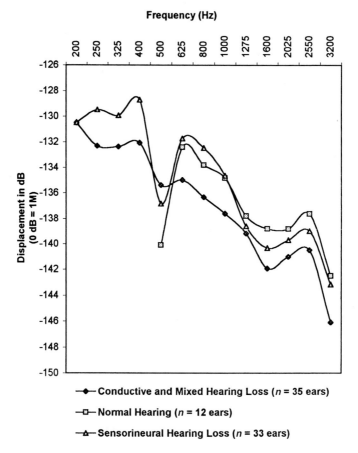

Fig. 3. Umbo displacement versus frequency. The averaged displacement data from the three groups of subjects is shown for the specific frequencies evaluated. Data below 500 Hz could not be obtained in normal ears below 500 Hz due to software limitations. The input chirp signal was presented at 80 dB SPL.

Normal ears

The H_1 transfer function in 12 normal ears is shown on an absolute scale on Figure 4. Based on the variance of the data, there was no remarkable difference in H_1 as frequency increased above 500 Hz. Coherence, defined as the ratio of transfer functions (H_2/H_1), was relatively flat for the control normal ears in the study (Fig. 5). The coherence value was close to 1.0, indicating that the HLV measurement system of these normal ears was functioning optimally.

The voltage from the probe microphone (input signal) and velocity of the umbo (output signal) for the frequencies studied are shown in Figure 6 for a normal hearing individual. A close correlation between input voltage and out-

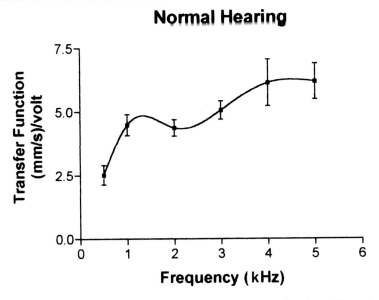

Fig. 4. Transfer function of normal ears. The averaged H$_1$ (±SEM) for the audiometric frequencies studied is shown for normal hearing ears (*n*=12). This represents a normalized response as the output (velocity) is adjusted for the input voltage (SPL).

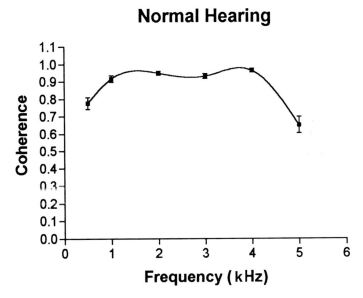

Fig. 5. Coherence of normal ears. The averaged coherence
and H$_1$ transfer function are shown for the spectrum of normal hearing ears (*n*=12). A value of
1.0 represents perfect coherence. Most ears approached perfect coherence except at the higher
frequencies.

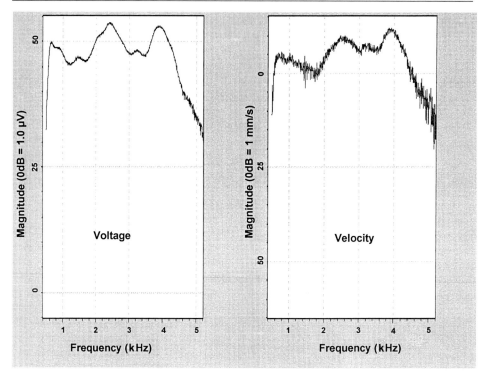

Fig. 6. HLV input-output relationship in normal hearing. A comparison of the input voltage (recorded by the probe microphone) and output velocity is shown for a normal hearing individual.

put velocity was seen. Figure 7 shows the H_1 and coherence functions from this same normal subject. Such data were observable at the time of acquisition (five seconds), as shown on these computer screen images. This allowed the clinician to discern the quality of his acquisition for immediate rejection or acceptance of the data.

Pure conductive hearing loss/mixed hearing loss

The four ears with an audiometrically-verified pure conductive hearing loss and normal underlying sensorineural function showed a statistically significant negative correlation between the umbo transfer function (H_1) and the degree of conductive hearing loss ($p=0.019*$, $r=-0.518$). There was a decline in umbo transfer function as the degree of conductive loss increased in these subjects (Fig. 8). A similar negative correlation was observed between transfer function and conductive hearing loss in individuals with mixed hearing impairment and no history of prior middle ear surgery ($p=0.0019**$, $r=-0.432$, $n=8$ ears; Fig. 9). Individuals with history of persistent conductive hearing loss following middle ear surgery ($n=21$ ears), on the other hand, did not show a significant correlation between transfer function and conductive hearing loss ($p=0.482$).

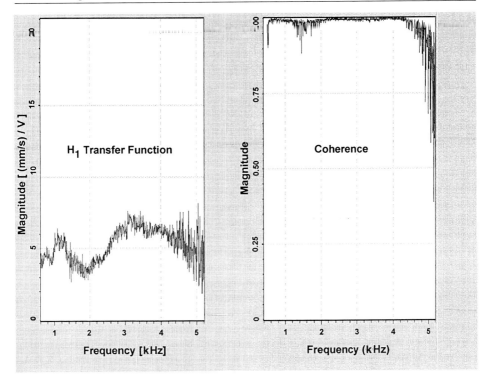

Fig. 7. HLV transfer function and coherence in normal hearing. The velocity transfer function, a normalized measure of middle ear mechanics, is shown with coherence in a normal hearing individual. These data and those in Figure 6 represent the HLV standard for normal hearing in the present study.

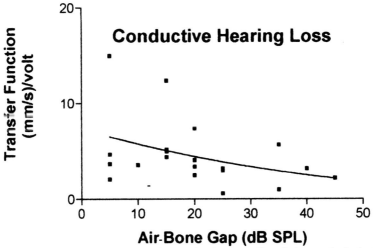

Fig. 8. HLV and audiometry: correlation for conductive loss. Correlation analysis depicting the declining transfer function with increasing audiometric air-bone gap. There was a significant inverse correlation between middle ear transfer function (H_1) measured by the HLV and air-bone gap measured audiometrically in four subjects with pure conductive hearing loss. Each point represents a pairing of an audiometrically-determined air-bone gap at either 250, 500, 1000, 2000 or 4000 Hz and the H_1 measured at the same frequency in that ear.

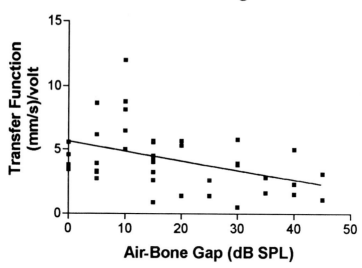

Fig. 9. HLV and audiometry: correlation for mixed loss. Correlation analysis depicting the declining transfer function with increasing audiometric air-bone gap. There was a significant inverse correlation between middle ear transfer function and air-bone gap in eight subjects with mixed hearing loss.

Intraoperative measurements

One individual (EW) with a history of otosclerosis, underwent HLV evaluation in the operating room during total stapedectomy, using the Hough posterior crus preservation technique. The speculum and laser/sound delivery adapter were gas sterilized prior to the intraoperative data acquisition. Three different measurements of the umbo were performed: an initial control measurement prior to lifting the tympanomeatal flap, a surgical control, after elevation (and replacement) of the tympanomeatal flap, and a postoperative measurement following stapedectomy. The postoperative measurements were made after removal of the footplate, interposition of the posterior crus into the oval window, and replacement of the tympanomeatal flap. Figures 10 and 11 show a notable improvement in umbo velocity following reconstruction of the ossicular chain, compared with the surgical control condition. A slight improvement in H_1 was noted in the lower frequencies, but this was difficult to appreciate due to the auto-scaling feature of the graph software package.

   In the operating room, the HLV workstation provided immediate outcome information and documented a 12-15 dB increase (three frequency average) in ossicular mobility in the lower frequency region, 5-25 msec into the chirp signal. This estimated improvement could be measured by observing the improved umbo velocity or displacement data. An 80 dB SPL input signal was utilized for control and post-surgical data acquisitions, although this SPL was not mea-

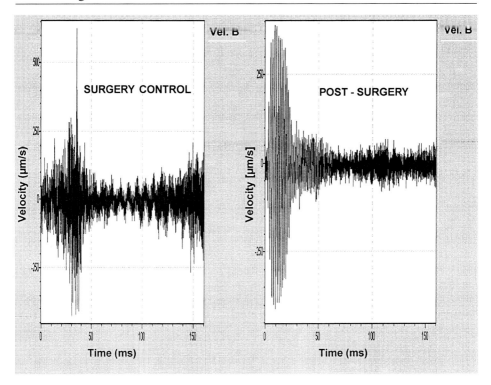

Fig. 10. Intraoperative velocity measures. A patient undergoing stapedectomy was evaluated intraoperatively using the HLV workstation. A comparison of umbo velocity was made after elevation of the tympanomeatal flap both before (surgery control) and following stapedectomy (post-surgery). Improvement in velocity was easily seen on the computer screen display, especially in the lower frequencies, by as much as 100 μm/sec.

sured at the tympanic membrane (TM) surface. This patient experienced complete closure of the air/bone gap days following surgery and her audiometric outcomes were consistent with the HLV data obtained in the operating room.

Discussion

Vlaming and Feenstra[9] first assessed the middle ear mechanics of temporal bone preparations using laser Doppler interferometry. They noted that displacement and velocity measurements were both reliable and accurate in a temporal bone model. Others, such as Gyo *et al.*[10] and Kurokawa and Goode[11] have further established the efficacy of interferometry in evaluating middle ear function in a temporal bone model. Tonndorf and Khanna[12] were the first to utilize laser interferometry for measuring small tympanic membrane vibrations *in vivo*.

The mechanical function of the middle ear transformer can be estimated by measuring the degree of conductive hearing loss present on routine audiometry. However, even ears with 'normal' middle ear function on routine audio-

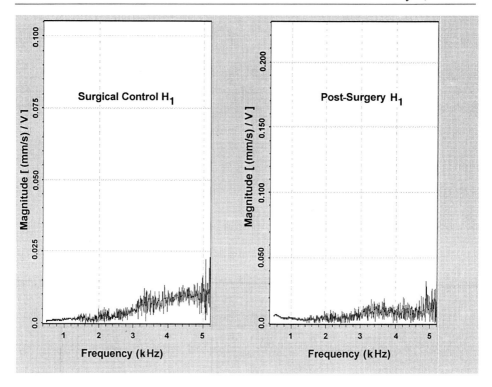

Fig. 11. Intraoperative transfer function. A patient undergoing stapedectomy was evaluated intraoperatively using the HLV. A comparison of umbo transfer function is shown prior to (left) and following (right) total stapedectomy with posterior crus preservation. An increase in transfer function in the lower frequencies was noted following stapedectomy. The ordinate scales are different due to the auto-scaling feature of the software package.

gram may have subtle differences in middle ear mechanics which impact hearing significantly, as described by Goode *et al.*[13]

An ideal method of measuring transfer of sound energy across the middle ear is to compare displacement and/or velocity at the umbo with a simultaneous interferometric measurement taken at the stapes footplate following presentation of a controlled acoustic stimulus. By measuring both targets, the middle ear transfer function for that ear can be determined. This dual interferometric measurement of the middle ear transfer function was recently performed in fresh temporal bones by Gan et al.[14]. Two-point laser middle ear mechanical analyses can only be performed in temporal bones or possibly at the time of middle ear surgery.

We have proposed that single measurement of the umbo dynamic response via laser Doppler interferometry may be useful in assessing middle ear mechanics in individuals with normal hearing, as well as those with conductive hearing loss. If it is assumed that the ossicular chain is intact, umbo velocity and displacement measurements provide an indirect method of evaluating stapes movement. Our analysis of umbo velocity in individuals with pure conductive hearing loss and those with mixed hearing loss pathology who had no history of previous ear surgery showed significant negative correlation between transfer function and conductive hearing loss. A decline in transfer function was observed as the degree of conductive hearing loss increased in these two groups. No correlation could be found between transfer function and conductive loss in individuals with conductive hearing impairment and a history of previous middle ear surgery.

Stasche et al.[15] noted a correlation between umbo velocity and conductive hearing loss following various experimentally induced alterations of middle ear transmission in a temporal bone model, using laser Doppler interferometry. A decline in umbo velocity was noted following stapes fixation, malleus head fixation, disruption of the ossicular chain, and when a middle ear effusion was present. Our in vivo results support the hypothesis that a relationship exists between middle ear mechanics and velocity transfer function measured at the umbo. However, a much larger sample size will be needed to make any firm conclusions about this complex relationship.

Most individuals with normal hearing by audiogram showed a nearly flat transfer function and a coherence factor close to 1.0. These individuals would correspond to the 'gold' ears described by Goode[16]. Figures 6 and 7 describe voltage, velocity, H_1 and coherence data from an individual whose HLV data represent the typical pattern seen in 'gold' ears. Other 'normal hearing' ears showed a drop in transfer function at certain frequencies, which may be indicative of poorer middle ear mechanics.

In the past, umbo displacement has been used as the primary method of characterizing tympanic membrane and middle ear performance. We have proposed that velocity transfer function be considered as an additional standard for evaluating middle ear performance, since transfer function measurements correct for variations in signal (SPL) input if the microphone has been properly calibrated. One of the limitations of the study was that the reference microphone was not calibrated for probe tube position either in amplitude or phase. In order for the H_1 to have total validity, such a calibration must be done. Several modifications of the HLV system have been suggested to improve its performance, such as decreasing the volume of the speculum adapter chamber and positioning the probe tube closer to the TM surface in order to enhance sound delivery and eliminate microphone calibration problems.

The single patient evaluated with the HLV prior to and immediately following a corrective stapedectomy showed a documented improvement in umbo velocity and velocity transfer function. These objective measures of middle ear performance predicted the improvement in conductive hearing loss seen with tuning fork testing in the operating room and later confirmed by audiometry. This surgical application of laser Doppler interferometry has potential promise for the otologist interested in optimizing the hearing outcome following surgical manipulation of the tympanic membrane or ossicular chain.

Conclusions

The HLV allows potentially objective and rapid (less than five minutes) *in vivo* measurements of umbo vibration to be performed in a clinic or operating room setting. HLV measurements of 80 ears were performed during this beta testing of the system. Preliminary results showed that normal hearing ears differ from each other in absolute transfer function values, but transfer function curves are similar in individuals with no conductive hearing loss pathology. Among normal ears, slight differences in transfer function may correlate with variations in middle ear mechanics, although more data are needed for true validation of the technique. Among individuals with conductive hearing loss who had no history of previous ear surgery there was a significant inverse correlation between transfer function and the degree of conductive hearing loss. In the future, a larger number of subjects will be required to further examine this correlation between hearing threshold levels and dynamic umbo response. The improvement in middle ear transfer function noted following corrective stapedectomy in one individual suggests that HLV may have a role in predicting a successful hearing outcome during middle ear surgery.

Acknowledgments

The technical and audiometric assistance of Ronald Voights, MS, Don Nakmali, BSEE, Helmut Selbach, PhD, Andrew Lewin, PhD and Bernd Ambruster, PhD is gratefully recognized. These individuals from the Hough Ear Institute and Seagate Technologies, Oklahoma City, and Polytec GmbH, Waldbronn, Germany, contributed to and made this study possible.

References

1. Decraemer WF, Khanna SM: Modelling the malleus vibration as a rigid body motion with one rotational and one translational degree of freedom. Hearing Res 72:1-18, 1994
2. Huber A, Asai M, Ball G, Goode RL: Analysis of ossicular vibration in three dimensions. In: Hüttenbrink KB (ed) Proceedings of the International Workshop on Middle Ear Mechanics in Research and Otosurgery. Univ. of Technol., Dresden, Germany, pp 82-87. 1996
3. Nishihara S, Goode RL: Measurement of tympanic membrane vibration in 99 human ears. In: Hüttenbrink KB (ed) Proceedings of the International Workshop on Middle Ear Mechanics in Research and Otosurgery, Univ. of Technol., Dresden, Germany, pp 91-94. 1996
4. Vogel U, Zahnert T, Hofmann G, Offergeld C, Hüttenbrink KB: Laser vibrometry in the middle ear: opportunities and limitations. In: Hüttenbrink KB (ed) Proceedings of the International Workshop on Middle Ear Mechanics in Research and Otosurgery, Univ. of Technol., Dresden, Germany, pp 128-133. 1996
5. Gan R, Dormer K, Wood MW, Ball GR, Dietz TG: Implantable hearing device performance measured by laser Doppler interferometry. ENT J 76(5):297-309, 1997
6. Lewin A, Mohr F, Selbach H: Heterodyn interferometer und vibrationsanalyse. Techniches Messen 57(9):335, 1990

7. Lewin A, Siegmund G: Implications of system sensitivity and resolution on an ultrasonic detecting LDV vibration measurements using laser techniques: advances and applications. SPIE Vol 2358 Vibration measurements, 292, 1994

8. Hudde H, Engel A: Eardrum impedance and drum coupling region. In: Hüttenbrink KB (ed) Proceedings of the International Workshop on Middle Ear Mechanics in Research and Otosurgery, Univ. of Technol., Dresden, Germany, pp 48-55. 1996

9. Vlaming M, Feenstra L: Studies on the mechanics of the reconstructed human middle ear. Clin Otolaryngol 11:411-422, 1986

10. Gyo K, Goode R, Miller C: Effect of middle ear modification on umbo vibration. Arch Otolaryngol Head Neck Surg 112:1262-1268, 1986

11. Kurokawa H, Goode R: Sound pressure gain produced by the human middle ear. Otolaryngol Head Neck Surg 113(4):349-355, 1995

12. Tonndorf J, Khanna S: Submicroscopic displacement amplitudes of the tympanic membrane (cat) measured by a laser interferometer. J Acoust Soc Am 6:1546-1554, 1968

13. Goode RL, Ball G, Nishihara S: Measurement of umbo vibration in human subjects-method and possible clinical applications. Am J Otol 14(3):247-251, 1993

14. Gan RZ, Wood MW, Dormer KJ: Middle ear transfer function measured by dual laser Doppler interferometry in human temporal bones. ARVO Abstracts 23:115, 2000

15. Stasche N, Foth HJ, Hormann K, Baker A, Huthoff C: Middle ear transmission disorders-tympanic membrane vibration analysis by laser Doppler vibrometry. Acta Otolaryngol (Stockh) 114:59-63, 1994

16. Goode RL: Middle ear function, biologic variation, and otosurgical alchemy: can we turn tin ears into gold? Arch Otolaryngol Head Neck Surg 112:923-924, 1986

INDEX OF AUTHORS